Artificial Intelligence in Medicine and Surgery - An Exploration of Current Trends, Potential Opportunities, and Evolving Threats - Volume 1

Edited by Stanislaw P. Stawicki

Published in London, United Kingdom

Artificial Intelligence in Medicine and Surgery - An Exploration of Current Trends, Potential Opportunities, and Evolving Threats - Volume 1
http://dx.doi.org/10.5772/intechopen.108661
Edited by Stanislaw P. Stawicki

Contributors
Latafat Abbas Gardashova, Yusif Aliyarov, Shamil A. Ahmadov, Stanislaw P. Stawicki, Thomas J. Papadimos, Michael Salibi, Scott Pappada, Ryan Yimeng Lee, Alyssa Imperatore Ziehm, Lauryn Ullrich, Juan Manuel Román-Belmonte, Hortensia De la Corte-Rodríguez, Beatriz Adriana Rodríguez-Damiani, Emérito Carlos Rodríguez-Merchán, Thomas Wojda, Carlie Hoffman, Jeffrey Jackson, Traci Conti, John Maier, Rohith Mohan, Alexandra King, Sarma Velamuri, Andrew Hudson, Vanessa Reese, Raivat Shah, Martin Oselkin, Parampreet Kaur, Naitik Patel, Aaron Alexander Mack, Amit Pal, Rajwinder Singh, Molly Mulflur, Allincia Michaud, Subba Rao Bhavaraju, Tania María Blanchar Martinez, Fernando Pio de la Hoz Restrepo, Manuel Cossio, Gabriel Szydlo Shein, Yoav Mintz, Ronit Brodie, Qian Dong, Wenli Xiu, Xiwei Hao, Nan Xia, Yongjian Chen, Haitao Niu, Noor us Saba, mohd Faheem, Xianjun Zhou, Chengzhan Zhu, Bin Wei

First published in London, United Kingdom, 2023 by IntechOpen
IntechOpen is the global imprint of INTECHOPEN LIMITED, registered in England and Wales, registration number: 11086078, 5 Princes Gate Court, London, SW7 2QJ, United Kingdom

British Library Cataloguing-in-Publication Data
A catalogue record for this book is available from the British Library

Additional hard and PDF copies can be obtained from orders@intechopen.com

Artificial Intelligence in Medicine and Surgery - An Exploration of Current Trends, Potential Opportunities, and Evolving Threats - Volume 1
Edited by Stanislaw P. Stawicki
p. cm.

This title is part of the Artificial Intelligence Book Series, Volume 19
Topic: Applied Intelligence
Series Editor: Andries Engelbrecht
Topic Editor: Carlos M. Travieso-Gonzalez

Print ISBN 978-1-83768-272-0
Online ISBN 978-1-83768-273-7
eBook (PDF) ISBN 978-1-83768-906-4
ISSN 2633-1403

For EU product safety concerns:
IN TECH d.o.o., Prolaz Marije Krucifikse Kozulić 3, 51000 Rijeka, Croatia,
info@intechopen.com or visit our website at intechopen.com.

IntechOpen Book Series

Artificial Intelligence

Volume 19

Aims and Scope of the Series

Artificial Intelligence (AI) is a rapidly developing multidisciplinary research area that aims to solve increasingly complex problems. In today's highly integrated world, AI promises to become a robust and powerful means for obtaining solutions to previously unsolvable problems. This Series is intended for researchers and students alike interested in this fascinating field and its many applications.

Meet the Series Editor

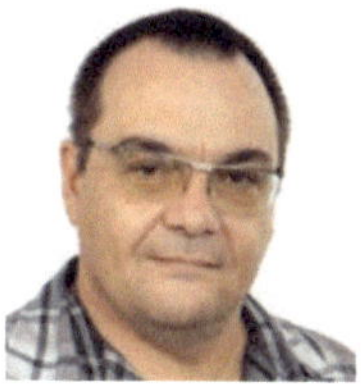

Andries Engelbrecht received the Masters and Ph.D. degrees in Computer Science from the University of Stellenbosch, South Africa, in 1994 and 1999 respectively. He is currently appointed as the Voigt Chair in Data Science in the Department of Industrial Engineering, with a joint appointment as Professor in the Computer Science Division, Stellenbosch University. Prior to his appointment at Stellenbosch University, he has been at the University of Pretoria, Department of Computer Science (1998-2018), where he was appointed as South Africa Research Chair in Artifical Intelligence (2007-2018), the head of the Department of Computer Science (2008-2017), and Director of the Institute for Big Data and Data Science (2017-2018). In addition to a number of research articles, he has written two books, Computational Intelligence: An Introduction and Fundamentals of Computational Swarm Intelligence.

Meet the Volume Editor

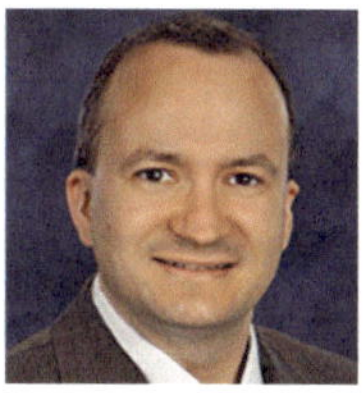

Dr. Stawicki is a Professor of Surgery and Chair of the Department of Research and Innovation, St. Luke's University Health Network, Pennsylvania, USA. A specialist in general surgery, traumatology and surgical critical care, he has co-authored more than 685 scholarly works, including more than 30 books. In addition to national and international medical leadership roles, Dr. Stawicki is a member of numerous editorial boards and grant review committees. His many areas of expertise include academic leadership, mentorship, patient safety, injury and critical care, point-of-care sonography, blockchain technology, Internet of Things (IoT), and artificial intelligence/machine learning applications.

Contents

Preface

Human history is full of instances where new inventions have created a sudden, significant, and lasting disruption. In a somewhat gradual and even stealthy way, artificial intelligence (AI) and machine learning (ML) are becoming part of our everyday lives, changing things in both predictable and unpredictable ways. This "randomly systematic" adoption process is putting humanity face to face with something never previously directly known to our civilization: an intelligence that may (and likely will) exceed our own.

It is fair to say that most people are not fully aware of current (and thus future) benefits, limitations, and threats related to AI/ML adoption. Within healthcare and medicine in general, there is little awareness of what AI/ML actually entails and what it is capable of at this time. It is this current state that will serve as our "starting point" in the emerging debate on AI/ML in medicine, including its integration, projected influence, and a variety of other considerations that are not all that different from other past technology adoption paradigms.

Like all other transformational human inventions, the emergence of AI/ML is a culmination of various simultaneous developments, often parallel and co-dependent, but also unpredictably synergistic, that ended up amalgamating to facilitate computational processes that approximate the "functional outcomes" of various human logical processes. Among the advances that were required for AI/ML to enter the mainstream were modern integrated circuits, higher computer processing speeds, ability to deploy parallel-processing capabilities, greater amounts (and lower cost) of computer memory, software engineering knowledge, and the ability to harness the power of the Internet to gather vast amounts of high-density data in an efficient and highly structured manner.

This new "artificial intelligence" phase in human history represents a confluence of multiple factors uniquely coming together to change our civilization forever. Although significant threats and opportunities exist in relation to real-life implementations of AI/ML in health care and beyond, a tremendous amount of promise and positive developments may also be realized. We are at a crossroads, and the outcome of any decisions made "right now" will heavily depend on whether we (i.e., humanity) make the right collective decision, at the right time, and for the right reasons. Although the gravity of this historic moment may not have yet become apparent, we will have to live with its consequences.

When implemented optimally, AI/ML has the potential to result in vast improvements in healthcare efficiency, workflows and other related processes, patient safety, and overall clinical outcomes. Specific benefits of AI/ML in the clinical realm include better, more accurate, and faster diagnostics; early disease detection, especially as it applies to cancer, cardiovascular, and genetic conditions; dynamically updated clinical guidelines, informed by actual patient outcomes and supplemented by real-time outcome data; and many other as yet undefined enhancements and advances. Specific threats related to AI/ML include workforce displacements (due to redundancies created by AI-based efficiencies); loss of human autonomy (due to "outsourcing of decision-making" to AI-based systems); and the propagation of various deleterious systemic biases (due to AI system reliance on potentially biased data feeding its ML algorithms).

As the early, more rudimentary capabilities of AI/ML continue to grow and mature, so will the diversity of the associated clinical applications. With further enhancements in hardware, software, and implementation infrastructure, increasingly complex areas (and problems) will become amenable to AI's general "scope of abilities" and influence. This will gradually expand into highly sophisticated systems and areas, such as social sciences and health care. In this collection of chapters, we discuss current trends and future developments related to AI and ML across medical and surgical specialties.

Stanislaw P. Stawicki, MD, MBA, FACS, FAIM
Department of Research and Innovation,
St. Luke's University Health Network,
Bethlehem, PA, USA

Section 1

Introduction

Chapter 1

Introductory Chapter: Artificial Intelligence in Healthcare – Where Do We Go from Here?

Stanislaw P. Stawicki, Thomas J. Papadimos, Michael Salibi and Scott Pappada

> *"When you outsource the production of something, you will gradually lose the knowledge and skills to make or produce it. What then, one might ask, will happen when we 'outsource' intelligence to another entity?"*
>
> *- Stanislaw P. Stawicki*

1. Introduction

The human history is full of examples where new inventions have created a significant disruption, dividing people into three broadly defined groups – proponents or early adopters, those who oppose, and those who are ambivalent [1]. When looking back at the relatively recent history of the great industrial revolution in Europe, it was not uncommon for opponents to attack and destroy new factories and new machines, with the perpetrators believing that the technological advances would eventually lead to the loss of their jobs and even entire professions [2]. As recently as in the mid-1980s, a group of mathematics teachers held a protest against the use of calculators in schools [3]. Fast-forwarding to today, calculators are now an integral part of our students' mathematics armamentarium!

Not surprisingly, our approach to artificial intelligence (AI) seems to be following a similar path. It is probably fair to say that most people are not fully aware of current (and thus future) benefits, limitations, and threats related to AI. Within medicine in general, there is little awareness of what AI actually entails, and what it is capable of at this time. It is this current state that serves as our "starting point" in the emerging debate on AI in medicine, including its integration, projected influence, and a variety of other considerations that are not dissimilar to past technology adoption paradigms.

In a very gradual and stealthy way, artificial intelligence (AI) and machine learning (ML) are becoming part of our everyday lives. This "randomly systematic" adoption process is putting humanity face-to-face with something never previously directly known to our civilization – An intelligence that may (and likely will) exceed our own. With the advent of modern computing capabilities, AI has evolved to a point where it can be integrated into everyday applications. Not surprisingly, it has been gradually introduced into various subdomains within the healthcare industry in recent years [4]. As a result, we will likely see significant shifts in education, clinical treatments and approaches, stakeholder expectations, and responsibilities – both in terms of type and scope, as well as potentially redefinition of jobs and other typical employee characteristics across the healthcare space [4, 5].

In this chapter, we will focus on some of the most profound challenges facing humanity as the "human-AI relationship" approaches the so-called "technological singularity" – A term based on the astrophysical concept of "black hole" that denotes a point beyond which there is "no way back" to the previous state of affairs. In the case of a "black hole," the gravitational force surrounding the super-massive object becomes so powerful that not even light can escape. In the case of AI, "singularity" refers to a point where "AI-based technology" is sufficiently evolved to essentially take over "control operations" of the human civilization [6, 7]. Alternative views describe both "integration" and "plurality" as possible scenarios, where humans and AI either co-exist synergistically (plurality) [8, 9] or even integrate successfully (e.g., human-machine hybridization) [10, 11].

As we explore the realities of this new world, with omnipresent AI and the growing need for human adaptation, change and caution, the issues at hand will likely become less and less "technological" but will rather gravitate toward the ethical and spiritual domains.

1.1 Destructive potential of AI

There are many science fiction movies highlighting the potential dangers of improperly implemented AI – just a few examples of such messaging include the "Terminator" series, "Star Trek Voyager," "The Matrix" trilogy, and "I, Robot." The most common themes across these artistic works include machines "taking over" for humans as a form of "misguided stewardship," the objectivization of humans as "destructive and dangerous" followed by active control efforts, and finally, the most extreme form of "AI dominance" where highly evolved AI "machine hives" determine that humanity needs to be eliminated in its entirety [12–16].

At a less physically destructive level, but perhaps equally problematic in its extent and implications, the use of AI / ML in misdirected "societal control" efforts may represent another formidable challenge. For example, what would be required to stop a malignant governmental and/or regulatory entity that possesses powerful AI /ML tools, combined with omnipresent social media platforms, from abusing the tremendous power to misinform, manipulate, and eventually subdue entire populations? [17–22]. Such concerns have been highlighted by Elon Musk and associates in their open letter, "Pause Giant AI Experiments," which now has nearly 6000 signatories from all walks of life [23]. This open letter is blunt in stating that AI systems with human-competitive intelligence pose a risk to our civilization. It goes on further to emphasize that the risks of powerful AI systems are likely unmanageable at this time. Appropriate oversight, tracking and regulatory frameworks must be put into place. The letter specifically addresses the inception of systems that are substantially more powerful that the more widely known GPT-4 (generative pretrained transformer 4) [24].

A further concern involves AI being used in the political and social influence spheres. Here there are ominous tidings regarding truth and transparency. In one instance, researchers at Stanford University examined whether AI could influence citizens regarding political issues such as assault weapons, a carbon tax, and parental leave...and it certainly did [25]. When looking at the case of ChatGPT in the setting of higher education, the AI-based system was able to readily pass exams at prestigious law and business schools, not to mention the United States Medical Licensing Examination [26–29]. Such issues are more than concerning, and they clearly constitute potential threats to civilized society and the ascent of man.

1.2 Potential benefits of AI

As much as there are negatives to wider AI implementation, there are certainly amazing potential benefits that can be derived from properly harnessed AI capabilities, from reaching previously unimaginable levels of efficiency within our established processes and workflows, to human-AI hybridization that could actively enable much longer functional (and meaningful) longevity, new disease cures, and solutions to both physical and mental disability [11, 30]. Furthermore, AI will allow the simulation of unusual or theoretical situations such as legal cases before judges and negotiations with business competitors. In fact, there are multiple domains in which AI will benefit us (**Table 1**) [31]. There are also estimates that AI-driven innovation may contribute nearly $13 trillion dollars to the world's economy by 2030 [32].

Perhaps the most significant benefits of AI will be realized in medicine and healthcare. Today's society faces staffing shortages of healthcare professionals [33–35]. In absence of sufficiently staffed healthcare organizations and institutions, current healthcare practitioners will require support to achieve optimal patient safety and levels of care provision. To this end, machine learning and AI-based systems will offer the potential to improve monitoring and alerting of healthcare providers such that patients who are in the greatest need are appropriately resourced.

It is important to note that although machine learning and AI are used interchangeably, they are not one and the same. Machine learning involves data science and the development of models based on large datasets to serve a particular function, for example, supporting diagnosis [36], time series prediction of therapeutic set points, predicting patient outcomes [37] such as readmission [38] or mortality [39]. AI, refers to an artificially intelligent system in that it can 'think and act' on its own with some degree of autonomy. While machine learning is closely related to AI, machine learning feeds into AI-based systems to leverage its results to perform some autonomous tasks. AI is best explained by looking at some of its initial use in video games, where antagonists (characters) in video games are programmed with AI to complete a primary task (e.g., stop the player from achieving some goal). AI in medicine and healthcare is the ultimate end goal, where patient data can be monitored continuously over time, and some aspects of treatment and care can be automated by AI. An example of this would be leveraging machine learning to support prediction of glucose in patients with type 1 diabetes [40] and leveraging predictions to automatically and dynamically adjust

Automation
Productivity
Solving Complex Problems
Decision-Making
Economy
Managing Repetitive Tasks
Defense
Disaster Management
Personalization
Lifestyle

Table 1.
Potential benefits of AI in our lives and work [31].

insulin delivery to maintain tight glycemic control. AI can be incorporated into this system to learn patterns in lifestyle, activity, and other pertinent variables to automatically adjust and adapt insulin delivery to further optimize glycemic control overtime given a patient's chaotic and unpredictable lifestyle. This is only one example of an application illustrating the power of machine learning and AI in healthcare.

2. Important considerations regarding AI in healthcare

Digital bias is an important concept that is bound to become a mainstream consideration in the still very young AI era [41]. In this context, biases that are already present in various types and channels of "source data" have the potential to perpetuate existing healthcare disparities, resulting in a system that may be technologically more advanced but also one that continues to disenfranchise entire segments of the population [42]. Some applications of AI and machine learning in healthcare are starting to come to the forefront. Primary healthcare education and training, as well as the area of continuing education and training are also important areas where machine learning and AI can play a role. Currently, medical education involves a one-size-fits-all curriculum approach where everyone is given the same set of training/education (simulation-based, didactic, and otherwise) regardless of real-world clinical experiences and proficiency/competency levels. To this end, machine learning and AI in medicine can be used in different ways including personalizing training/education of healthcare professionals [43]. In this context, optimal training and education of healthcare professionals is a "big data" problem and via prediction of performance and knowledge/skill acquisition, maintenance and decay over time, it will be possible to personalize training for an individual provider [44–49].

With the advent of AI and machine learning in any field, there is always the worry that it will replace the jobs of professionals in the field. Although there has been tremendous growth and advancement of AI and machine learning in healthcare, bedside care providers are not at risk of replacement any time soon. In the near term, AI and machine learning in healthcare will primarily offer the potential to augment the performance of healthcare providers and simplify or support their clinical decision-making processes and clinical workflows. This will likely result in a reduction of workload by identifying patterns and trends in large electronic medical records databases and bringing to the forefront key information that will assist the provider in diagnostics and making the best treatment decisions for their patients. AI and machine learning will become extremely important in our fast-changing world and our continually evolving society, where staffing shortages of medical professionals are likely to remain a significant issue, with demographic trends working "against us" well into the future. Having AI and machine learning-based technologies which ultimately optimize the performance and efficiency of healthcare professionals is therefore urgently needed.

3. Artificial Intelligence in academic medicine

The topic of AI in academic medicine is certainly a heated one. It is becoming evident that the introduction of AI into medical education will likely prompt significant rethinking, and likely rebuilding, of our medical curriculums. This will help ensure that both our medical schools and the new generation of medical trainees are sufficiently prepared to optimize the positive aspects of AI while minimizing any potentially negative aspects and considerations [5]. For the current, fairly traditional medical school curricula, the introduction of ML and AI applications will be both transformational and hugely challenging. Similarly, the increasing presence of ML/AI in clinical medicine will force many changes in clinical information management, patient care workflows, the broad range of diagnostics, and many other related areas [50, 51]. The optimal end-product will be the advent of true "precision medicine" where each patient can be treated using highly individualized and much more optimized approaches.

For all of the above to happen seamlessly, without undue disruptions, the incorporation of AI applications into medical education will require unique curricular modifications. It is likely that the current evidence-based medicine (EBM) guidelines will quickly become obsolete and instead may be replaced by dynamically updated AI-based recommendations (AIBRs). Consequently, how we train our next generation of physicians and other healthcare professionals will likely become unrecognizable in the next 10–20 years. Moreover, the issues of "black box" interpretability, data security, and decision liability are bound to present us with problems not addressed by traditional curricula [52].

It is reassuring to know that research in this area has been ongoing and that a significant amount of expertise is available and continues to grow [5, 52]. Our collective perception of AI is also likely to evolve over time. According to recent data, a large proportion of medical students perceived AI as an assistive technology that could facilitate physicians' access to information, and patient access to healthcare, all while reducing the number and impact of medical errors [53]. In parallel, more and more medical students are expressing the need for updates in the current medical school curriculum, accommodating the need for adaptation to AI-facilitated healthcare industry transformation [54, 55]. Curricular updates should revolve around equipping future physicians with the knowledge and skills to effectively harness the power of AI-based applications, minimize potential harms related to the misuse of AI, and ensure that their professional values and rights are protected.

At the same time, implementing the right plan and appropriately re-setting professional requirements and boundaries is not an easy task. All clinicians, students, and AI professionals alike should understand the social, ethical, legal, and regulatory issues that will determine whether AI-based tools will narrow or widen health disparities, affect professional independence, and potentially influence any existing healthcare gaps. A multi-pronged approach should involve the development of novel teaching models, the recruitment of qualified and experienced content specialists (to design and teach ML/AI curricula), and subsequently, the facilitation of communication challenges relative to any existing and/or perceived knowledge gaps between physicians and engineers [53].

Parallel to the issue of medical education reform, another set of critical issues will arise pertaining to intellectual property, content attribution, and content originality (e.g., plagiarism) [56]. Within this context, we must remember that ML, AI, and other advanced tools like "chatbots" and "ChatGPT" are not inherently "good or bad," and that any inappropriate uses of said technological capabilities will stem from misuse by individuals whose intentions lack ethical and/or moral grounding. The educational setting in general, and higher education in particular, is largely based on the presence of academic integrity as an essential component of the system. While AI-based technologies have the potential to greatly enhance our lives and improve our efficiency across various areas of society [6], it is not unreasonable to speculate that such highly sophisticated tools could easily "fool an expert" into giving credit for effort that should have never been attributed to a particular individual, in effect propagating intellectual fraud [57, 58].

In addition to the potential for difficult-to-detect plagiarism, AI-based technologies also have the potential to be used for other nefarious purposes, such as cheating on assignments, using 'deep fake' or other unethical practices to gain an unfair advantage, and even assisting unscrupulous individuals in actively lying on their resumes and job applications [59, 60]. As modern technology continues to advance relentlessly, it becomes increasingly difficult to determine whether a piece of writing is truly original or if it has been generated by a machine [61]. This raises questions about the value of originality and the importance of properly crediting sources in the digital age. It also highlights the need for individuals to be more critical of the information they consume and follow, as well as the importance of careful consideration of the sources of the information being actively shared, especially in the context of omnipresent social media [19]. Finally, we must always remember that AI-generated content will be inherently limited by the quality of data inputs utilized during the generative process.

4. Synthesis and conclusion

Similar to all other transformational human inventions, the emergence of AI/ML is a culmination of various simultaneous advances – often parallel and co-dependent – that synergistically combine to facilitate computational processes that approximate the "functional outcomes" of various human logical processes. Among the advances that were required for AI/ML to enter the mainstream were modern integrated circuits, higher computer processing speeds, greater amounts of computer memory, software engineering knowledge, and the ability to harness the power of the Internet to gather vast amounts of high-density data in a very efficient manner.

As the early, more rudimentary capabilities of AI/ML grew, so did the diversity of their applications. With further growth in hardware, software, and implementation infrastructure, increasingly complex areas (and problems) became amenable to AI's general "scope of abilities." This gradually expanded into highly sophisticated systems and areas, such as social sciences and healthcare. In this collection of chapters, we will discuss current trends and future developments related to artificial intelligence and machine learning across medical and surgical specialties.

Author details

Stanislaw P. Stawicki[1*], Thomas J. Papadimos[2], Michael Salibi[3] and Scott Pappada[4]

1 Department of Research and Innovation, St. Luke's University Health Network, Bethlehem, Pennsylvania, USA

2 Department of Anesthesiology, The University of Toledo, Toledo, Ohio, USA

3 Department of Emergency Medicine, St. Luke's University Health Network, Richard A. Anderson Campus, Easton, Pennsylvania, USA

4 Department of Bioengineering, Healthcare Technology and Innovation Laboratory, The University of Toledo, Toledo, Ohio, USA

*Address all correspondence to: stawicki.ace@gmail.com

References

[1] Juma C. Innovation and Its Enemies: Why People Resist New Technologies. Oxford: Oxford University Press; 2016

[2] Gera I, Singh S. A critique of economic literature on technology and fourth industrial revolution: Employment and the nature of jobs. The Indian Journal of Labour Economics. 2019;**62**(4):715-729

[3] Hochman A. Math Teachers Stage a Calculated Protest [cited 2023 April 29, 2023]. 1986. Available from: https://www.washingtonpost.com/archive/local/1986/04/04/math-teachers-stage-a-calculated-protest/c003ddaf-b86f-4f2b-92ca-08533f3a5896/

[4] Çalışkan SA, Demir K, Karaca O. Artificial intelligence in medical education curriculum: An e-Delphi study for competencies. PLoS One. 2022;**17**(7):e0271872

[5] Chan KS, Zary N. Applications and challenges of implementing artificial intelligence in medical education: integrative review. JMIR Medical Education. 2019;**5**(1):e13930

[6] Upchurch M. Robots and AI at work: the prospects for singularity. New Technology, Work and Employment. 2018;**33**(3):205-218

[7] Good IJ. Speculations concerning the first ultraintelligent machine. In: Advances in Computers. New York, USA: Elsevier; 1966. pp. 31-88

[8] Plebe A, Perconti P. Plurality: The end of singularity? In: The 21st Century Singularity and Global Futures. Cham, Switzerland: Springer; 2020. pp. 163-184

[9] Barr J, Cabrera LF. AI gets a brain: New technology allows software to tap real human intelligence. Queue. 2006;**4**(4):24-29

[10] Bloom P, Bloom P. Heading toward integration: the rise of the human machines. In: Identity, Institutions and Governance in an AI World: Transhuman Relations. Cham, Switzerland: Palgrave Macmillan; 2020. pp. 67-92

[11] White JJ. Artificial Intelligence and People with Disabilities: a Reflection on Human–AI Partnerships. In: Humanity Driven AI: Productivity, Well-being, Sustainability and Partnership. Cham, Switzerland: Springer; 2022. pp 279-310

[12] Arney C. Our final invention: artificial intelligence and the end of the human era. Mathematics and Computer Education. 2016;**50**(3):227

[13] Francis A, Davies J, Data LC. The Measure of a Machine: The Psychology of Star Trek's Artificial Intelligence. New York, USA: Sterling Publishing; 2017, pp. 251-265

[14] Garvey C. Testing the 'Terminator Syndrome': Sentiment of AI News Coverage and Perceptions of AI Risk. 2018. Available at SSRN 3310907

[15] Bennett E. Deus ex machina: AI apocalypticism in terminator: the sarah connor chronicles. Journal of Popular Television. 2014;**2**(1):3-19

[16] Cheng X. AI vs Nuclear Weapons: Which Is More Dangerous?. Available online at: http://large.stanford.edu/courses/2018/ph241/cheng1/ [Last accessed June 6, 2023]

[17] Eke D et al. Nigeria's Digital Identification (ID) Management Program: Ethical, Legal and

Socio-Cultural Concerns. Journal of Responsible Technology. 2022;**11**:100039

[18] Plaza M et al. The use of distributed consensus algorithms to curtail the spread of medical misinformation. International Journal of Academic Medicine. 2019;**5**(2):93

[19] Stawicki SP, Firstenberg MS, Papadimos TJ. The use of blockchain in fighting medical misinformation: A concept paper. In: Blockchain in Healthcare: From Disruption to Integration. Cham, Switzerland: Springer; 2023. pp. 225-239

[20] Conti K et al. The evolving interplay between social media and international health security: a point of view. In: Contemporary Developments and Perspectives in International Health Security-Volume 1. London, UK: IntechOpen; 2020

[21] Papadimos TJ, Stawicki SP. Hannah Arendt's Prognostication of Political Animus in America: Social Platforms, Asymmetric Conflict, and an Offset Strategy. Open Journal of Philosophy. 2020;**11**(1):85-103

[22] Farrell H, Newman A, Wallace J. Spirals of delusion: How AI distorts decision-making and makes dictators more dangerous. Foreign Affairs. 2022;**101**:168

[23] Letters FO. Pause Giant AI Experiments: An Open Letter. Future of Life Institution; 2023 Available from: https://futureoflife.org/open-letter/pause-giant-ai-experiments

[24] Nori H et al. Capabilities of gpt-4 on medical challenge problems. arXiv preprint arXiv:2303.13375, 2023.

[25] Myers A. AI's Powers of Political Persuasion [cited 2023 April 17, 2023]. 2023. Available from: https://hai.stanford.edu/news/ais-powers-political-persuasion

[26] Mbakwe AB et al. ChatGPT Passing USMLE Shines a Spotlight on the Flaws of Medical Education. San Francisco, CA USA: Public Library of Science; 2023. p. e0000205

[27] Ryznar M. Exams in the Time of ChatGPT. Washington and Lee Law Review Online. 2023;**80**(5):305

[28] Gilson A et al. How does CHATGPT perform on the United States Medical Licensing Examination? the implications of large language models for medical education and knowledge assessment. JMIR Medical Education. 2023;**9**(1):e45312

[29] Choi JH et al. ChatGPT Goes to Law School. SSRN; 2023

[30] Lillywhite A, Wolbring G. Coverage of artificial intelligence and machine learning within academic literature, Canadian newspapers, and twitter tweets: The case of disabled people. Societies. 2020;**10**(1):23

[31] Lateef Z. Top 10 benefits of artificial intelligence [cited 2023 April 17, 2023]. 2023. Available from: https://www.edureka.co/blog/benefits-of-artificial-intelligence/

[32] Szczepanski M. Economic impacts of artificial intelligence (AI) - European Parliament Briefing [cited 2023 April 17, 2023]. 2019. Available from: https://www.europarl.europa.eu/RegData/etudes/BRIE/2019/637967/EPRS_BRI(2019)637967_EN.pdf

[33] Harp JJ. The shortage of Healthcare Workers in the United States: A Call to Action. In: Assessing the Need for a Comprehensive National Health

System in the United States. Hershey, Pennsylvania, USA: IGI Global; 2023. pp. 123-138

[34] Chervoni-Knapp T. The staffing shortage pandemic. Journal of Radiology Nursing. 2022;**41**(2):74-75

[35] Butler CR, Webster LB, Diekema DS. Staffing crisis capacity: A different approach to healthcare resource allocation for a different type of scarce resource. Journal of Medical Ethics. 2022;**2022**. DOI: 10.1136/jme-2022-108262. [Published Online First: 01 July 2021]

[36] Ragab M et al. Ensemble deep-learning-enabled clinical decision support system for breast cancer diagnosis and classification on ultrasound images. Biology. 2022;**11**(3):439

[37] Du Y et al. An explainable machine learning-based clinical decision support system for prediction of gestational diabetes mellitus. Scientific Reports. 2022;**12**(1):1170

[38] Huang Y et al. Application of machine learning in predicting hospital readmissions: a scoping review of the literature. BMC Medical Research Methodology. 2021;**21**(1):1-14

[39] Thorsen-Meyer H-C et al. Dynamic and explainable machine learning prediction of mortality in patients in the intensive care unit: a retrospective study of high-frequency data in electronic patient records. The Lancet Digital Health. 2020;**2**(4):e179-e191

[40] Pappada SM et al. Neural network-based real-time prediction of glucose in patients with insulin-dependent diabetes. Diabetes Technology & Therapeutics. 2011;**13**(2):135-141

[41] Packin NG. Disability discrimination using artificial intelligence systems and social scoring: Can we disable digital bias? Journal of International and Computer Law. 2021;**8**:487

[42] Celi LA et al. Sources of bias in artificial intelligence that perpetuate healthcare disparities—A global review. PLOS Digital Health. 2022;**1**(3):e0000022

[43] Pappada S et al. Personalizing simulation-based medical education: the case for novel learning management systems. International Journal of Healthcare Simulation. 2022;**2022**:1-8

[44] Patel UK et al. Artificial intelligence as an emerging technology in the current care of neurological disorders. Journal of Neurology. 2021;**268**:1623-1642

[45] Poly TN et al. Artificial intelligence in diabetic retinopathy: Bibliometric analysis. Computer Methods and Programs in Biomedicine. 2023;**231**: 107358

[46] Itchhaporia D. Artificial intelligence in cardiology. Trends in Cardiovascular Medicine. 2022;**32**(1):34-41

[47] Makhni EC, Makhni S, Ramkumar PN. Artificial intelligence for the orthopaedic surgeon: an overview of potential benefits, limitations, and clinical applications. JAAOS-Journal of the American Academy of Orthopaedic Surgeons. 2021;**29**(6):235-243

[48] Vearrier L et al. Artificial intelligence in emergency medicine: benefits, risks, and recommendations. The Journal of Emergency Medicine. 2022;**62**(4):492-499

[49] Benke K, Benke G. Artificial intelligence and big data in public health. International Journal of Environmental Research and Public Health. 2018;**15**(12):2796

[50] Mintz Y, Brodie R. Introduction to artificial intelligence in medicine. Minimally Invasive Therapy & Allied Technologies. 2019;**28**(2):73-81

[51] Ahmed Z et al. Artificial intelligence with multi-functional machine learning platform development for better healthcare and precision medicine. Database. 2020;**2020**:1-35

[52] Savage TR. Artificial intelligence in medical education. Academic Medicine. 2021;**96**(9):1229-1230

[53] Civaner MM et al. Artificial intelligence in medical education: A cross-sectional needs assessment. BMC Medical Education. 2022;**22**(1):772

[54] Hu R et al. Insights from teaching artificial intelligence to medical students in Canada. Communication & Medicine. 2022;**2**(1):63

[55] Pucchio A, Eisenhauer EA, Moraes FY. Medical students need artificial intelligence and machine learning training. Nature Biotechnology. 2021;**39**(3):388-389

[56] Francke E, Bennett A. The potential influence of artificial intelligence on plagiarism: A higher education perspective. In: European Conference on the Impact of Artificial Intelligence and Robotics (ECIAIR 2019). 2019;**31**:131-140

[57] Dehouche N. Plagiarism in the age of massive Generative Pre-trained Transformers (GPT-3). Ethics in Science and Environmental Politics. 2021;**21**:17-23

[58] Taswell SK et al. The hitchhiker's guide to scholarly research integrity. Proceedings of the Association for Information Science and Technology. 2020;**57**(1):e223

[59] Campbell C. AI by Design: A Plan for Living with Artificial Intelligence. Boca Raton, Florida, USA: CRC Press; 2022

[60] Maras M-H, Alexandrou A. Determining authenticity of video evidence in the age of artificial intelligence and in the wake of Deepfake videos. The International Journal of Evidence & Proof. 2019;**23**(3):255-262

[61] King MR. and ChatGPT, A conversation on artificial intelligence, chatbots, and plagiarism in higher education. Cellular and Molecular Bioengineering. 2023;**16**(1):1-2

Section 2

Artificial Intelligence and Machine Learning: General Considerations

Chapter 2

Unlocking the Potential of Artificial Intelligence (AI) for Healthcare

Parampreet Kaur, Aaron Alexander Mack, Naitik Patel, Amit Pal, Rajwinder Singh, Allincia Michaud and Molly Mulflur

Abstract

This book chapter examines the potential of artificial intelligence (AI) to improve healthcare. AI has become increasingly prominent in healthcare, providing the capability to automate tasks, analyze large patient data sets, and deliver quicker and more cost-effective healthcare. We focus on its various applications in healthcare including vital sign monitoring, glycemic control, radiology, and emergency room triage with point of care ultrasound (POCUS). We also address AI's ethical, legal, and privacy implications in healthcare such as data protection and safeguarding patient privacy. Finally, we explore the potential of AI in healthcare improvement in the future and investigate the current trends, opportunities, and evolving threats posed by AI in healthcare, as well as its implications for human-AI interfacing and job security. This book chapter provides an essential and comprehensive overview of the potential of AI in healthcare, providing a valuable resource for healthcare professionals and researchers in the field.

Keywords: artificial intelligence (AI), healthcare clinical management, AI in healthcare, vital sign monitoring, glycemic control, radiology, point of care ultrasound (POCUS), ER triage, AI data security, human-AI interfacing, machine learning (ML), neural networks (NNs), deep learning (DL), AI ethical concerns, AI healthcare benefits

1. Introduction

AI has been rapidly increasing in popularity and application within the healthcare industry over the past decade. AI has the potential to greatly increase the efficiency and accuracy of healthcare, resulting in improved patient care, better decision-making, and overall cost savings. AI allows for complex and rapidly growing datasets to be evaluated and analyzed with unprecedented accuracy and detail, using machine learning (ML), neural networks (NNs), deep learning (DL), and large language models (LLM).

AI and ML are two distinct but related branches of computer science. The two are related in that AI requires data to be used in order to make decisions, and ML provides the tools to do so. Artificial intelligence is a spectrum of intelligence, learning, and analytical proficiency. Machine learning and deep learning are related applications within the artificial intelligence space with varying aptitudes and capabilities (see **Figure 1**). Machine learning (ML) can understand relationships from the data without the need to define them a priori and can derive predictive models without a need for strong assumptions about the underlying mechanisms. In other words, ML converts the inputs of an algorithm into outputs, using statistical tools [1, 2]. It can change when exposed to new data and can improve from experience.

In contrast, deep learning (DL) uses multilayered neural networks to compute large volumes of data and accept multiple data types (heterogenicity). This feature has proven applicability in healthcare, that is. the EHR system. Of the deep learning algorithm, convolutional neural networks (CNN) processes data exhibiting natural spatial invariance (clinical images) [1]. Compared to ML, DL requires considerably less human guidance, and the overall difference is how DL interprets and presents raw data.

The level of analysis, sophistication, and detail exhibited by AI would be impossible for humans to do alone. This can help healthcare organizations to gain insights and identify trends that would otherwise be difficult to detect. In addition, AI can provide real-time recommendations and feedback to healthcare professionals, helping them make better, more informed decisions.

As AI technology advances and becomes more integrated into healthcare systems, healthcare organizations can leverage its many advantages to become more efficient and effective such as automating mundane and repetitive tasks freeing up healthcare professionals to concentrate on more critical aspects of patient care. AI can also improve the accuracy and timeliness of diagnosis and treatment decisions, reducing the risk of medical errors, and potentially saving lives. Additionally, AI can be used to monitor patient health, alert healthcare professionals to potential issues before they become serious, predict future health outcomes, and help healthcare organizations

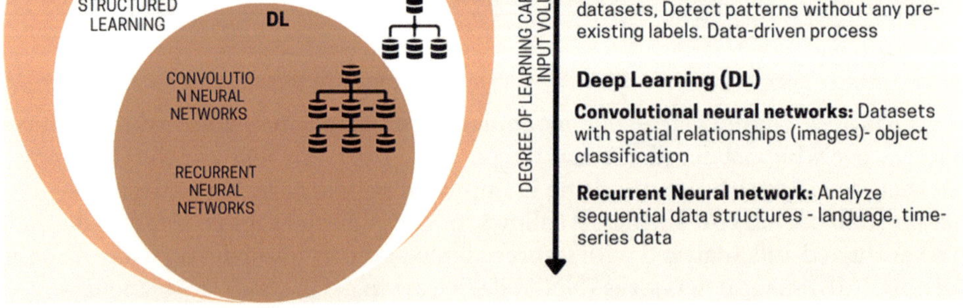

Figure 1.
Artificial intelligence (AI) hierarchical relationship.

better plan for potential scenarios. The recent arrival of conversational AI systems based on LLM such as ChatGPT has opened a plethora of potential uses including but not limited to preauthorization, automatic generation of medical reports, summarizing the electronic health record, and interactive computer-aided diagnosis (CAD) [3]. These applications are possible because LLM is efficient in a wide variety of tasks including summarization, machine translation, and quickly answering questions. Ultimately, AI applications enhance communication between healthcare professionals and patients, providing more personalized care and optimizing processes such as appointment scheduling and prescription refills. However, studies need to be performed and validated to confirm whether utilizing these resources brings ultimate value to patient care. See **Table 1** for acronyms and abbreviations.

2. Methodology

We conducted a literature search of articles on AI in various healthcare fields in English over the last five years on search engines: PubMed and Google scholar.

Acronyms and abbreviations	Meaning
AI	Artificial intelligence
AI-ML	Artificial intelligence-machine learning
AUC	Area under the receiver operating characteristic (ROC) curve
CAD/CADe	Computer-aided diagnosis
CGM/rtCGM	Continuous glucose monitors/real-time CGM
CNN	Convolutional neural networks
CT	computed tomography scan
CXR	Chest X-ray
DL	Deep learning
DNN	Deep neural network
ER/ED	Emergency room/department
ESI	Emergency severity index score
IVC	Inferior vena cava
LLM	Large language models
MEWS	Modified early warning score
MI	Myocardial infarction
ML	Machine learning
MRI	Magnetic resonance imaging scan
NNs	Neural networks
POCUS	Point of care ultrasound
SIRS	Systemic inflammatory response syndrome
SOFA/qSOFA	Sequential organ failure assessment score/Q = quick

Table 1.
Acronyms and abbreviations.

The following key terms were used to generate the search: "artificial intelligence (AI)" in healthcare, vital sign monitoring, glycemic control, radiology, point of care ultrasound (POCUS), ER triage, AI data security, human-AI interfacing, machine learning (ML), neural networks (NNs), deep learning (DL), AI ethical concerns, and AI healthcare benefits. For the first review, two team members manually went over articles. For the next step, various topics of artificial intelligence on different subjects, such as radiology, vital signs monitoring, glycemic control, point of care ultrasound, and ER triage, were divided among the authors with relevant specialties. Each author then wrote the section with following themes: its utility, challenges, liabilities, implications on job security, and future education.

3. Utility of AI in radiology

AI is increasingly being used in radiology to improve diagnostic accuracy, efficiency, and decision-making. Some of the most common applications of AI in radiology include image analysis, computer-aided diagnosis (CADe), image segmentation, automated image interpretation, and automated reporting [4–6].

AI-based systems can be trained to detect and identify specific structures or abnormalities on medical images such as tumors, blood vessels, or organ abnormalities [5, 7, 8]. This can improve diagnostic accuracy and efficiency by highlighting potential abnormalities that may have been missed by radiologists [9]. Additionally, AI-based systems can be used to assist radiologists in the diagnostic process by classifying different types of tumors or identifying specific patterns on medical images, which can help radiologists make more accurate, specific diagnoses, and guide treatment decisions [4, 5, 8]. AI-based systems can also be used to generate automated reports and summaries that include relevant information and analysis, which can save time, reduce the workload and errors caused by manual reporting, and improve communication with other healthcare providers [4, 6, 10].

AI applications have the protentional to be used in radiology for detection and characterization in many body systems [8, 9]. Recent advances in AI for thoracic applications have focused on using deep learning techniques to assist with a lung cancer diagnosis and pulmonary nodule detection on CT scans. In abdominal and pelvic applications, AI has been used to assist with liver lesion analysis and the detection of abnormalities on CT and MRI scans. General lesion analysis using AI typically involves training a model on a large dataset of images to identify and classify various types of lesions [11]. This can include detecting and characterizing tumors, identifying and measuring anatomic structures, and determining the presence of certain disease states.

3.1 How is AI utilized in radiology?

AI in radiology utilizes the expertise of experienced radiologists to supply predefined criteria for properly programming the algorithm [4, 8]. Radiologists with specialized knowledge in chest, abdominal, or musculoskeletal radiology can offer the essential insight and direction required to train AI algorithms to identify and locate specific structures or anomalies on medical images. This involves providing the algorithm with a set of "ground truth" or baseline images that have been annotated by radiologists to indicate the presence and location of specific structures or abnormalities. The algorithm can then learn to identify these structures or abnormalities based on the patterns and features that are present in the images.

AI algorithms can also learn from a large volume of data with supervised or unsupervised strategies. Supervised learning is when the algorithm is provided with labeled data, where each image is associated with a specific diagnosis or label [4, 12]. This allows the algorithm to learn from the data and make predictions about new images. Unsupervised learning is when the algorithm is provided with unlabeled data, where the algorithm must learn to identify patterns and features in the data without any prior knowledge [4, 12]. This can be useful for identifying new or previously unknown patterns or features in the data. The algorithm can also be trained to extract information *via* patterns and share deep insights that can be used to improve diagnostic accuracy, efficiency, and decision-making [4].

3.2 How can AI transform the work of a radiologist?

AI can play a transformative role to help unlock the solutions to many challenges of radiology such as increasing workload and staff shortages. AI can also transform the work of a radiologist by mainly following steps in image analysis, which includes detection, characterization, and monitoring in several ways [5, 11, 13] (see **Figure 2**). One of the most important areas where AI is used in radiology is **image analysis,** where AI-based systems can be trained to detect and identify specific structures or abnormalities on medical images such as tumors, blood vessels, or organ abnormalities. This can improve diagnostic accuracy and productivity by highlighting potential abnormalities that may have been missed by the human eye [5, 11].

Another important area is **characterization,** where AI-based systems can be trained to classify and characterize different types of abnormalities or lesions [5, 11]. For example, AI algorithms can be used to differentiate benign from malignant tumors or to classify different types of liver lesions. This can help radiologists to make more accurate and specific diagnoses and guide treatment decisions [5, 8]. This can also reduce the need for additional imaging or biopsies, which can save time and money.

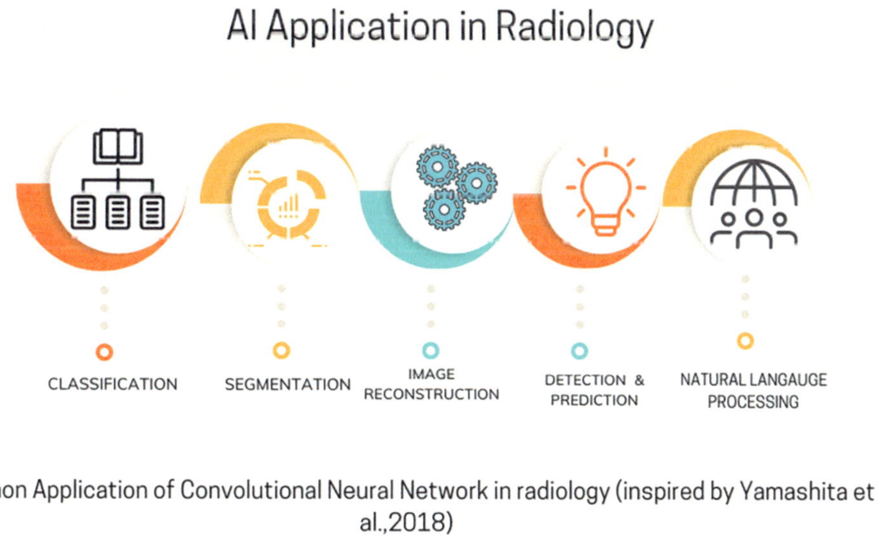

Figure 2.
AI applications in radiology.

Monitoring is another area where AI is being used in radiology, where AI-based systems can be used to monitor changes in lesions over time [5]. For example, AI-based systems can track the growth of a tumor or the response to treatment [11], which can help radiologists to make more informed decisions about patient care. This can also help to identify patients who need additional monitoring or treatment and can lead to improved patient outcomes.

AI is also being used in **image acquisition** by deep learning-based reconstruction algorithms that can reduce scan time and improve image quality, especially in MR imaging. MR imaging can take anywhere from 30 and 60 minutes and occasionally longer depending on the protocol. Some patients, particularly elderly patients, can become uncomfortable and claustrophobic lying in a confined space for this period of time. Being able to obtain high-quality imaging in a shorter time can help alleviate this issue and reduce the presence of motion artifact. This can ultimately improve the diagnostic confidence in the images and prevent unnecessary repeating sequences [14].

Additionally, AI can assist radiologists by providing them with **automated reports and summaries** that include relevant information and analysis, which can save time, reduce the workload and errors caused by manual reporting, and improve communication with other healthcare providers [8]. AI can also support radiologists by integrating with other healthcare systems, providing them with comprehensive patient information and data from other sources such as electronic health records, lab results, and previous imaging studies, which can provide a more comprehensive view of the patient's condition and assist in the diagnostic process.

It is important to note that AI in radiology still requires human interpretation and oversight, as AI algorithms are not perfect, they can make errors or miss certain findings. It is anticipated that AI in radiology will become increasingly more precise and reliable over time as more data is acquired and technology advances.

3.3 Challenges of AI and liabilities around wrong and missed diagnosis

Though AI has the promise to improve diagnostic accuracy and efficiency, it also poses certain liabilities related to wrong and missed diagnoses [9]. One potential liability is that AI systems may produce incorrect or unreliable results due to factors such as poor image quality, incorrect data input, or errors in the algorithms used to analyze the images [15]. This could lead to wrong, delayed, or missed diagnoses, or unnecessary treatments [9].

Another potential liability is that AI systems may not be able to detect certain types of lesions or diseases, particularly those that are rare or atypical. Additionally, there are concerns about the lack of standardized benchmarks to compare and validate AI models for practical implementation. This could lead to missed diagnoses, which can be particularly dangerous if the condition is serious or life-threatening.

AI systems also require proper validation and testing before they are used in clinical practice. Validating data sets is time-consuming, and thus can jam many machine-learning projects. Handling unexpected inputs such as artifacts and poor imaging can also pose a problem in high-quality data sets. Medical research on data sets can also act as a hurdle as many patients value their privacy [16, 17]. If they are not appropriately validated, they may not be suitable for the intended use or population, and this can lead to wrong or missed diagnoses as well.

Additionally, there is also a lack of reasoning and an inability to explain AI models [17]. There is the potential that AI systems could be used to override the judgment of

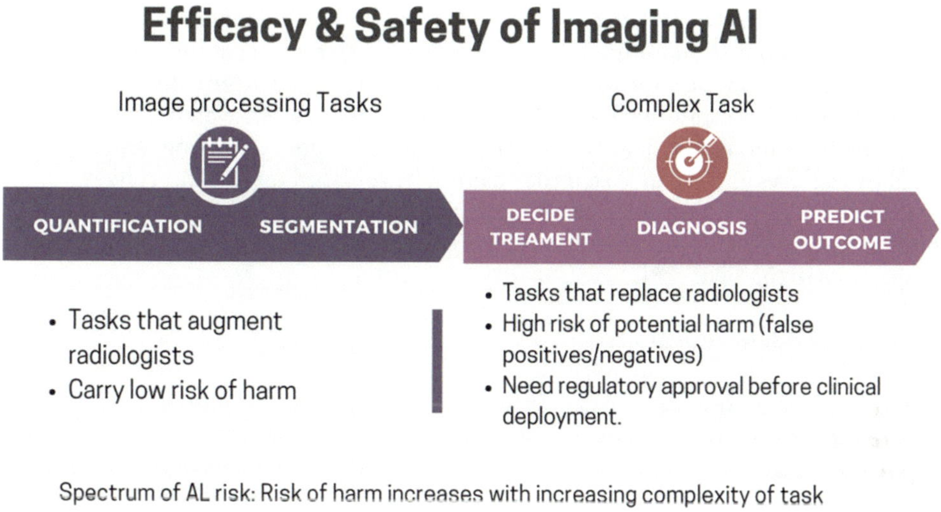

Figure 3.
Efficacy and safety of images.

radiologists, leading to an increased risk of wrong or missed diagnoses if the radiologist's judgment is ignored (see **Figure 3**).

To mitigate these liabilities, it is imperative to ensure that AI systems are properly validated and tested before they are used in clinical practice and that radiologists are properly trained in their use. Since investigating liability issues will require different skills from lawyers and additional evidence from technology along with medical expert opinion, we will need support from our technology law colleagues to design regulations [18]. It is vital to have proper governance, policies, and regulations in place for the use of AI in radiology.

3.4 Future implications for job security

AI has the potential to construct intelligent applications that can mimic the cognitive capabilities of humans, potentially revolutionizing the workforce in myriad ways. Some experts believe that AI could eventually replace certain tasks currently performed by radiologists and technologists [17] such as the interpretation of medical images. However, it is also possible that AI could augment radiologists' abilities and productivity, allowing them to spend more time on higher-level tasks such as consulting with other physicians, analyzing more complex cases, and providing follow-up to patients [19]. Though there are more than 80 approved algorithms in the US and Europe, only 40 of these have been approved by the FDA and only 34% of those were used for interpretation. The number of radiologists working in the US has risen by 7% in five years from 2015 to 2019 [20, 21].

Regarding job security, it is likely that radiologists and technologists who are trained and experienced in using AI systems will be in high demand. However, those who are not able or refuse to adapt to this new technology may face challenges in their job market [7, 10, 17]. Administrative staff may also be impacted as AI can automate some of the tasks they do, but this may also be a positive change as it can lead to more time for the staff to focus on patient care and other important tasks.

Overall, the effects of AI on the radiology workforce will depend on how the technology is adopted and implemented. Radiologists, standing at the leading edge of digital medicine, can provide support in the incorporation of AI into healthcare, their role in diagnostics communication, the incorporation of patient values and preferences, medical judgment, quality assurance, education, policy-making, and interventional procedures and ensures that they cannot be replaced by AI [22]. However, it is important for all radiologists, technologists, and administrative staff to stay informed about the latest developments in AI and work to develop the necessary skills to remain competitive in the field [23].

3.5 Future resident education

The increasing presence of AI applications in radiology necessitates educators to prepare trainees and radiologists as proficient users and stewards of AI technology. Yet, despite the controversy around if and to what extent AI should be incorporated into radiology residency programs, organized AI education and AI-ML curricula are still limited to a few institutions, with formal training opportunities lacking across the board.

AI has the potential to revolutionize radiology resident education by providing new tools and resources for teaching and learning and is likely to include a greater emphasis on AI-ML curricula and precision medical education [24, 25]. By incorporating AI and machine learning into radiology resident education, they can stay up to date with the latest techniques and technologies used to diagnose and treat patients and gain valuable experience with AI as it becomes increasingly important in healthcare.

One potential application of AI in radiology resident education is the use of AI-assisted image interpretation, which could help residents to develop their diagnostic skills and improve their understanding of complex medical images [25]. For example, AI systems can be used to identify and highlight certain features on an image such as tumors or blood vessels, which can help residents to identify these structures and improve their diagnostic accuracy more easily.

Another potential application of AI in radiology resident education is the use of virtual reality and simulation to provide hands-on training experiences [26, 27]. This technology can be used to create realistic simulations of medical scenarios such as a surgical procedure or an interventional radiology procedure, which can provide residents with an immersive and interactive learning experience.

AI can also be used to provide personalized and adaptive learning experiences to analyze each resident's progress and create personalized learning plans [24, 25]. For example, AI-based systems can be used to track residents' progress, provide feedback, and adjust the learning experience based on their strengths and weaknesses. This can include providing tailored feedback and resources to help them improve their diagnostic accuracy, as well as providing opportunities for hands-on training and simulation. By incorporating AI-ML curricula for radiology residents, the residency program can be at the forefront and focus on teaching residents the fundamental concepts and techniques of AI and machine learning such as data pre-processing, coding, model training, theory, and evaluation [28]. This would enable residents to understand how AI systems work and how to use them effectively in their practice. Precision medical education, which is an approach that aims to provide tailored education based on individual needs and characteristics, will also play an important role in and would involve using AI systems to personalize the learning experience for each resident, considering their strengths, weaknesses, and learning style [24, 28].

Additionally, AI can also be used for automated grading and feedback for radiology residents, which can save time for educators and provide more accurate and consistent feedback to the residents. Overall, the future of AI in radiology resident education will be closely tied to the development of AI-ML curricula and precision medical education encompassing the three learning theories (behaviorist, cognitive, and constructivist), which will enable residents to learn the latest techniques and technologies in an effective and efficient way and personalize the learning experience based on the residents' needs [24].

A recently developed elective in data science pathway (DSP) for fourth-year radiology residents at Brigham and Women's Hospital (BWH) in Boston has the potential to prepare the next generation of radiologists to lead the way in artificial intelligence and machine learning (AI-ML) [28]. The resident feedback from the pilot resulted in the establishment of a formal AI-ML curriculum for future residents, which included logistical, planning, and curricular considerations for DSP implementation at other institutions [28].

In summary, AI has the potential to greatly enhance radiology resident education by providing new tools and resources for teaching and learning, improving diagnostic skills, providing hands-on training experiences, and personalized learning experiences, as well as automated grading and feedback.

AI will impact radiology such asmany other medical fields, but radiologists can play a leading role in this forthcoming change by reducing the huge amount of data and information into the most relevant information.

4. AI and ML in emergency room triage and point of care ultrasound

Artificial intelligence in medical practice is shaping the way clinicians assess, analyze, and diagnose potentially life-threatening conditions, which will significantly impact the delivery of emergency care. The use of AI algorithmic systems may give the tools to possibly overcome previously ingrained limitations in care delivery strategies [29] thus extending the ability of emergency physicians to diagnose and treat acute and critical illnesses. Over the last 10 years, the U.S. Food Drug and Administration (FDA) has approved more than 500 AI and ML devices [30]. Of these, 100+ were radiology applications for devices used during an emergency.

This section will highlight the applications of artificial intelligence (AI), machine learning (ML), deep learning (DL), and convolutional neural networks (CNN) in emergency room triage and their use, specifically in point of care ultrasound testing. The applicability of these technologies has an obvious advantage in emergency medicine as every year the demands on the emergency medicine practitioner increase as the number of emergency room visits grows and physicians are expected to care for more patients with fewer resources. The ability to provide timely efficient and accurate life-saving interventions is crucial, and AI holds the potential to help physicians streamline processes, increase efficiency, and cognitively offload.

4.1 AI impact on emergency room care

Triage is the prioritization of the sick and injured based on their need for emergency treatment. Traditionally, in the emergency department clinical support staff gather primary patient demographic data, vital signs, and basic information about a patient's initial presenting problem. The patient then undergoes a brief evaluation by a clinician, usually a nurse, to determine the patient's acuity or need for emergent care or resources. Commonly during this process, a patient is assigned an emergency severity index (ESI) score, which is a common triage tool that provides a clinically relevant framework to stratify patients into five groups from one (most urgent) to five (least urgent) based on acuity and resource needs. This system essentially determines who receives care first. Subsequently, clinicians thoroughly assess presenting symptoms, perform appropriate physical examinations, order applicable laboratory studies, imaging studies, and consultations and either discharge the patient to home or admit them to the hospital as indicated [31]. With the growing number of emergency room visits annually and a growing shortage of nurses and emergency medicine practitioners, the ability to provide timely efficient and accurate life-saving interventions is crucial.

Effective triage is of the utmost importance to patient quality of care and outcome, especially as ER capacities are further and further stretched by increased volume and decreased resources, which have led to prolonged ED stays and wait time for care. Although ER wait times are multifactorial, convenient registration and the early identification of impending life-threatening conditions can obviate adverse patient outcomes and decrease mortality. One study that assessed the performance of a deep learning system, PatientFlowNet, in predicting patient flow in emergency departments found that the PatientFlowNet model prediction of patient arrival rates was higher, with substantially more accuracy in predicting treatment and discharge rates than the baseline methods used in the ER. The resulting mean absolute error was 4.8% lower than the leading baseline [32]. Applying AI tools that combine both clinical narratives (symptoms, pain scores, and ESI) and structured data (demographics and vitals), there is potential to positively influence outcomes.

The AI algorithmic tool (TriageGO) recently developed at Johns Hopkins aims to integrate patient medical health records with presenting symptoms, as well as vital signs to further risk stratify patients and predict morbidity and mortality [33]. Additionally, the DNN model with word embedding AI tool, which integrated clinical narratives and structured data, outperformed and better predicts patients' hospitalization and discharge when compared to the rapid emergency medicine score (REMS) [34]. Furthermore, rapid response is paramount with time-sensitive complaints such as chest pains. Goto et al. neural networks AI model predicts whether patients presenting to ER chest discomfort needs urgent revascularization 12-lead EKG. Their AI model detects the presence of specific EKG characteristics not recognized by physicians [35]. Than et al. developed their "MI3 clinical support tool" to predict the likelihood of myocardial infarction (MI) using machine learning which achieved a high AUC (0.963) for diagnosing MI, which outperformed the European Society of Cardiology 0/3-hour pathway [36]. In all these examples, the impact of AI on today's healthcare system has the potential to be transformational.

4.2 AI impact on point of care ultrasound

Over the last twenty years, ultrasound equipment has become more effective, economical, and compact because of this the applications and uses have broadened and the use of ultrasound at the bedside as a modality has become more ubiquitous. This is especially palpable in the world of emergency medicine (EM). In EM, there is an inherent need to arrive at a time-sensitive diagnosis and initiate potentially life-saving treatments, and the use of bedside ultrasound of point of care ultrasound is a crucial tool that facilitates this. POCUS is the medical use of ultrasound (US) technology for the bedside evaluation of acute or critical medical conditions. It is utilized for diagnosis, the guidance of procedures, monitoring of certain pathologic states, and as an adjunct to therapy. It has also demonstrated its utility as an adjunct in the resuscitation of the critically ill.

POCUS examinations are typically performed, interpreted, and integrated into care by the treating physician in real-time at the bedside making it distinct from traditional radiology-based applications [37]. Instead of performing a systems-based study designed to interrogate a particular anatomic area, POCUS seeks to help answer specific clinical questions that are often binary in nature (e.g. is there free fluid in the peritoneum, is there a pneumothorax, is there hydronephrosis, etc.). An additional factor that differentiates POCUS from the traditional use of medical ultrasound is the fact that POCUS practitioners are inherently diverse in their training and their ability. Ultrasound image acquisition is a user-dependent skill, and both because of this as well as the binary nature that drives POCUS use at the bedside, POCUS is an area that is ripe for the application of artificial intelligence (AI) and deep learning (DL) [37].

The use of DL in POCUS is varied as the model used depends on the problem it is trained to solve [37]. For example, DL in POCUS has been already used to help identify structures [37], for image enhancement [38], and for the classification of images [38]. In each different application, depending on the clinical question, the POCUS operator would "only need to provide an image, and the trained DL model would be able to immediately return the desired output, whether it be the outline of an organ, an enhanced US image, or the classification of the US image along with a confidence score [37]." The ability of DL application allows the practitioner to cognitively offload some elements of image acquisition and interpretation, and thus be able to concentrate more on real-time application and direct patient care [37]. The advantage of this is especially palpable in the world of emergency medicine (EM). In EM, there is an inherent need to arrive at a time-sensitive diagnosis and initiate potentially life-saving treatments.

AI and DL have demonstrated utility in several cardiac studies (e.g., estimation of ejection fraction, calculation of IVC caliber and collapsibility to predict fluid responsiveness, and the identification of cardiac tamponade), as well as pulmonary applications (AI-enhanced lung ultrasound in discriminating viral and bacterial pneumonia, estimation of size of pneumothorax based on location of lung point, and prediction of antibiotic response from US lung images using DL). These applications expand the EM practitioner's ability to risk stratify and implement treatment.

There is further potential, as AI ability evolves, to eventually achieve "real-time" image interpretation. This could in theory expand the number of POCUS practitioners beyond the ranks of physicians or EM-trained clinicians to first responders, EMTs, and those responding to mass-casualty events or real-time disasters. The ability to use POCUS in the "field" by untrained or novice user will allow those on site to potentially diagnose fractures, abdominal/thoracic free-fluid or hemorrhage, pneumothorax, or even cardiac standstill thus optimizing the triage response and subsequent allocation of resources. A similar conclusion can be drawn from those practicing in the global health realm, which is traditionally a lower-resource practice environment.

However, despite the obvious advantages, there are some limitations to the use of AI in POCUS. Imaging modalities, such as CXR, CT, and MRI, have standardized imaging protocols that are archived for later use/review leading to the construction of large persistent imaging datasets for AI to "mine." POCUS images and videos, on the other hand, are acquired and interpreted at the bedside, and findings are immediately applied with variable storage/archiving protocols depending on time limitations, patient acuity, machine capabilities, and institutional guidelines. Additionally, the large variation in POCUS user skill level, the order in which images are acquired, and the image acquisition technique create a great deal of "noise" or randomness which further complicates the building of large, standardized ultrasound datasets. Despite, this as AI advances and DL modeling and the creation of CNN becomes more sophisticated pathways are being found to navigate these limitations.

The impact of AI on today's emergency room can be transformational from its effects on triage to disease diagnosis and detection. AI can reintegrate and augment ER staff rather than replace the human workforce by decreasing the work burden and improving clinical outcomes.

5. AI and ML for vital sign monitoring

Today's healthcare, especially in the hospital setting, is complex, fast-paced, and busier than ever. Physicians make many individual decisions and treatment plans that are influenced by copious amounts of data that are collected and available for review in the EHR. Hospitalized patients are monitored frequently through vital signs and lab tests for signs of deterioration or instability. There is now a desperate need to automate this essential job and quickly alert clinicians if there are any signs of deterioration.

With the advancement of technology, artificial intelligence (AI) and machine learning (ML) algorithms are being used to analyze vital sign data and detect signs of disease in real-time, improving the accuracy and speed of diagnosis [39]. Conditions, such as sepsis, are commonly managed in the hospital setting and are the leading cause of inhospital death [40]. Traditionally, clinicians have relied on scoring systems such as the modified early warning score (MEWS), SIRS, Rothman index, sequential organ failure assessment score (SOFA), and quick SOFA (qSOFA) to identify patients at risk of deterioration. These scores utilize several data points from the patient's record to predict the risk of deterioration. However, due to their high sensitivity and low discriminatory ability, these scores may identify a larger number of patients at risk than present [39, 41].

Studies have concluded that individual machine learning models can predict sepsis onset ahead of time and with more accuracy compared directly with the traditional sepsis screening tools such as SIRS, MEWS, and SOFA scores [39, 41]. From a clinical perspective, ML models are particularly useful as they could trigger earlier detection of sepsis and allow for early antibiotic administration leading to decreased mortality. Some additional studies have also highlighted earlier predictions of severe deterioration in sepsis utilizing only vital signs. For instance, Mao et al. developed a gradient tree boosting model using data from only six vital signs: systolic BP, diastolic BP, heart rate, respiratory rate, peripheral capillary oxygen saturation, and temperature. This model was able to predict sepsis at the onset with high AUC (0.92) and septic shock 4 hours in advance with a high AUC (0.96). The model was also able to predict severe sepsis 4 hours in advance with a higher AUC (0.85) than the onset time for statistically calculated SIRS AUC (0.75) [42].

Additionally, AI-based monitoring incorporated into the EHR can facilitate the use of large volumes of data for the prediction of mortality in hospitalized patients. Shickel et al. used a modified recurrent neural network model on temporal intensive care unit data to develop DeepSOFA, a real-time mortality risk prediction score based on the traditional SOFA score [43]. This model compared the traditional SOFA scores to deep learning technology in augmenting a clinician's decision-making by generating accurate real-time prognostic data relating to mortality [43]. The DeepSOFA model was more accurate than baseline SOFA models for predicting inhospital mortality among ICU patients with baseline SOFA models significantly underestimating the probability of death, especially among non-survivors [43]. Recognition of mortality risk earlier in the disease course has the potential of aiding clinicians in taking preventative measures earlier and with more accuracy resulting in improved outcomes.

The COVID-19 pandemic demonstrated the utility of AI and ML for prehospital and posthospital management of patients. For instance, remote patient monitoring (RPM) came to the forefront during the pandemic as hospital systems became overwhelmed with patients. RPM is a healthcare technology that uses digital devices, wearable sensors, and wireless communication to collect and transmit medical data from patients outside of traditional clinical settings. Traditionally, RPM has been utilized to monitor chronic diseases; however, the pandemic accelerated the use of this technology for acute monitoring and management of patients with COVID-19 infections. RPM is achieved through use of smart devices such as blood pressure meters, thermometers, glucometers, and pulse oximeters utilizing an ecosystem known as the internet of health things (IoHT). IoHT refers to the interconnectivity of medical devices, wearables, and healthcare systems that allow for the exchange of health-related data between patients and healthcare providers.

ML techniques applied to enormous data sets generated through continuous monitoring of cardiac- and respiratory-related signals, coughing, body temperature, and patterns of activity collected from COVID-19 patients help predict the health status of a patient or individual easily [44]. Consequently, based on these measurements, the appropriate medication can be administered, or people can be transferred to the hospital when necessary. Crotty et al. utilized RPM capabilities to monitor 5367 patients with COVID-19 infection and found a substantial reduction in ICU utilization, reduced length of stay, and lower 30- and 90-day mortality when compared to patients who did not participate in active monitoring [45]. RPM has the potential to improve patient engagement and health literacy by providing real-time information that can improve outcomes, such as pruning education, which likely led to improvement in oxygenation requirements and improved outcomes [45].

AI and ML are also improving cardiovascular health through predictive analytics. Predictive analytics is the use of data, statistical algorithms, and machine learning techniques to identify the likelihood of future outcomes based on historical data. In the case of cardiovascular health, predictive analytics can be used to identify patients who are at high risk of cardiovascular disease [46, 47]. By using data from EHR, wearable devices, and other sources, healthcare professionals can identify patterns and trends such as low heart rate variability (HRV) that may indicate a higher risk of subsequent cardiovascular events (14). AI and ML algorithms can be also used to analyze HRV signals to track and evaluate the effectiveness of therapeutic interventions such as HRV biofeedback. Burlacu et al. outlined a systematic review on the beneficial effects of HRV-biofeedback, a slow breathing technique, on different cardiovascular diseases such as arterial hypertension, heart failure, and coronary artery disease. HRV modulation can be implemented in high-risk patients to significantly reduce stress levels and improve autonomic nervous system function and cardiovascular endpoints [48].

5.1 Challenges of AI *in vital* sign monitoring

With the increasing utilization of smart medical devices, there is a growing risk of sensitive medical data being accessed [49] or stolen. To address this concern, it is necessary to implement robust security measures such as encryption and access controls to ensure that personal information is properly protected. Rajasekaran proposed that the IoHT must include several key features such as trust ability, low transmission latency, security, confidentiality, integrity, and availability [50]. They proposed a blockchain-based anonymous privacy-preserving authentication scheme to preserve the key features outlined above.

Additionally, the lack of interoperability of the different wearable devices is one of the biggest hurdles that we need to overcome. By enabling different devices to share data, interoperability opens the door to new possibilities for personalized healthcare. For example, a wearable health device that tracks a user's physical activity can share data with another device that monitors their heart rate. This data can then be combined to create a more complete picture of the user's health, helping healthcare providers make more informed decisions about treatment and care. Interoperability will also help generate high-quality data that can be used to train ML algorithms.

For machine learning algorithms to work effectively, they require a large amount of high-quality data to train on. ML algorithms can be biased if the training data contains systematic inaccuracies or overrepresents one group. Straw et al. demonstrated one such bias when they reviewed Indian Liver Patient Dataset (ILPD), which is the open source data set used extensively to create algorithms that predict liver disease. Due to the under representation of females in the data set, the model demonstrated a higher false negative rate in women leading to lower disease detection in females [51]. To minimize the risk of bias, it is important to carefully select training data by using diverse and representative data sets. Additionally, the development and deployment of ML models should be guided by ethical and inclusive principles. Mccradden et al. outlined ethical principles of nonmaleficence, relevance, accountability, transparency, and justice as the foundation for the regulation of healthcare ML algorithms [52].

In inference, AI and ML have the potential to revolutionize the way healthcare is delivered. With the ability to collect vast amounts of patient data in real-time, AI algorithms can provide valuable insights into patients' health, improve the accuracy of diagnosis, detect health issues early, and improve patient engagement and health literacy. While there are still challenges to overcome such as security, interoperability of wearable devices, and ML bias, AI and ML have the potential to significantly improve patient outcomes and transform the way healthcare is delivered. Clinicians and policymakers, however, must ensure that the technology is accessible and affordable for all patients, regardless of their socioeconomic status. While there have been significant advancements in RPM technology in recent years, many patients, particularly those living in rural or underserved areas, may not have access to these tools due to cost or limited availability.

6. AI in diabetes and Glycemic control

Artificial intelligence is a fast-growing field with its applications for persons living with many chronic diseases such as diabetes. There has been global concern about the ever-increasing incidence rate of diabetes with one in two persons undiagnosed and untreated [53]. The total number of people living with diabetes is likely to rise to 643 million by 2030 and 783 million by 2045 [53]. A recent study of 300,000 patients with type 2 diabetes on medical therapy found that after 3 months, 31% of patients had discontinued their diabetes medications that number was widened to 44% by 6 months, and to 58% by 1 year [54]. Besides, about 75% of diabetic adults live in low- and middle-income countries with only 5% of those receiving thorough treatment according to guidelines [55]. The best care for diabetes is mostly hindered by lack of real-time crucial health information required to make necessary choices with diabetes control and therapy.

Today, advances in AI have introduced a shift in diabetes care from conventional management approaches to targeted data-driven precision care. There is a spectrum of interventions spread across different care processes in diabetes. AI is not only being applied to predict diabetes risk utilizing genetic data and to diagnose diabetes *via* electronic health record data in clinical decision support but it is also transforming diabetic care and predicting the potential sequelae of diabetes such as nephropathy and retinopathy. Such solutions have enhanced the workflow of both medical staff and patients.

6.1 How is AI utilized in diabetic care?

To help fight diabetes disease and improve its management, AI can play a vital role in diabetic care at many different levels discussed below that can benefit both providers and patients in a team-oriented approach.

6.1.1 Diabetes prediction

AI can help diagnose diabetes noninvasively and proactively by identifying a subset of populations with the highest risks at a pre-illness stage. Though diabetes prediction models have been generated by conventional statistics, machine learning (ML) can maximize the predictive performance of conventional models to the next level [56]. Algorithms built by ML can do risk stratification by analyzing genomics, lifestyles, mental and physical health, and social media activity. Earlier detection and intervention for at-risk individuals could decrease the incidence of diabetes, and the financial costs associated with uncontrolled diabetes.

6.1.2 Lifestyle guidance for diabetes patients

Monitoring glucose levels in real-time is being done using wearable devices and continuous glucose monitoring systems of patient symptoms and biomarkers. Continuous glucose monitors (CGM), which are now frequently used by diabetics, acquire a large amount of data that has previously been underutilized. The amount of glucose in the fluid inside the body is measured by CGM. In certain circumstances, the sensor is glued to the back of the arm or is implanted under the skin of the belly rapidly and painlessly. The information is then sent to a wireless-pager-like monitor through a transmitter on the sensor [57].

CGM sensors can be divided into two main categories: Professional CGM sensors and real-time CGM sensors (rtCGM) [58]. Professional CGM sensors are prescribed by healthcare professionals usually for limited periods of time, they record glucose concentration data in blinded modalities (i.e., the patient cannot visualize the data in real-time), and they allow the healthcare professional to retrospectively review the patient's glycemic trends and make therapy adjustments. Conversely, with real-time CGM sensors (rtCGM) the recorded data are accessible in real-time to the patient, who can use these data for improved decision-making in the daily management of Type 1 diabetes. AI can enable patients to decide what to eat or drink and what level of physical exercise is suitable.

6.1.3 Insulin injection guidance

AI can be used to provide personalized recommendations for insulin dosage besides meal planning based on glucose levels, physical activity, and other factors. The CGM sensors provide in real-time, every 1–5 minutes, the current blood glucose concentration, and its rate-of-change, two key pieces of information for improving the determination of exogenous insulin administration and the prediction of forthcoming adverse events such as hypo−/hyper-glycemia.

The most popular rtCGM sensors are minimally invasive electrochemical sensors that measure interstitial glucose concentration by a small transcutaneous electrode placed under the skin of the abdomen, or the arm. Some insulin pumps can be integrated with rtCGM sensors into the so-called closed-loop system in which a control algorithm automatically adjusts the insulin dose based on the glucose concentration measured [58]. A recent randomized controlled trial using an automated AI-based decision support system for insulin showed statistically no difference in the percentage of time spent within the target glucose range with no adverse events reported in patients on remote AI arm versus three adverse events in patients on remote adjustments by physicians' arm [59].

6.1.4 Glycemic adverse events detection

Particularly, pediatric and geriatric patients are at risk of severe hypo- and hyperglycemic events. Many noninvasive techniques using AI-based algorithms are being proposed and tested to detect glycemic events. Scientists have developed an AI system that will detect hypoglycemia or low glucose through data collected *via* CGM, which is employed for detecting low glucose levels using a noninvasive wearable sensor.

Glycemic events, using ECG signals collected through noninvasive devices, are also being tested [60]. ECG-based glucose detection can be more practical for diabetic patients with comorbidities who are more familiar with ECG monitoring for other clinical monitoring [61]. It could also be more favorable for prediabetics who might be more aware due to commercial use in fitness or sports applications. Such AI assistants also provide statistics and communicate with the care provider in the case of an emergency.

6.1.5 Monitoring diabetes complications

Progress in AI for improving screening and detection of diabetic retinopathy, macular edema, and foot ulcers can transform the gaps in clinical care. The cost of screening and limitation on human and equipment resources is still challenging despite adoption of telemedicine especially in developing countries. The early detection of complications can protect patients from dangerous stages that may later cause blindness and foot amputations. Providers are successfully leveraging deep learning to automate the diagnosis of retinopathy with high accuracy and specificity levels [62].

6.1.6 Patient engagement

Improving patient engagement and self-management through immersive technology, virtual coaching, and educational programs can shift disease courses to better outcomes. Face-to-face educational programs are followed in less than 10% of newly diagnosed people, but the emergence of digital health has given them the opportunity to overcome the challenges of lower engagement and participation from patients [63]. A statewide survey study in Indianapolis found that about 50% of people use technology to communicate with providers [63]. Telemedicine, *via* various telehealth portals, is now accepted as the necessary new normal and is expected to grow by 33% from 2019 to 2026 thus reaching $ 185.6 billion by 2026 [64]. Patients involved in their healthcare will experience better long-term health outcomes and incur lower costs, so there is a push toward promoting greater patient engagement.

6.2 Challenges in AI of diabetic care

Though there are many diabetic AI apps and devices everywhere, however, there has been a lower uptake in the long-term engagement of digital health technologies [65]. Even with a slower understanding of technologies, digital data collected from diabetic patients is growing exponentially. Data is the key to creating better AI insights, but it can be very easy to get exhausted by big data. Besides, data collected by wearables has constraints around their integration into existing systems. It also raises concerns about data privacy, security, and even legal hurdles.

Our ambition should be to create comprehensive and relevant solutions to enhance the usability of AI-based tools with evidence-based models in collaboration with all stakeholders including patients. Effectiveness will depend on the rapidity of con struction and modification of new apps, devices, and sensors according to improve diabetes experience for patients and organizational needs. The resolution of such challenges will depend on adequate scientific research and regulation.

7. Conclusion

In conclusion, artificial intelligence (AI) has the potential to revolutionize healthcare management and provide tremendous benefits to healthcare organizations and patients alike. AI can help healthcare organizations gain insights into data that would otherwise be difficult to obtain, provide real-time decision support and recommendations, automate mundane tasks, improve diagnosis and treatment accuracy, monitor patient health, predict future health outcomes, and improve communication between healthcare professionals and patients. As AI continues to advance, healthcare organizations must take advantage of its many benefits and integrate the technology into their systems to ensure they are staying competitive in an ever-changing healthcare landscape.

Author details

Parampreet Kaur[1,2,3,4*], Aaron Alexander Mack[5], Naitik Patel[6], Amit Pal[7], Rajwinder Singh[7], Allincia Michaud[5] and Molly Mulflur[8,9]

1 Research and Quality Improvement, SLUHN Anderson Campus, Easton, PA, USA

2 GME Data Management and Outcomes Assessment, SLUHN, Bethlehem, PA, USA

3 SLUHN Institutional Review Board, SLUHN, Bethlehem, PA, USA

4 Lewis Katz School of Medicine at Temple University, Bethlehem, PA, USA

5 Department of Research and Innovation, St. Luke's University Health Network, Bethlehem, PA, USA

6 Internal Medicine, SLUHN Anderson Campus, Easton, PA, USA

7 Radiology, St. Luke's University Health Network, Bethlehem, PA, USA

8 Emergency Medicine, SLUHN—Anderson Campus, PA, USA

9 Adjunct, Lewis Katz School of Medicine at Temple University, Bethlehem, PA, USA

*Address all correspondence to: parampreet.kaur@sluhn.org

References

[1] Esteva A et al. A guide to deep learning in healthcare. Nature Medicine. 2019;**25**(1):24-29

[2] Miotto R et al. Deep learning for healthcare: Review, opportunities and challenges. Briefings in Bioinformatics. 2018;**19**(6):1236-1246

[3] Shen Y et al. ChatGPT and other large language models are double-edged swords. Radiological Society of North America. 2023;**2023**:230163

[4] Hosny A et al. Artificial intelligence in radiology. Nature Reviews Cancer. 2018;**18**(8):500-510

[5] Makary MS. Artificial intelligence in radiology: Current applications and future technologies. The Journal. 2021;**21**(4):205-208

[6] Santos MK et al. Artificial intelligence, machine learning, computer-aided diagnosis, and radiomics: Advances in imaging towards to precision medicine. Radiologia Brasileira. 2019;**52**:387-396

[7] AI in Radiology. 2022

[8] Gandhi Y. 8 applications of AI in Radiology. Analytics Steps. 31 Mar 2022. Available from: https://www.analyticssteps.com/blogs/8 applications ai radiology

[9] Oren O, Gersh BJ, Bhatt DL. Artificial intelligence in medical imaging: Switching from radiographic pathological data to clinically meaningful endpoints. The Lancet Digital Health. 2020;**2**(9):e486-e488

[10] Will AI. Replace radiologists? Intelerad, in Interlerad. May 13, 2022

[11] Jin D, Harrison AP, Zhang L, Yan K, Wang Y, Cai J, et al. Chapter 14 - Artificial intelligence in radiology. In: Xing L, Giger ML, Min JK, editors. Artificial Intelligence in Medicine. Academic Press; 2021. pp. 265-289. DOI: 10.1016/B978-0- 12-821259-2.00014-4. ISBN 9780128212592. Available from: https://www.sciencedirect.com/science/article/pii/B9780128212592000144

[12] Hosny A, Parmar C, Quackenbush J, Schwartz LH, Aerts HJWL. Artificial intelligence in radiology. Nature Reviews Cancer. Aug 2018;**18**(8):500-510. DOI: 10.1038/s41568-018-0016-5. PMID: 29777175; PMCID: PMC6268174

[13] Bi WL et al. Artificial intelligence in cancer imaging: Clinical challenges and applications. CA: A Cancer Journal for Clinicians. 2019;**69**(2):127-157

[14] Wang S, Xiao T, Liu Q, Zheng H. Deep learning for fast MR imaging: A review for learning reconstruction from incomplete k-space data, Biomedical Signal Processing and Control. 2021;**68**:102579. DOI: 10.1016/j.bspc.2021.102579. ISSN 1746- 8094. Available from: https://www.sciencedirect.com/science/article/pii/S1746809421001762

[15] T., N., Top ten issues on liability and regulation of Artificial Intelligence (AI) systems. Top Ten Issues on Liability and Regulation of Artificial Intelligence (AI) Systems, A.o.C.C. (ACC), Editor. August 2, 2021

[16] Bak M et al. You can't have AI both ways: Balancing health data privacy and access fairly. Frontiers in Genetics. 2022;**13**:1490

[17] Sajid H. Ai in radiology: Pros & cons, applications, and 4 examples, in V7. 2023

[18] Korngiebel DM, Solomonides A, Goodman KW. Ethical and Policy Issues. In: Cohen TA, Patel VL, Shortliffe EH, editors. Intelligent Systems in Medicine and Health. Cognitive Informatics in Biomedicine and Healthcare. Cham, Springer; 2022. DOI: 10.1007/978-3-031-09108-7_18

[19] Ahuja AS. The impact of artificial intelligence in medicine on the future role of the physician. PeerJ. 2019;7:e7702

[20] AAMC, Number of people per active physician by specialty

[21] Smith G, Funk J. Ai has a long way to go before doctors can trust it with your life in Quartz. June 4, 2021

[22] Pesapane F, Codari M, Sardanelli F. Artificial intelligence in medical imaging: Threat or opportunity? Radiologists again at the forefront of innovation in medicine. European Radiology Experimental. 2018;**2**:1-10

[23] Hardy M, Harvey H. Artificial intelligence in diagnostic imaging: Impact on the radiography profession. The British Journal of Radiology. 2020;**93**(1108):20190840

[24] Duong MT et al. Artificial intelligence for precision education in radiology. The British Journal of Radiology. 2019;**92**(1103):20190389

[25] Biswas S. Artificial intelligence in radiology education. International Journal of Radiological Radiational Therapy. 2023;**10**(1):1-3

[26] Spear LG et al. Rethinking clinical trial radiology workflows and student training: Integrated virtual student shadowing experience, education, and evaluation. Journal of Digital Imaging. 2022;**35**(3):723-731

[27] Uppot RN et al. Implementing virtual and augmented reality tools for radiology education and training, communication, and clinical care. Radiology. 2019;**291**(3):570-580

[28] Wiggins WF et al. Preparing radiologists to lead in the era of artificial intelligence: Designing and implementing a focused data science pathway for senior radiology residents. Radiology: Artificial Intelligence. 2020;**2**(6):e200057

[29] Lai L, Wittbold KA, Dadabhoy FZ, Sato R, Landman AB, Schwamm LH, et al. Digital triage: Novel strategies for population health management in response to the COVID-19 pandemic. Healthcare (Amsterdam, Netherlands). 2020;**8**(4):100493. DOI: 10.1016/j.hjdsi.2020.100493

[30] Ebrahimian S et al. FDA-regulated AI algorithms: Trends, strengths, and gaps of validation studies. Academic Radiology. 2022;**29**(4):559-566

[31] Estrada EG. Triage systems. Nursing Clinics of North America. 1981;**16**(1):13-24

[32] Sharafat AR, Bayati M. PatientFlowNet: A deep learning approach to patient flow prediction in emergency departments. IEEE Access. 2021;**9**:45552-45561

[33] Tool Developed to assist in Triage in the Emergency Department in John Hopkin news and publication. 2022

[34] Chen C-H et al. Emergency department disposition prediction using a deep neural network with integrated clinical narratives and structured data. International Journal of Medical Informatics. 2020;**139**:104146

[35] Goto S et al. Artificial intelligence to predict needs for urgent

revascularization from 12-leads electrocardiography in emergency patients. PLoS One. 2019;**14**:e0210103

[36] Than MP et al. Machine learning to predict the likelihood of acute myocardial infarction. Circulation. 2019;**140**(11):899-909

[37] Tayal V, Raio C. ACEP Policy Statement-Ultrasound Guidelines: Emergency. Point-of-Care, and Clinical Ultrasound Guidelines in Medicine. 2016

[38] Shokoohi H et al. Enhanced point-of-care ultrasound applications by integrating automated feature-learning systems using deep learning. Journal of Ultrasound in Medicine. 2019;**38**(7):1887-1897

[39] Fleuren LM et al. Machine learning for the prediction of sepsis: A systematic review and meta-analysis of diagnostic test accuracy. Intensive Care Medicine. 2020;**46**:383-400

[40] Murphy SL, Xu J, Kochanek KD. Deaths: final data for 2010. National Vital Statistics Reports. 8 May 2013;**61**(4): 1-117. PMID: 24979972

[41] Islam MM et al. Prediction of sepsis patients using machine learning approach: A meta-analysis. Computer Methods and Programs in Biomedicine. 2019;**170**:1-9

[42] Mao Q et al. Multicentre validation of a sepsis prediction algorithm using only vital sign data in the emergency department, general ward and ICU. BMJ Open. 2018;**8**(1):e017833

[43] Shickel B et al. DeepSOFA: A continuous acuity score for critically ill patients using clinically interpretable deep learning. Scientific Reports. 2019;**9**(1):1879

[44] Saeed U et al. Machine learning empowered COVID-19 patient monitoring using non-contact sensing: An extensive review. Journal of Pharmaceutical Analysis. 2022;**12**(2):193-204

[45] Crotty BH et al. Hospitalization outcomes among patients with COVID-19 undergoing remote monitoring. JAMA Network Open. 2022;**5**(7):e2221050-e2221050

[46] Huang J-D et al. Applying artificial intelligence to wearable sensor data to diagnose and predict cardiovascular disease: A review. Sensors. 2022;**22**(20):8002

[47] Fang S-C, Wu Y-L, Tsai P-S. Heart rate variability and risk of all-cause death and cardiovascular events in patients with cardiovascular disease: A meta-analysis of cohort studies. Biological Research for Nursing. 2020;**22**(1):45-56

[48] Burlacu A et al. Influencing cardiovascular outcomes through heart rate variability modulation: A systematic review. Diagnostics. 2021;**11**(12):2198

[49] DeepMind faces legal action over NHS data use Oct 2021

[50] Rajasekaran AS et al. Blockchain enabled anonymous privacy-preserving authentication scheme for internet of health things. Sensors. 2022;**23**(1):240

[51] Straw I, Wu H. Investigating for bias in healthcare algorithms: A sex-stratified analysis of supervised machine learning models in liver disease prediction. BMJ Health & Care Informatics. 2022;**2002**:29

[52] McCradden MD et al. Patient safety and quality improvement: Ethical principles for a regulatory approach to bias in healthcare machine learning. Journal of the American

Medical Informatics Association. 2020;**27**(12):2024-2027

[53] Federation I. IDF Diabetes Atlas, tenth. International Diabetes. 2021

[54] Latts L. ADA/IBM Watson Health Study (N> 300,000) finds that nearly 60% of people with T2D discontinue therapy after one year. American Diabetes Association 78th Scientific Session. 2018

[55] Flood D et al. The state of diabetes treatment coverage in 55 low-income and middle-income countries: A cross-sectional study of nationally representative, individual-level data in 680 102 adults. The Lancet Healthy Longevity. 2021;**2**(6):e340-e351

[56] Nomura A et al. Artificial intelligence in current diabetes management and prediction. Current Diabetes Reports. 2021;**21**(12):61

[57] A., P. How predictive models of AI & Machine Learning Can Transform Diabetes Care. mddionline.com. 15 June 2022

[58] Vettoretti M et al. Advanced diabetes management using artificial intelligence and continuous glucose monitoring sensors. Sensors. 2020;**20**(14):3870

[59] Nimri R et al. Insulin dose optimization using an automated artificial intelligence-based decision support system in youths with type 1 diabetes. Nature Medicine. 2020;**26**(9):1380-1384

[60] Andellini M et al. Artificial intelligence for non-invasive glycaemic-events detection via ECG in a paediatric population: Study protocol. Health and Technology. 2023;**2023**:1-10

[61] Porumb M et al. Precision medicine and artificial intelligence: A pilot study on deep learning for hypoglycemic events detection based on ECG. Scientific Reports. 2020;**10**(1):170

[62] Nanegrungsunk O, Ruamviboonsuk P, Grzybowski A. Prospective studies on artificial intelligence (AI)-based diabetic retinopathy screening. Annals of Translational Medicine. 2022;**2022**:24

[63] Health & Social Care Information Centre. National Diabetes Audit – 2013-2014 and 2014-2015: Report 1, Care Processes and Treatment Targets [Internet]. NHS Digital. 2015

[64] globenewswire.com, Telemedicine Market to Reach USD 185.66 Billion by 2026 June 2022

[65] Pal K et al. Digital health interventions for adults with type 2 diabetes: Qualitative study of patient perspectives on diabetes self-management education and support. Journal of Medical Internet Research. 2018;**20**(2):e40

Chapter 3

Types of Artificial Intelligence and Future of Artificial Intelligence in Medical Sciences

Noor Us Saba and Mohd Faheem

Abstract

Artificial intelligence (AI) is the machine-based approach for processing various communications and data in computers for defining their actions in future performances. Different types of machine learning are described in medical sciences for proceedings in medical education, medical research, and clinical trials and in treatment of the diseases after appropriate diagnosis. These require less time and efforts of medical professionals and bring a more efficient way to fulfill the standards of medicine. The clear understanding of the workforce accomplishments is required for the future doctors to perform well, alongside the AI. Awareness of AI in the field of medicine is needed for general population to give them an idea for utilization of all new technologies, thus enlightening the feasibility of machine learning at consumer level as well. In future, AI will enhance the efficiency and effectiveness of healthcare delivery in all sectors of medicine and surgery.

Keywords: artificial intelligence, future medical science, healthcare, medical education, medical research, robotic surgery

1. Introduction

Artificial intelligence, AI, is the process of developing perspicacious machines from already existing statistics and data. Past experiences of the different events are learned by these machines to perform human like activities including decision making on their own. This type of complicated technique can be used in almost every sector of the societies like transportation, healthcare, banking, and entertainment [1].

An English mathematician, computer scientist and theoretical biologist, Alan Turing, has been widely considered to be the father of Artificial intelligence. Term artificial intelligence was first coined in the Dartmouth college conference, in 1955. AI program MYCIN was the first use of AI in medicine, developed to identify the treatments of blood infections, in 1970s [2, 3].

Here authors describe various types of AI and role of this machine-based technology in medical sciences along with future perspective of AI for the budding doctors.

2. Methodology of the chapter

The wide range of classifications have been described in different researches [4–7]. We have classified AI based on the need in medical sciences. The aim of present classification is predominantly focused on the understanding of this evolving technology for the scholars of the medical field and the clinicians [8]. This method of categorization makes AI easy to understand to all the personnel concerned with their practices in every sector of the medicine.

To explore the future of AI in medical sciences various scholars in their study had focused individually on the criteria of medical education [9], innovations and researches [10], and disease diagnosis and treatments [11, 12]. Here, we have incorporated all the research details collectively and analyzed them for further use at multi-disciplinary level. Publications of AI on medical curriculum and research were few in comparison to the AI discussions on diagnostic methods and treatments of the diseases.

Here in this chapter, importance of AI in medical curriculum and innovative research are also stressed, along with the use of AI in delivery of medical services. Key word 'artificial intelligence' was used to search references on PubMed and on Google. Further literature was procured by exemplification of primary articles.

3. Types of artificial intelligence

Artificial intelligence in medical sciences is divided into two main categories [8]:

- Virtual
- Physical

3.1 The virtual component

Machine learning delineates the virtual part, which helps to control health management systems by electronic records of health and actively guides the physicians for decision making. It is a neural network-based system using deep learning of information for different approaches of the clinicians. This machine learning or deep learning has three types of mathematical algorithms (**Table 1**).

S.No	Type	Applications
1	Unsupervised learning	Previously undetected patterns are grouped in a logical way
2	Supervised learning	Previous existing patterns are used to compare the given samples
3	Reinforcement learning	Machine learns from its own experiences
		Model based- advanced control of the planning from the learning
		Value based- deep networks represent the functions
		Policy based- more complex neural networks exemplify the functions

Table 1.
Virtual component of artificial intelligence.

- Unsupervised learning (UL)
- Supervised learning (SL)
- Reinforcement learning (RL)

3.1.1 Unsupervised learning (UL)

Unsupervised learning identifies the patterns that are undetected previously. Machines classify them without any guidance from any source. It groups the information in a logical way after comparing and categorizing the unlabeled data, thus performs more complicated process compared to other forms of deep learning. UL is an auto-correction technique based on interpretation and identification to amend the issues of unpredictability. A more commodious AI aid can be developed by taking unsupervised learning principles to ameliorate the effectiveness and precision of health systems. Priority for the health in new generations causes a great number of clinicians to focus specifically on the use of UL to upgrade the efficiency of applications in medical sciences [4].

3.1.2 Supervised learning (SL)

Supervised learning uses the already existing labeled data to generate the correct conclusions from the samples given. Machines becomes more accurate to give conclusions as number of the samples increases. Machines in SL have already been trained by the previously labeled correct and appropriate input data. This data input helps the machine to further plan a correct output when new unsolved tasks are subsequently given to it. Various algorithms and computational methods are used in SL techniques. Some frequently used learning methods in SL are Neural Networks, Naïve Bayes, Linear Regression, Logistic Regression, Support Vector machine, K-nearest neighbor, and Random Forest for accurate data predictions [5].

3.1.3 Reinforcement learning (RL)

Reinforcement learning is the science of creating verdict, which is akin to the process that appeared previously to focus in animal behavioral psychology. In this deep learning method, positive and negative reinforcement plays a key role to give reward for machine learning. Unlike supervised learning, in RL, machine is always bound to learn from its own experiences and does not use already labeled correct data for any favorable outcome (**Figure 1A**). RL gives output based on its own exploration of data with a balance between scrutiny of a given data and exploitation of the basic knowledge of machine for that data [6].

Three main approaches are there to apply in Reinforcement Learning [6]: policy based, value based and model based (**Figure 1B**).

3.1.3.1 Policy based

Policy is the core element of RL. Policy of RL has been made when an agent's behavior at a particular time mapped by the machine and perceived by the environment.

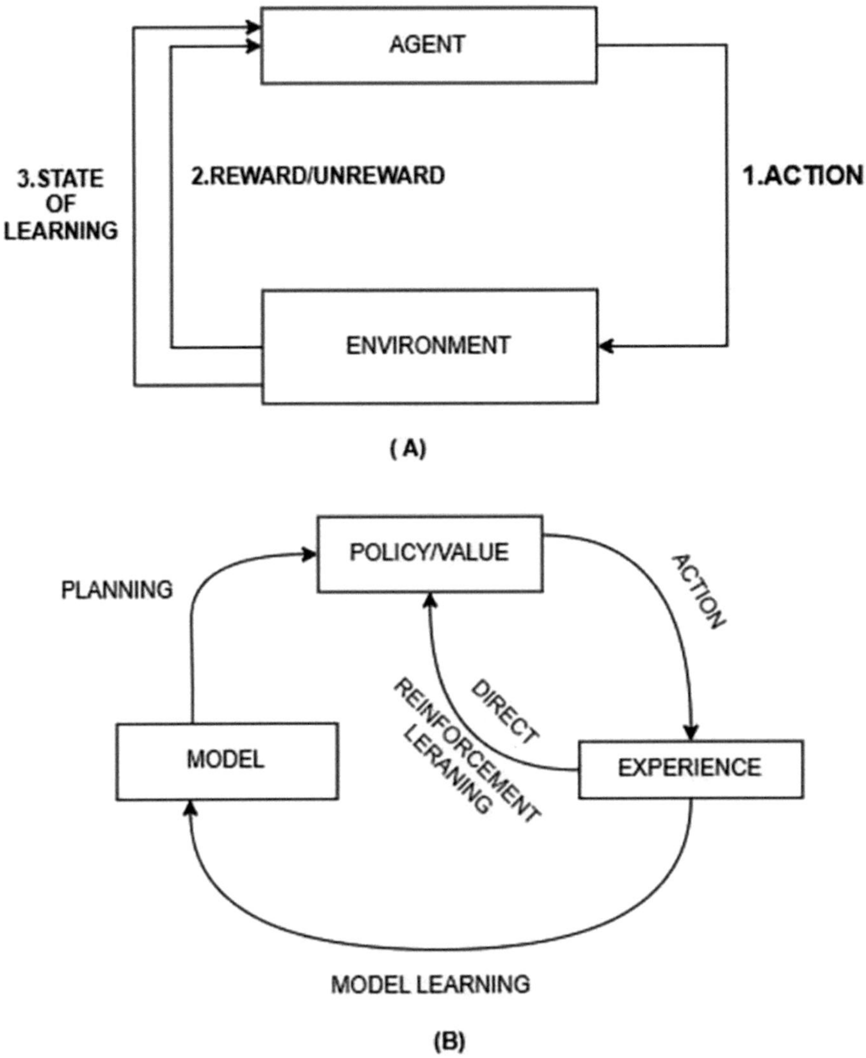

Figure 1.
Reinfiorcement learning. (A) Steps of reinfiorcement learning. (B) Model based, value based, and policy based reinfiorcement learning.

3.1.3.2 Value based

Value based approach gives an idea about the favorable and unfavorable situations to reward or un-reward the agent and depends on the signals for all good and bad steps. It predicts value of a behavior when measured by reward, whereas it counts no value when behavior has been finalized without any reward by the machine.

3.1.3.3 Model based

Model based approach is especially useful for further planning of the ways to take the set of tactics in consideration with all the future circumstances. It acts to make machines in learning process with a goal of having forward thinking in deep learning.

Complex objective after many steps can be attained by these neural network-based learning [6].

3.2 The physical component

Robots, nanorobots, physical objects, medical equipment and many futuristic robots meant to deliver proper care to the patients, come under physical components of AI (**Table 2**). They assist to perform surgeries and help handicapped and aging population to deal with day-to-day challenges in their life [2].

Diagnosis of a disease is frequent and time draining process due to applications of various diagnostic procedures and their interpretation by a limited number of expert doctors. It brings the medical fraternity under a lot of stress for saving the patient's life within limited initial golden hours of the treatment. Digitalized automatic diagnosis of diseases by complex algorithms of machine learning makes a cost effective and time saving measure for doctors as well as for patients. Standard algorithms for diagnoses can benefit consistently with the main quality of their universality in the form of assessment with same team of top experts globally on a low price and within seconds. AI also provides treatment alternatives for the specific diseases, which have been diagnosed by the machines [13].

Earliest detection of impending autism in children can be detected by the eye tracking technology in psychiatry [13]. Robotic characteristics of communication and teaching have created the most impressive example of AI utility in autistic children in future [14–16]. Facial emotion recognition (FER) is a separate area in AI to analyze patient's emotions by comparing images with the available database in the system. This systematic database has already been fed with the patient's data, who had undergone with the same disorders and treatments [13].

Robotic systems which can be used in surgeries are robotic surgery, computer assisted surgery and robotically assisted surgery. Open surgeries have now been improved in the form of minimally invasive surgeries when they are assisted by robots. Tele manipulator devices provide the possibility of distant surgeries in the areas where no surgeons are available. A remote control, governed by the doctor, potentiates the real surgeries on patients without the presence of specialist surgeon on the site of operation [13].

S.No	Type	Applications
1	Digital devices	Early detection of some diseases (autism, stroke, lung cancers, neurological malignancy)
		Digital diagnosis
		Care of elderly people
		Treatment of autism
2	Robots, nano robots, remote control devices	Robotic surgeries
		Computer assisted surgeries
		Remote surgeries
		Robotic solo performance

Table 2.
Physical component of artificial intelligence.

Da Vinci surgical system and AXSIS robot of the Cambridge advisors are well acquainted robots in surgery [13]. Da Vinci surgical system is commonly used for gynecologic surgeries and for prostate surgeries. Cardiac valve repair is the newer and propitious development by this machinery system. Most recent forms of robotic devices are highly evolved to give solo performance in advanced surgeries [14–16].

Benign and malignant tumors of the central nervous system and lung cancer detection by low dose computer tomography (LDCT) for high-risk individuals are some other applications of AI in medicine. Support vector machine (SVM) and convolutional neural network (CNN) are expert machinery system for identification and classification of stroke even before the episode of stroke. Direct analysis of stroke can be notified to the hospital team with in minutes. It helps the clinicians for early detection and treatment of such a medical emergency causing brain damage of the patient if there is any delay in the treatment [13]. Robots also has become promising to take care of elderly individuals and are becoming most emerging medical devices to help aging population on their own [14–16].

4. Future of artificial intelligence in medical sciences

Medical science enfolds various courses which describe the anatomy and functions of human body. Basic biology like anatomy, physiology, and biochemistry with many other graduate subjects in medicine come under medical sciences. Today, AI technology and machine learning (ML) have developed ahead of biological sciences to apply on a vast majority of medical specialties such as radiology, screening, psychiatry, primary medical care, diagnosis of the disease and telemedicine [17, 18].

Future of AI in medical sciences can be discussed in three forms (**Table 3**).

- Medical education
- Medical research and innovations
- Diagnosis and treatment of diseases

4.1 AI in medical education

Curriculum of medical education now emphasize more on e-learning methods which are yet to adopt in many countries. AI helps to see the bridge between the availability of digital resources and utilization of the resources by medical students and teachers. Integration of many technologies akin to neural networks, expertise, deep learning, machine learning, speech, image, and language recognition simulate insightful behavior of humans. Lately, AI has gained vast application in medical education. Many research has been conducted to observe the cause of underutilization of e-content by the students and teachers to reach the conclusion for possible solutions of those problems [9].

Presumably, AI will help teachers to promote the students for self-directed learning and will help to give healthy discussions on case-based studies. The major hurdle is to face multiple distractions while finding knowledge about simple and small topics by the students through e-learning platforms. In near future, as the technology advances, there might be a possibility of level wise distribution of digital

S.No	Category	Methods	Future expectations
1	Medical education	Availability of standard and best quality digital resources	Consumer friendly E learning platforms
			E content utilization by medical students and teachers
			Promotion of self-directed learning of medical students
			Level wise distribution of digital content for graduate, postgraduate and researcher scholars
			Digital synchronization of topic understanding between medical student and faculty
		Monitoring the use of digital content	Quality based efficiency of the electronic data for students and teachers can be measured
		Digital assessment program	Self-assessment methods to shape the right direction of student's learning
2	Medical research and innovations	Research exploration through machine learning	Time saving and cost-effective clinical trials
			Fair and ethical innovations by the diverse teams making universally acceptable data
3	Diagnosis and treatments	image analysis	Interpretation of radiological and pathological images
		Wide spread clinical practices	Digital clinical notes by speech recognition and text identification of the patient
			Integration of medical professionals with newer technology
		Prediction of high-risk situations	Stroke, sepsis, and heart failure
		Digital recording of genetic outlines in different tumors	Early detection and treatment of cancers
		Message alert and provocative action devices for the patient	Personalized and contextualized care of the patient
		Documentation of health records and claims processing	Administration, health insurers and other stakeholders time will be saved

Table 3.
Future of artificial intelligence in medical sciences.

content based on the understanding of graduate and post graduate students, as well as researcher and scientists. This distribution of content in digital library will be time saving for the teachers, students as well as for researchers [19].

Moreover, standard and quality along with the accessibility of the content will be considered the double edge sword for any digital content to make it available for the students. Digital files will be more consumer friendly whether for teachers or for medical students, filling the gap between physical and digital resources. AI can be used to monitor the efficiency of e-resources to be used by the consumer on frequent basis and enhances the scope of improvement in medical education system globally in the universal form. It can make a synchronized understanding of the subjects between students and the medical faculty [20].

As the teaching is always followed by the assessment of students for different subjects, development of various digital platforms will make the assessment methods more convenient and user friendly. These platforms will save much time for the assessment as compared to the conventional methods. It will make formative evaluation easier for the teachers. Students can also evaluate themselves on different steps of learning by the newly developed assessment methods, giving them more confidence for development in the correct direction during their stay in medical schools. A digital self-assessment program can be developed for the students to judge themselves as to where they stand overall throughout the medical studies. These types of assessments will be helpful and time saving for the challenging newly applied competency based medical education curriculum, which is promising for creating competent physicians and surgeons to embark in health care system globally [21, 22].

4.2 AI in medical research and innovations

Implementation of machine learning (ML) to expedite clinical exploration are sporadically discussed on intellectual ground. Medical research is an extensive field, with investigations and observational evaluation, guiding traditional trials with realistic elements which in turn encourage clinical registries and additional implementation work. Clinical research is invaluable to improve the health care and outcomes. It has been proved as complicated, demanding in terms of labor, expensive and vulnerable to unexpected errors. ML has the possibility to help and improve the accomplishments, universality, patient focusing and effectivity of clinical trials, preventing the loss of years as well as dollars of expenditure as have been done in many conventional settings of analysis [10, 23].

Functional and metaphysical barriers in ML can do well in clinical research in future after précised focus on them. The prospective applications of ML to medical research recently overtake its existing use, because few potential studies are available about the reasonable effectiveness of ML in contrast to the conventional approaches. Conversion of traditional methodology to ML needs time, enthusiasm, and collaboration for effective adoption. Communication and cooperation are crucial for application of this favorable technology for the future application in medical research and innovations [24].

The future goal for application of ML in research is to create fair and ethical innovations that will be universally acceptable. Vigorous and integrative collaborations can reduce chances of bias in clinical research with ML. More diverse teams may offer innovative insights for de-biasing ML models [2].

4.3 AI in diagnosis and treatment of diseases

For healthcare delivery of the future AI has a very important role. At the beginning, efforts to provide diagnosis and treatment are challenging but expectations to pick up in this area is anticipated in the future (**Table 2**). In radiology and pathology most images will be analyzed and examined by the machines at some point. Usage of already working speech recognition and text identification for communication with the patients and getting clinical notes will increase [11]. A widespread challenge for the use of AI in health domain is the ensured adoption in clinical practices rather than proven capability of technology itself. This provocation can overcome by integration with the system, approval by the regulators, sufficient standardization, awareness to the clinicians and getting updated (both medical professionals and consumers) over time-to-time basis. Overcoming the challenges will take longer time compared to the time taken by technologies to mature [12].

There will be more use of technologies in next 10 years but not within 5 years due to this time constraints in adoption of something new in medical field. On a substantial scale, it is very clear that AI methods will not supersede the human physicians, but rather will boost their endeavors for patient's care. Human physicians gradually may proceed towards the job motif that makes them capable on unique soft skills like empathy, and the integration with unique understanding on the big scale. Conceivably, the healthcare personnel who deny to work next to the artificial intelligence will no longer have a job in near future [12].

It is important to consider the development of our health care systems in terms of AI. These technologies potentially transform various aspects of patient care better than humans, most importantly the diagnosis of disease. But replacing humans by computer's AI for a vast medical domain will take many years due to multiple barriers [25]. To achieve the human level performance in terms of cognition, intelligent behavior of a computer has been used since year 2016, a well-known time to show highest investments in AI for healthcare applications [26].

As we already are familiar with "virtual" and "physical" subtypes of AI [8]. The physical part deals with the performance of robots in various surgeries, care of handicapped individuals and elderly people. The virtual part deals with a range of information data from digital records of the patient's health to the guided neural network in treatment decisions of the patients. It describes the diagnosis of the patients via two wide techniques: Flowchart based and Database [2].

The flowchart-based method translates the sequence of questions of a physician for taking history to reach a most likely diagnosis after amalgamation of complex presented symptoms. A large amount of data, containing multidirectional clinical features of diseases, is the main requirement into cloud-based machinery networks. A major challenge in ML is inability to gather patient's cues which can only be observed directly by a doctor during consultation. This results in a belief that AI can assist the physicians in future but cannot replace the human physicians in health care [2].

The database uses recognition of different images of a specific group to apply for answering the questions related to a particular diagnosis. A decade ago, google project "artificial brain" was designed on the principle of deep learning by database approach. This approach was used to match and mismatch various images in radiology and pathology for diagnosis of distinct sets of diseases [2].

MYCIN, Watson and some free open source such as Tensor Flow on Google are systems developed to incorporate in healthcare system. The strict rule oriented clinical opinion making machinery systems are not easy to maintain on medical ground due to constant change in medical knowledge. A big amount of data handling too is a big challenge for the healthcare system in ML. Statistically based ML framework leading the way in a period of evidence-based medicine, which is reflecting a positive change in broad term, but has many challenges such as ethical issues of the patients. Google now a days collaborates with health delivery channels to make prediction designs from big data to alert the physicians for high-risk situations, like sepsis and heart failure [12].

Various firms are also there to focus more on investigation and treatment protocols of different cancers based on their genetic outlines. Foundation medicine and Flatiron health are specialized firms for complex understanding of all the genetic variants of cancers and their response to new treatment protocols. These rules-based, algorithmic diagnosis and treatment methods are many times challenging to get embedded in clinical fields. Majority of AI techniques address only one aspect of medical care thus standalone in nature. Such incorporation issues have possibly been a substantial barrier to broaden the application of AI than accuracy and effectiveness of the technique itself [27].

Patient's cooperation is the final need for making any method to give good or bad outcomes. Better outcome has been observed as the participation of patients increases when they become more active to owe well-being and good health. For the better health outcomes, AI will be developed in such a way which personalize and contextualize the care. This can be supplemented by message alerts and provocative actions for the concerned patients [12].

Administration uses the AI less potentially, but it provides substantial efficiency in management of revenue cycle, clinical notes, claims processing and medical records documentation. False insurance claims can be identified easily and help the health insurers and governments to save time, finance, and lot of efforts of stakeholders [12].

To the best of all outcomes by using AI, it is believed that no jobs will be eliminated in health care working in parallel with the AI. Jobs pertaining to the direct patient interaction will have less impact to fade itself. In AI systems, radiology and pathology perform a single task such as specific nodule detection in chest computed tomography and specific specimen findings in a biopsy result. Only a few of pathology and radiology findings have been identified by AI till date, thus showing the role of human pathologist and radiologist to be there for a longer time before technology fully replace all the possible tasks done by the medical specialists. It is likely to create more jobs for the individuals having knowledge to work with AI which can further develop the effective use of AI in future [11].

In public health area, AI has a well-established role, which causes reduction in time of the doctors given on diseases already observed and treated many times, augmenting their work on more complicated and rare cases. Reshaping of various aspects of medical services are possible by these developing technologies and many patients can take advantages of taking alternative medications and follow-up care without much efforts. AI is expanding to have a significant impact on every angle of primary health care, reducing physician's labor and increasing their efficiency, precision, and effectivity. But AI cannot replace medical experts completely in the tactful branch of mankind [2].

5. Limitations of artificial intelligence in medical sciences

Data availability for construction of well executed artificially intelligent models consult the large quantities of high-quality data. Patient's confidentiality and public right to privacy issues restrict the data availability [14–16, 24], making compromised framework with limited potential (**Table 4**). This fragmented data limits the predictability of a model for successful application of AI within and between the organization. Biased data processing with or without biased data collection in terms of population specificity for distinct race, age, and gender result in the distorted

S.No	Limitations	Causes of the limitations
1	Data availability	Ethical issues
		Biased data collection
		Biased data processing
2	Complex mathematical algorithm	Burdensome for the medical users
		Obstinate to adapt the constant change in medical sciences
3	Human social skills	Not possible by machines and robots
		Medical professional assistance needed

Table 4.
Limitations of artificial intelligence in medical sciences.

collection of data, fabricating defective algorithm. Thus, it is invariably difficult to find elite algorithm matched for upcoming task to accomplish. Basic information is constantly needed to understand, for the building of AI prototypes, by a user. These details help them to interpret the correct or incorrect output and execution of preferable use of the output. But, despite having some latest studies in this direction, complex black boxes of mathematical algorithms are burdensome to approach and decipher precisely by the medical users [24].

Machines can be able to construe human behavior, but many human characteristics such as rational thinking, interactive and social skills, emotional understanding, and ingenuity cannot be acuminated by the machines and robots. The qualities for humanity present in the doctors cannot be replaced absolutely by AI. It is required for the medical neophyte to learn the notions and relevance of AI and how to ramify well organized work along with machines for greater advantages alongside plowing soft skills in them [8]. A wide range of skills are needed in future physicians to accommodate the constant changing technology-based healthcare delivery. An adequate understanding of technical concepts, basics of AI, data management and treatment oriented ethical issues are some newer expertise to incorporate in upcoming medical generations apart from the mastering medicine. These abilities will equip the doctors to identify the accuracy of machines, reducing the chances of error. Thus, a supervisor of AI tools will always be needed even with a well-established source of treatment modality and robots [28, 29].

6. Conclusion

Artificial Intelligence is an expanding science. The types of AI come under two categories, including virtual and physical components. Virtual components have many subdivisions in the applications of AI. The combinations of these Machine-based learning can be utilized in medical sciences including medical education, medical research and innovations along with the diagnosis and treatment of diseases. Some freely openable sources have already been developed in the field of health care, but need many modifications to define the uniqueness of AI for incorporation in the medical field effectively. Various research signals that AI is an intrinsically developing trade in the area of medicine. It can be safely concluded, there will be massive benefit to the healthcare care system by the application of AI under the supervision of medical professionals.

Acknowledgements

I am thankful to my family for the support they have provided in writing this chapter.

Conflict of interest

"The authors declare no conflict of interest."

Author details

Noor Us Saba[1*] and Mohd Faheem[2]

1 Department of Anatomy, King George's Medical University, Lucknow, U.P, India

2 Department of Neurosurgery, Uttar Pradesh University of Medical Sciences, Saifai, U.P, India

*Address all correspondence to: noorussaba83@gmail.com

References

[1] Jiang F, Jiang Y, Zhi H, Dong Y, Li H, Ma S, et al. Artificial intelligence in healthcare: Past, present and future. Stroke and Vascular Neurology. 2017;**2**(4):230-243. DOI: 10.1136/svn-2017-000101

[2] Amisha MP, Pathania M, Rathaur VK. Overview of artificial intelligence in medicine. Journal of Family Medicine and Primary Care. 2019;**8**:2328-2331

[3] XSOLIS Insights [Internet]. 2021. Available from: https://www.google.com/search?q=the+evolution+of+artificial+intelligence+in+healthcare [Accessed: April 7, 2023].

[4] Wang J, Biljecki F. Unsupervised machine learning in urban studies: A systematic review of applications. Cities. 2022;**129**:103925

[5] Sarker IH. Machine learning: Algorithms, real-world applications and research directions. SN Computer Science. 2021;**2**:160

[6] GeeksforGeeks [Internet]. 2023. Available from: https://www.geeksforgeeks.org/what-is-reinforcement-learning/ [Accessed: April 8, 2023]

[7] Sarker IH. AI-based modeling: Techniques, applications and research issues towards automation, intelligent and smart systems. SN Computer Science. 2022;**3**(2):158. DOI: 10.1007/s42979-022-01043-x

[8] Hamet P, Tremblay J. Artificial intelligence in medicine. Metabolism. 2017;**69S**:S36-S40

[9] Civaner MM, Uncu Y, Bulut F. Artificial intelligence in medical education: A cross-sectional needs assessment. BMC Medical Education. 2022;**22**:772. DOI: 10.1186/s12909-022-03852-3

[10] Weissler EH, Naumann T, Andersson T. The role of machine learning in clinical research: Transforming the future of evidence generation. Trials. 2021;**22**:537. DOI: 10.1186/s13063-021-05489-x

[11] Davenport TH, Kirby J. Only Humans Need Apply: Winners and Losers in the Age of Smart Machines. New York: Harper Business; 2016

[12] Davenport T, Kalakota R. The potential for artificial intelligence in healthcare. Future Healthcare Journal. 2019;**6**(2):94-98

[13] George J, Bijimol TK. AI in medical field. In: International Conference on Intellectual Property Rights. International Journal of Science and Research. 2021:70-73

[14] Cornet G. Robot companions and ethics a pragmatic approach of ethical design. Journal International de Bioéthique. 2013;**24**(4):49-58 [179-80]

[15] Larson JA, Johnson MH, Bhayani SB. Application of surgical safety standards to robotic surgery: Five principles of ethics for nonmaleficence. Journal of the American College of Surgeons. 2014;**218**(2):290-293

[16] Knight BA, Potretzke AM, Larson JA, Bhayani SB. Comparing expert reported outcomes to National Surgical Quality Improvement Program risk calculator–predicted outcomes: Do reporting standards differ? Journal of Endourology. 2015;**29**(9):1091-1099

[17] The school of health [Internet]. Available from: https://www.schoolofhealth.com/be-better/natural-health-definitions/medical-sciences/ [Accessed: May 3, 2023]

[18] Gillett G. Medical science, culture, and truth. Philosophy, Ethics, and Humanities in Medicine. 2006;**1**:13. DOI: 10.1186/1747-5341-1-13

[19] Paranjape K, Schinkel M, Nannan Panday R, Car J, Nanayakkara P. Introducing artificial intelligence training in medical education. JMIR Med Educ. 2019;**5**(2):e16048. DOI: 10.2196/16048

[20] Imran N, Jawaid M. Artificial intelligence in medical education: Are we ready for it? Pakistan Journal of Medical Sciences. 2020;**36**(5):857-859. DOI: 10.12669/pjms.36.5.3042

[21] Lee Juehea W, Siyu A, David L, Mahan KK. Artificial intelligence in undergraduate medical education: A scoping review. Academic Medicine. 2021;**96**(11S):S62-S70. DOI: 10.1097/ACM.0000000000004291

[22] Jia K, Wang P, Li Y, Chen Z, Jiang X. Lin C-L and Chin T (2022) research landscape of artificial intelligence and e-learning: A bibliometric research. Frontiers in Psychology. 2022;**13**:795039. DOI: 10.3389/fpsyg

[23] Buch VH, Ahmed I, Maruthappu M. Artificial intelligence in medicine: Current trends and future possibilities. The British Journal of General Practice. 2018;**68**(668):143-144. DOI: 10.3399/bjgp18X695213

[24] Basu K, Sinha R, Ong A, Basu T. Artificial intelligence: How is it changing medical sciences and its future? Indian Journal of Dermatology. 2020;**65**(5):365-370. DOI: 10.4103/ijd.IJD_421_20

[25] Mintz Y, Brodie R. Introduction to artificial intelligence in medicine. Minimally Invasive Therapy & Allied Technologies. 2019;**28**:73-81

[26] CB Insights Research. Healthcare remains the hottest AI category for deals. 2017. Available from: https://www.cbinsights.com/research/artificial-intelligence-healthcare-startups-investors/. [Accessed: April 9, 2023]

[27] Low LL, Lee KH, Ong MEH. Predicting 30-day readmissions: Performance of the LACE index compared with a regression model among general medicine patients in Singapore. Biomed Research International. 2015;**2015**:169870

[28] Park SH, Do K, Kim S, Park JH, Lim Y. What should medical students know about artificial intelligence in medicine? Journal of Educational Evaluation for Health Professions. 2019;**16**:18. DOI: 10.3352/jeehp.2019.16.18

[29] Wartman SA, Combs CD. Medical education must move from the information age to the age of artificial intelligence. Academic Medicine. 2018;**93**(8):1107-1109. DOI: 10.1097/acm.0000000000002044

Chapter 4

Artificial Intelligence in Healthcare: Doctor as a Stakeholder

Subba Rao Bhavaraju

Abstract

Artificial Intelligence (AI) is making significant inroads into healthcare, as in many other walks of life. Its contribution to clinical decision making, to achieve better outcomes, image interpretation especially in radiology, pathology and oncology, data mining, generating hidden insights, and reducing human errors in healthcare delivery is noteworthy. Yet there are physicians as well as patients and their families, who are wary of its role and its implementation in routine clinical practice. Any discussion on AI and its role in healthcare brings into consideration issues like hype and hope associated with any new technologies, uncertain understanding of who the stakeholders are, patients' views and their acceptance, validity of data models used for training and decision making at the point of care. These considerations must be accompanied by thorough policy discussions on the future of AI in healthcare and how the curriculum planners in medical education should train the medical students who are the future healthcare providers. A deliberation on the issues on the issues that are common to Information Technology (IT) like cybersecurity, ethics and legal aspects, privacy, and transparency is also needed.

Keywords: artificial intelligence, data at point of care, stakeholders, annotation, anonymisation, ethical and legal issues, privacy and security, trust, concerns, explainability, medical education, emotions and behaviour, disability, negative impact

1. Introduction

Artificial Intelligence (AI) is making significant inroads into healthcare, as in many other walks of life. Its contribution to clinical decision making, improved outcomes, image interpretation especially in radiology, pathology and oncology, data mining, new insights generation and elimination of human errors creeping in healthcare delivery is noteworthy. Yet there are physicians as well as patients who are wary of its role and its implementation in routine clinical practice.

Data is key for successful AI and machine learning (ML) and more is not always better. Statistics and artificial intelligence need to analyse large data sets to discover useful information and the data should be accurate, appropriate, and clean. Care of the data in healthcare at its generation—the point of care and its value in AI and the healthcare provider's role cannot be overemphasised. Is AI a totally computer scientists' dominion? What is the doctor's role in it? Are they just the beneficiary.

Any discussion on AI and its role in healthcare brings into consideration the issues like hype and hope associated, who are the stakeholders, healthcare personnel and the patients' views and their acceptance, data at its generation—at the point of care, the future of AI in healthcare and how would the curriculum planners in medical education train the medical students, who are the future healthcare providers. Also needed is a deliberation on the issues that are common to Information Technology (IT) like cybersecurity, ethics and legal aspects, privacy, and transparency. This also brings into review various issues the developers of AI solutions in healthcare need to bear in mind. The gaps in the current knowledge and databases also need a thought. Do the AI database and the EHR cover the global scenario adequately. Many areas in the world do not follow the EHR. Are the ethnic and regional differences in health and disease well represented in the Database?

2. Methodology

This chapter is a review of the literature relevant to the medical profession and their concerns as stakeholders on a subject that is not primarily their dominion. The important search engines used are Google, Microsoft Bing, Google Scholar, and PubMed. The Search words used are: Artificial Intelligence, Data at point of care, Stakeholders, Annotation, Anonymisation, Ethical and Legal Issues, Privacy and Security, Trust, Concerns, Explainability, Medical Education, Emotions and behaviour, Disability, Negative Impact, and loss of Jobs.

The search included blogs, articles, reports and publications in peer reviewed journals referring to AI in healthcare. The ultimate beneficiary of AI in healthcare is the patients. The concerns of the patients as well as healthcare professionals with reference to trust and possible ethical and legal issues are covered. The claims of the AI are not without certain negative impacts. An attempt is made to cover the pros and the cons of AI in healthcare. The technical work concerned with the development of the AI/ML platforms and algorithms is beyond the scope of this review and are excluded. A number of tools applying AI/ML are currently in use in healthcare. A few of them are in pipeline. The purpose of this review is not to evaluate the AI/ML tools that are currently in use or in pipeline in healthcare (**Table 1**).

Pros	Cons
Precision in Diagnosis: Computer Vision	Absence of Trust: Lack of Human Touch
Elimination of Human Error	No Peer Review of Processes
Efficient performance of Repetitive tasks: No Fatigue	Absence of Research Protocol—Double blind Study
Decision Support	Scare of Job Loss
Speed of Action	Explainability
Digitalisation	Not Universally Accepted
Newer Insights	Reliability
Costs: Claim reduction	Expensive to implement

Table 1.
AI in healthcare—Pros and Cons.

3. The Hype and The Hope

In today's world of data intensive computing [1–3], we seem to live in a state of hype and hope for the role of artificial intelligence in every walk of life. A hope that AI is the panacea or cure all to a mistrust, and scepticism exist in several fields. The doctor patient relationship is a type of bond, much beyond the factual clinical relation of diagnosis, intervention, and outcome. The patients as well as doctors are circumspect and wary of the ability of AI to substitute that relationship [4, 5].

The ability of creating AI and to let an algorithm take over the human function is not preferred by many. The patients have a significant hesitation in handing over their health issues to a machine. Can the machine match the subtleties of communication, eye contact, personal touch and the empathy that is expected from a human? Can the AI manage a situation end to end in patient care? The complexities of healthcare are thought to be beyond the capability of a machine. Is the AI too standardised and not flexible enough to the individual needs of a patient. Decision support systems in vogue are accepted by the patient but want the decision making is preferred to be left to humans [6, 7].

The doctor performs a number of duties in the doctor patient relationships. Does the AI promise to replace the doctor in every aspect? As a clinician, he does interpret the difficulties the patient has, elicits certain signs suggestive of a diagnosis and orders relevant investigations. It is possible that humans err in judgement, may not be fully equipped with all the knowledge and is prone to have his own bias. AI certainly promises to cover these deficits of a human. However, does the AI take over the functions as a team leader, comfort the patient when needed, help the patient in risk assessment and make right decisions in contrasting and compromising situations. One of the most important duties of the doctor is in terminal illness, palliative care, empathy, psychological support and even conveying the sad news of a near one's death [8]. Is the AI equally competent to humans in these functions?

4. The stakeholders

Is AI a computer scientists' dominion– the theoreticians, the analysts, the developers [9]? Who are all the stakeholders? Is the end user in healthcare—the patient or the provider a stakeholder? The healthcare provider is an important stakeholder. The doctor, nurse and other parties involved in the healthcare are responsible as a generator of the data at the point of care and as a beneficiary of the final product in AI. The patient too is a stakeholder. Some of the data unless provided by the patient does not contribute to the database under consideration in AI. Needless to mention, the patient is a beneficiary too of the improved outcome and error prevention. What is the stakeholder's responsibility. They all are accountable, liable, and blameworthy [10].

5. The data at the point of care

The data is the most important resource in the AI process. Efficient and effective management of this data by AI depends on many factors. The data in healthcare consists of the details of the patients—personal demographic details, historical aspects of the illness, clinical observations, diagnostic evaluation, reports generated, treatment including medication, outcomes, and financial data like costs, billing. For effective analytics, be it descriptive, predictive, prescriptive, or cognitive, the data shall be accurate and comprehensive. The healthcare providers play a major role.

Much of the data that forms the basis of AI development is generated at the time the patient is at the healthcare provider, at the point of care. The importance of recording the data at the point of care cannot be overemphasised, once the opportunity of recording an event is lost, the data could be lost forever [11].

How careful are the clinicians, the laboratory staff, and others in the health care team while recording the data at the stage of its occurrence? Do they record the deficiencies, errors, personal bias in ordering tests and their interpretation? Are the complications and untoward reactions reported and recorded? One should know the value of data and the vigilance to be maintained at the point of care—where it is generated. The details, the quality, its reliability, and totality, including a report on the unexpected events, complications and interpretations need proper documentation.

Digital case records like electronic health records (EHR) have significantly enhanced the scope of the data collection [12]. The EHR is a health record that keeps the demographic data, clinical details including symptomatic, historical, clinical, diagnostic, therapeutic and outcome data, nurses' notes, pharmacy, other therapists like physical therapists, insurance, and billing data. Healthcare providers and organisations collect, track, store, and transmit personal health information. With so much data accumulating, what is important and what is not in the perspective of AI is an issue. What goes into the databases is important [13]. The responsibility of the health care personnel is noteworthy. The comments of the former editor of New England Journal of Medicine [14] reflect the rather unfortunate situation. He regrets to note that the published work does not represent the true state with significant data unpublished. True picture of the illness, its presentation, features, outcomes and complications and untoward reactions may go unrepresented in the database. With the policy of insisting on publication for academic recognition, doubts are cast on the validity of the published work [15, 16]. One should remember the old saying, "If an event is not documented, it did not occur." The value-based care depends on the validity of the database and its true reflection of knowledge base [17]. Many countries are making electronic health records mandatory. These include Australia, Belgium, Canada, Denmark, the United Kingdom, and United States. The goal of these initiatives in health information technologies is to digitally transform the collection, display, transmission, and storage of patient leading to a steady increase in data at the point of care [18–20].

Two other dimensions need consideration when EHR is discussed. The EHR is not followed universally in all countries. Paper case records and data entry in non-digital format is common. The inadequacies that are incidental in paper records and their reflection in the database need consideration. The EHR or the paper case records talk of the patient data while he is in doctor's office or in the hospital. Modern technology offers a different dimension to the data.

With advances in mobile technology, digital patient monitoring, tele-healthcare, ambulatory care and wearable devices, the data is generated while the patient is away from the hospital, at home, work or elsewhere. These data provides the status of the patient during the period intervening the doctor's visits, contextual and historical data that influence the outcomes and insights that the AI generates. The providers have an obligation to incorporate this data in the patient records. Transfer of this self-collected data to the AI database and its influence on the insights provided by AI in healthcare is to be ensured. The mobile technology and the wearables generating data also lead the concerns of patient privacy, transparency, interoperability, and data sharing across all platforms [21, 22]. The actual time when the event occurred and the uploading of the data is also important as the data is likely to change with times, especially in acute care situations.

6. Annotation

One of the most important steps in AI is Annotation. Data Annotation is the process of categorising and labelling individual elements of the data for AI applications. The data can be in image, a video, audio, graphic or a text format. The annotation is to convert the data into a machine-readable format. The annotation was being done manually to start with, but machine read annotations are available currently. Manual annotators are currently creating the data sets helping the computers using Natural Language Processing (NLP) and Computer Vision to detect the text and images in interpreting images in radiology, pathology, oncology, retinopathy, biometrics, and data insights. Uniformity in description and standardisation of the data annotation detectable by NLP or computer vision forms the basics of annotation. Healthcare provider has an obligation to use the right machine-readable word for the text and description of an image or video. The AI interpreted annotation is one of the future probabilities. Even for the AI interpreted annotations, the algorithms. Need to consider manual data annotation to start with [23–28].

7. The AI and legal issues

A detailed discussion on the various legal issues relevant to AI and healthcare is beyond the scope of the current note and the reader shall look elsewhere. A brief account of the legal issues in relation to the healthcare is presented for awareness of the doctor as a user and stakeholder, especially in case of untoward reaction and damages occurring during the course of one's actions using the AI. As per the common law, a person of unsound mind is not responsible for his actions. It means only a person with sound mind is responsible for his actions. The common law also talks of subjective element of criminal intent. Is the computer which lacks the human mind and intent held responsible for its actions. The AI is considered as a technological tool with ability to simulate human brain and perform some of the duties that require human intelligence [29–33]. In case of wrong decisions, adverse reactions and untoward outcomes resulting after usage of AI, what is the liability of the AI and the healthcare team? The machine does not have its own identity but there are multiple persons involved finally in AI in healthcare—the vendor, the owner of the company, the designer, the hardware or the software developer, the persons who evaluates and tests the tool, the person who supplies the data or the database itself, or the doctor who uses the AI platform on a patient. Who is responsible or accountable for the damages caused in using the AI? The legal issues that arise in addition to adverse reaction or the outcome are—a foreseeable damage, a human rights violation, violation of privacy, a criminal intent, cybercrime, and risk of a hacker laying his hands on the data. While the machine is not responsible in itself, can the person behind the machine be held responsible? To what extent is the doctor accountable as a user. Are the people who built it and use it responsible. Lack of accountability raises concerns about the possible safety consequences of using unverified or unvalidated AI in clinical settings.

Awareness of the potential of AI, responsible use of the AI and the insights provided, potential harms, taking an informed consent from the patient while using AI interpreted results, is the responsibility of the doctor [34–38]. The interesting case of Google vs. Information Commission (UK) shows the issues that need consideration. Issues in handling sensitive data like privacy, transparency need attention. A code of ethics has to be developed [39–41].

Explainability is an issue that needs consideration [42–44]. How do the AI driven algorithms arrive at a prediction or a conclusion in a given situation? Should the process of AI be a part of the informed consent? Is it necessary to explain the process? Ethically the medical doctor is accountable for his actions. The informed consent one obtains shall be really informed. When using the AI driven clinical decision support systems, the doctor has to be aware of the reasoning behind such decisions. Four principles are considered when we talk of explainability of AI—the algorithms used in a language the user understands, the evidence and reasoning behind the conclusions drawn, the reliability of the processes used, and the proof for the outcomes or insights. Doctor patient relationship involves mutual trust. The doctor has to explain his actions and decisions and they shall be transparent, patient centred and holistic. Are the processes and algorithms involved in reaching the conclusions in AI systems explainable to a doctor?

8. Privacy and security of data

The AI in healthcare deals significant sensitive personally identifiable information (PII) consisting of demographic and health data of the patient. Apart from the doctors, the nurses, pharmacists, diagnostic lab personnel, other therapists, some statutory bodies like regulatory authorities and the patients themselves access the digital platform in healthcare at various stages. This data generated is accessed at the point of care, at data analysis, deep mining, and when looking for insights. The data necessarily has to be transparent and portable and is stored cloud. This scenario is a hacker's haven. Whose responsibility is its security? When in a specific case the AI fails or is misused, the ethical principles of privacy, autonomy, and justice could be violated. Data theft and misuse are common threats in any computer program, and it is the responsibility of the user to protect the privacy, and security of the owner of the data. All the stakeholders who have access to the data have to be careful of the data in such a situation. The AI developer and user has to keep a watch on the impact of the misuse or discrimination. What processes should we implement to monitor the impact and how to overcome the unintended clinical outcomes. What skills does a developer, or a user has to acquire to enable performance of these tasks. A dialogue between all the stakeholders is necessary on these issues to protect the rights of those involved against direct or indirect coercion. Should the doctor as a user of the AI systems, and as a person involved in the management of the patient, the ultimate beneficiary, be involved in the various processes of AI [45–47]?

9. Anonymisation and encryption

Most countries have regulatory procedures to protect the privacy of the data. The Digital Personal Data Protection Bill 2022, The European Union's new General Data Protection Regulation (GDPR), The California Consumer Privacy Act (CCPA) and Digital Information Security in Health Care Act (DISHA) [48–51] are some of the acts concerned with the data protection. Anonymisation and encryption are the two methods of protecting the identity of personal data when large databases are created and stored in places accessed in AI or other computer programs. Encoding, anonymization, pseudonymisation, generalisation, masking, data swapping, data perturbation are some of the methods of removing or coding the words that connect the data to its owner, whereby the personal identity. Encrypted data storage in cloud and use of Internet of Things for remote access is in practice. Blockchain based secure sharing of data in healthcare is another form of secure data handling [52–55].

10. The promise and challenges of AI in healthcare

The AI in healthcare promises a bright future. The functions of AI can be summarised as relieving, splitting, replacing, and augmenting the role of healthcare personnel [56]. The AI helps streamlining of the work, front office management, the EHRs, human error prevention, administrative work, and provides the expert systems, decision making algorithms, and new insights. The contribution of AI in the diagnostic work especially the interpreting the images in radiology, retinopathy, pathology, and oncology is striking. Help in analysis and mining of large cohorts is a great boon to the epidemiologist. The speed and accuracy of the data processing and predictions are more efficient than humans. Stroke prediction and cardiovascular risk assessment are some of the newer algorithms available. Robotics processes automation are used in healthcare, for repetitive tasks like prior authorisation, updating patient records and billing [57–59].

The challenge of acceptance by the patients remains. The value of the databases used and updating is always problematic. The ownership of the data, portability and sharing across all data sets need clarity. The ethical and legal issues of responsibility and accountability for adverse outcomes of use or rejection of expert advice of AI need clearer understanding. Informed consent is another area when AI based expert systems are used or not used. How informed is informed consent? It is necessary to inform the patient if the clinician is basing his decision as per the recommendations of AI [60].

There are some problems in AI [61]. Unlike much of the research publications and recommendations, the AI data and inferences are not peer reviewed and blinded on evaluation. Who is responsible and accountable for the insights it provides—the developer, the tech company, the regulator, or the clinician? Can the emotional component of the doctor patient relationship be simulated? Who among the developer, the tech company, regulator, the doctor, or other stakeholders are accountable for any mishaps that happen when AI system recommendations are followed? The AI in healthcare has on one side systematised the various tasks and made available the information at the click of a button, does it with confidence dispense away the human supervision, assure safety and security? Not all human qualities are easy to digitise, and machines may not succeed in copying the sensitive and realistic relationship between the patient and the doctor. The quality AI depends on the quality data. One is aware of the old colloquial saying "garbage in and the garbage out".

11. Emotions and AI

Anxiety and emotions play a significant role in healthcare. The patients exhibit emotional reaction to the situation they are in. The suffering form pain is not equal in all and is significantly subjective. Reaction to hearing an unpleasant news like a diagnosis of cancer, prognosis of a permanent disability or even news of death have a variable emotional component. Doctors and other healthcare personnel on the other hand, are expected to provide the emotional support to the patient. An arm around the shoulders, empathy, communication, the eye contact, and the body language while sharing the unpleasant news have significant influence on the patient and the family. The patients' expectations and the helpers' perceptions influence the emotional support. The support has to be customised often. Where do the machines stand in this context [62, 63]?

The computers need to recognise and respond to the emotions and show empathy. They need to be ethical too. AI chatbots, intelligent healing platforms, therapeutic intelligence, communicative AI, emotion AI or affective AI are some of the AI tools that tend to simulate human emotions [64–70]. Software used is computer vision and natural language processing with facial recognition and voice recognition. The chatbots are becoming popular, earning the trust and engage the subjects in conversation either verbal or in the text format. While these were not rated as poor, opinion generally is in favour of a human over a machine proving the support. Simulating cultural differences in body language and communication pose problems of misinterpretation. Affective AI and Human Behaviour—Change Project (HBCP) [71, 72] deal with human behaviour. Bringing about a change in the human behaviour like mental health issues and therapy in addiction are the areas the AI is stepping into. AI and the HBCP are creating an open-access online knowledge system of behaviour change interventions. The use of natural language processing and sentiment analysis another branch of AI, has permitted interpretation of verbal communication and helped understand human expressions. Emotion and behavioural assessment is possible through the sentiment analysis [73, 74].

12. AI and differently abled

AI empowers the differently abled. The disability could be physical, restricting the access or mental, restricting the cognition. Smart devices provide support in the activities of daily living. Assistance to the disabled is showing promise. The AI is stepping into help communication and cognition. Assistive technologies are showing lot of promise and a positive outlook for the differently abled. AI is into the diagnosis of cognitive disabilities like autism and such disorders. However, there are issues that need consideration and scope for improvement [75–77]. ABIDE (Autism Brain Imaging Data Exchange) is one of the AI projects for Autism and it helps the diagnostic evaluation to be less time consuming, more efficient, and accurate. It even identifies certain phenotypes that respond better for therapeutic interventions [78].

13. Medical education and future scope

The current curriculum in most institutes offering graduate and post graduate studies does not expose the students to AI and its importance in patient care. While the clinicians use AI platforms like clinical decision support systems, expert systems, outcome scores and special AI programs developed to help clinical judgements and gain insights, what knowledge of AI is being imparted to the students, postgraduates, and those already in practice. Medicine is a lifelong pursuit and need continuous learning. With the projections showing a great potential of AI in healthcare, is it not necessary to prepare the future healthcare force to be prepared for this growth? A basic information of AI and its impact in practice, and its promise is desirable. The healthcare personnel need not know the intricacies of AI and its development. They should at least know how the AI is used, interpret, and explain its utility to the patients. When ethical issues like privacy and autonomy are involved, the students shall know the legal standing as well. The medical doctor is a team leader in the healthcare, and he needs to know the future trends and possibilities. While at the current undergraduate program, an introduction to AI in the form of electives are offered to introduce the concepts of AI, the postgraduate needs to know more of AI. Integration into the curriculum short courses in data science, informatics, importance of data entry at the point of care, ethical and legal implications along with the use and interpretation of AI in healthcare in their curriculum is essential. Continuing education programs, refresher courses and workshops in AI in virtual or physical mode to current practitioners are to be planned. There are two categories of doctors: those who need basic knowledge and those who show interest and wish to involve themselves in the promotion of AI in healthcare. The institutes shall identify the tech savvy faculty who can take the leadership and design a short course on computers, data and its importance and even assess the competence of the data entry at the point of care [79–82]. Certain published surveys [83, 84] indicate a mixed response from positive acceptance to totally negative fear.

14. Negative impact of AI

The developers of AI are striving continuously to make the computers simulate the human brain and visualise a day, computers outperform humans. There are many areas where the AI claims success. Recent advances have shown successful attempts to enter the emotional domain of human brain. The elimination of human error and fatigue factor in repetitive tasks, decision making algorithms, speed of action, and precision are some of the advantages. Yet there are concerns of the negative impact of AI.

The foremost concern is the lack of trust. The user perceptions and reliability of AI are two issues that influence the trust. The computers act on the inputs and function as a rule-based machine. The AI/ML tools are built on the database and as algorithms. With the concept of patient centred health care delivery gaining importance, the explainability, validity and reliability of the AI decision support systems are of great concern. Situations unexpected or unusual, are often met in clinical practice. Does the database reflect the real-world situation and ethnic variations. The influence of bias in sample selection, variations in the disease patterns, false negatives and false positives influencing the clinical decisions is significant on what is essentially retrospective database that is used while training the AI/ML tools. How predictable is the AI when applied to a prospective situation? Does it cover adequately the drifts and data shifts possible in newer practices, populations, and lifestyles? The clinician is likely to ignore diagnostic challenges or alternatives when an easier option like decision support systems is available. The human bias in case selection contributing to the database may lead to erroneous insights [85–89].

The scare of loss of jobs when a computer takes over the human actions is a reality. Fatigue or distraction are common in humans performing repetitive tasks. The precision the computers achieve is well known. The scare one might be replaced by a computer that outperforms a human is a fear in many. A Gallup poll held in USA revealed that the jobs lost are more than created. The AI proponents argue creation of new jobs will compensate the losses of human jobs to machines. The new jobs need new skills. Skill sets required, shortages in healthcare personnel will keep the AI in forefront in job creations, the proponents of AI claim. The AI developers have to strive hard to gain the trust of users and other stakeholders [89, 90]. Those concerned with healthcare, instead of mistrust in AI, should exercise their stakes in this technology. The medical professional shall see the database is well represented covering all variations and contribute to the development of AI. Data at the point of care contributing to the database is the primary responsibility of the healthcare personnel on which the AI/ML tools are built.

15. Conclusions

The medical doctor is an important link in the AI ecosystem in healthcare. The profession has a significant role in the data generation that forms the basis for diagnosis, management, and treatment. Doctor is also the ultimate user and beneficiary of the AI platforms. Data generation at the point of care and the comprehensive database for development of AI are heavily dependent on healthcare profession. For us to understand the true impact of AI, adverse and unwanted effects and complications of all interventions must be recorded at the point of care. However much the promise of intelligent machines performing the duties of the human, at least, as of today and the foreseeable future, the personal touch and empathy provided by the doctors is irreplaceable. Further studies are needed to fully evaluate the potential and limitations of AI in healthcare. The medical profession instead of viewing the AI as a competitor, should collaborate and support actively this technology.

Artificial Intelligence is being promoted as the next major advance in healthcare delivery. AI is here to stay because of the promise, it offers across multiple fields of medicine. For the world to be able to see the true benefits of AI, new technologies using AI must also be developed and validated like any other technology in medicine. Development of AI based technologies must start with thorough evaluation of appropriate use cases, understanding of user needs, whether the user is a patient or the doctor, and comprehensive assessment of risks and benefits. Because the outcome of any AI driven tool depends so much on the data used for training the algorithms, adequate care must be taken in collecting, curating, and use of data. Governing and regulatory bodies and standard committees must work with technical matter experts and intended users (both physicians and patient advocates) to set policies and guidance that define the boundaries of use of this technology and establishing guardrails that prevent misuse or abuse of AI.

Conflicts of interest

Nil

Financial support

Nil

Originality

This is the original work of mine and has not been published or submitted for publication to any peer reviewed periodical.

Author details

Subba Rao Bhavaraju
GVP Institute of Healthcare and Medical Technology, Visakhapatnam, India

*Address all correspondence to: bhasurao@gmail.com

References

[1] Shamsi J, Ali M, Khoja Mohammad K, et al. Data-intensive cloud computing: Requirements, expectations, challenges, and solutions. Journal of Grid Computing. 2013;**11**(2):281-310. DOI: 10.1007/s10723-013-9255-6

[2] Patel S. Available from: https://www.powermag.com/Hype-and-Hope-Artificial-Intelligences-Role-in-the-Power-Sector/

[3] Zamorano A. Available from: https://www.Forbes.com/sites/cognitiveworld/2020/04/30/ai-hype-or-ai-hope-when-will-ai-disrupt-the-pharmaceutical-Industry/?

[4] Longoni C and Morewedge CK. AI Can Outperform Doctors. So Why Do not Patients Trust It?. Available from: https://hbr.org/2019.10/ai-can-outperform-doctors-so-why-don't-patients-trust-it

[5] Harvey H. Why AI will not replace radiologist. Available from: https://www.kdnuggets.com/2018/11/why-ai-will-not-replace-radiologists.html

[6] Yokoi R, Eguchi Y, Fujita T et al. Artificial intelligence is trusted less than a doctor in medical treatment decisions: Influence of perceived care and value similarity International Journal of Human-Computer Interaction: 2021.37(10).981-990 10.1080/10447318.2020.1861763

[7] Tamora H, Yamashina H, Mukai M, Mori Y, Ogasawara K: Acceptance of the use of artificial intelligence in medicine among Japan's Doctors and the Public: A Questionnaire Survey, JMIR Human Factors: 2022;9(1).e24680 10.2196/24680

[8] Liu X, Keane PA, Denniston AK. Time to regenerate: The doctor in the age of artificial intelligence. Journal of the Royal Society of Medicine. 2018;**111**(4):113-116. DOI: 10.1177/0141076818762648

[9] Price A, Harborne D, Brains D, et al. Stakeholders in Explainable AI. 2019. Available from: https://deepai.org/publication/stakeholders-in-explainable-ai

[10] Responsible AI and Its Stakeholders | DeepAI: . Available from: https://arxiv.org/pdf/2004.11434v1.pdf

[11] Wanga EO What is point of care documentation? Available from: https://experience.care/blog/what-is-point-of-care-documentation/2022

[12] Bhavaraju SR. From Subconscious to Conscious to Artificial Intelligence: A Focus on Electronic Health records. Neural India. 2018;**66**:1270-1275

[13] William VD. Meaningful use of patient-generated data in EHRs. Available from: http://library.ahima.org/doc?oid=106996#.W34S9S2B2qA

[14] Angell M. No longer possible to believe much of clinical research published. Available from: https://ethicalnag.org/2009/11/09/nejm-editor/

[15] Fung J. The corruption of evidence-based medicine—killing for profit. Available from: https://medium.com/@drjasonfung/the-corruption-of-evidence-based-medicine-killing-for-profit-41f2812b8704

[16] Enago Academy: Publish or Perish: What Are Its Consequences?. Available from: https://www.enago.com/academy/publish-or-perish/consequences/

[17] Cohen E. Available from: https://appian.com/blog/if-its-not-documented-did-it-happen?

[18] Available from: https://www.hhs.gov/hipaa/for-professionals/special-topics/hitech-act-enforcement-interim-final-rule/index.html

[19] Sittig DF, Singh H. Rights and responsibilities of users of electronic health records. Canadian Medical Association Journal. 2012;**184**:1479-1483

[20] Electronic Health Record (EHR) Standards for India. 2016 . Available from: https://mohfw.gov.in/basicpage/electronic-health-record-ehr-standards-india-2016

[21] Muzny M, Henriksen A, Giordanengo A, et al. Wearable sensors with possibilities for data exchange: Analysing status and needs of different actors in mobile health monitoring systems. International Journal of Medical Informatics. 2020;**133**:104. DOI: 10.1016/j.ijmedinf.2019.104017

[22] He J, Baxter SL, Xu J, et al. The practical implementation of artificial intelligence technologies in medicine. Nature Medicine. 2019;**25**:30-36

[23] Willemink MJ, Koszek WA, Martin J et al: Preparing medical imaging data for machine learning Radiology 2020. 295,192,224 10.1148/radiol.2020192224

[24] Bartolo M, Roberts A, Welbl A, et al. Beat the AI: Investigating adversarial human annotation for reading comprehension. Transactions of the Association for Computational Linguistics. 2020,**8**:662-678. DOI: 10.1162/tacl_a_00338

[25] Meskó B, Görög M. A short guide for medical professionals in the era of artificial intelligence. NPJ Digital Medicine. 2020;**3**:126. DOI: 10.1038/s41746-020-00333

[26] Kalir RH, Garcia A. Annotation. United Kingdom: MIT Press; 2021

[27] Zech J, Pain M, Titano J, et al. Natural language–based machine learning models for the annotation of clinical radiology reports. Radiology. 2018;**287**:570-580

[28] Krenzer A, Makowski K, Hekalo A, et al. Fast machine learning annotation in the medical domain: A semi-automated video annotation tool for gastroenterologists. Biomedical Engineering Online. 2022;**25**:21-33. DOI: 10.1186/s12938-022-01001-x

[29] Price WN II. Artificial Intelligence in Health Care: Applications and Legal Issues 2017. SciTech Lawyer. 2017;**14**:10. Available from: https://ssrn.com/abstract=3078704

[30] Sullivan HR, Schweikart SJ. Are current tort liability doctrines adequate for addressing injury caused by AI? AMA Journal of Ethics. 2019;**21**(2):E160-E166. DOI: 10.1001/amajethics.2019.160

[31] Schönberger D. Artificial intelligence in healthcare: A critical analysis of the legal and ethical implications. International Journal of Law and Information Technology. 2019;**27**:171-203. DOI: 10.1093/ijlit/eaz004

[32] Rodrigues R. Legal and human rights issues of AI: Gaps, challenges and vulnerabilities. Journal of Responsible Technology. 2020;**4**:100. DOI: 10.1016/j.jrt.2020.100005. https://www.sciencedirect.com/science/article/pii/S2666659620300056

[33] Gerke S, Minssen T, Cohen G. Ethical and legal challenges of artificial intelligence-driven healthcare. Artificial Intelligence in Healthcare. 2020:295-336. DOI: 10.1016/B978-0-12-818438-7.00012-5. Epub 2020 Jun 26. PMCID: PMC7332220

[34] Norton Rose Fulbright. Available from: https://www.insideteachlaw.com/publications/legal-risks#section1

[35] Bartoletti, I: AI in Healthcare: Ethical and privacy challenges. In: Riaño D, Wilk S, ten Teije, A. (eds) Artificial Intelligence in Medicine. 2019. Springer, Cham. 10.1007/978-3-030-21642-9_2

[36] Anderson M, Anderson SL. How should AI be developed, validated, and implemented in patient care? AMA Journal of Ethics. 2019;**21**(2):E125-E130. DOI: 10.1001/amajethics.2019.125

[37] Atkinson K, Bench-Capon T, Bollegala D. Explanation in AI and law: Past, present, and future. Artificial Intelligence. 2020;**289**:103387. DOI: 10.1016/j.artint.2020.103387. https://www.sciencedirect.com/science/article/pii/S0004370220301375

[38] Molnár-Gábor F. Artificial intelligence in Healthcare: Doctors, patients and liabilities. In: Wischmeyer T, Rademacher T, editors. Regulating Artificial Intelligence. Cham.: Springer; 2020. DOI: 10.1007/978-3-030-32361-5_15

[39] Boddington P. Introduction: Artificial intelligence and ethics. In: Towards a Code of Ethics for Artificial Intelligence. Artificial Intelligence: Foundations, Theory, and Algorithms. Cham: Springer; 2017. DOI: 10.1007/978-3-319-60648-4_1

[40] Miquido. 2020. Available from: https://www.miquido.com/blog/ai-legal-issues

[41] Available from: https://www.royalfree.nhs.uk/patients-visitors/how-we-use-patient-information/information-commission-office-ico-investigation-into-our-work-with-deepmind/2017

[42] Amann J, Blasimme A, Vayena E, et al. Explainability for artificial intelligence in healthcare: A multidisciplinary perspective. BMC Medical Informatics and Decision Making. 2020;**20**:310. DOI: 10.1186/s12911-020-01332-6

[43] Astromskė K, Peičius E, Astromskis P. Ethical and legal challenges of informed consent applying artificial intelligence in medical diagnostic consultations. AI & SOCIETY. 2021;**36**:509-520. DOI: 10.1007/s00146-020-01008-9

[44] McNamara M. 2022 . Available from: https://www.netapp.com/blog/explainable-ai/

[45] Kadircan H. Keskinbora: Medical ethics considerations on artificial intelligence. Journal of Clinical Neuroscience. 2019:277-282. DOI: 10.1016/j.jocn.2019.03.001

[46] Geis JR, Brady AP, Carol C, et al. Ethics of artificial intelligence in radiology: Summary of the Joint European and North American Multisociety Statement. Radiology;**293**(2):436-440. DOI: 10.1148/radiol/2019191586

[47] Martinho A, Kroesen M, Chorus C. A healthy debate: Exploring the views of medical doctors on the ethics of artificial intelligence. Artificial Intelligence in Medicine. 2021;**121**:102190. http://creativecommons.org/licenses/by/4.0/

[48] The Digital Personal Data Protection Bill. 2022. Available from: https://www.meity.gov.in/content/digital-data-protection-bill-2022

[49] General Data Protection Regulation (GDPR). 2016. Available from: EUR-Lex-32016R0679-EN-EUR-Lex (europa.eu)

[50] Bill Text—AB-375 Privacy: Personal information: businesses. (ca.gov). 2017. Available from: https://leginfo.legislature.ca.gov/faces/billtextclient.xhtml?bill_id20172018ab375

[51] Digital Information Security in Health Care Act (DISHA). 2018. Available from: https://mohfw.gov.in/newshighlights/comments-draft-digital-information-security-health-care-actdisha

[52] CFI Team: Data Anonymisation. 2022 . Available from: https://www/corporatefinanceinstitute.com/resources/business-intelligence/data-anonymization

[53] Elliot M, O'Hara K, Raab C, et al. Functional anonymisation: Personal data and the data environment. Computer Law & Security Review. 2018;**34**:204-221. DOI: 10.1016/j.clsr.2018.02.001

[54] Ghazal TM. RETRACTED ARTICLE: Internet of things with artificial intelligence for health care security. Arabian Journal for Science and Engineering. 2023;**48**:5689. DOI: 10.1007/s13369-021-06083-8

[55] Xi P, Zhang X, Wang L, Wenjuan W et al.: A review of blockchain-based secure sharing of healthcare data appl. Sciences. 2022;12(15):7912 10.3390/app12157912

[56] Aung YYM, DCS W, Ting DSW. The promise of artificial intelligence: A review of the opportunities and challenges of artificial intelligence in healthcare. British Medical Bulletin. 2021;**139**:4-15. DOI: 10.1093/bmb/ldab016

[57] Weins J, Shenoy ES. Machine learning for healthcare. On the verge of a major shift in Healthcare Epidemiology. Clinical Infectious Diseases. 2021;**66**:149-153. DOI: 10.1093/cid/cix731

[58] Keerthy AS, Manju Priya S.Artificial intelligence in healthcare databases. In: Suresh A, Paiva S, editors. Deep Learning and Edge Computing Solutions for High Performance Computing. EAI/Springer Innovations in Communication and Computing. Cham: Springer; 2021. DOI: 10.1007/978-3-030-60265-9_2

[59] Davenport T, Kalakota R. The potential for artificial intelligence in healthcare. Future Healthcare Journal. 2019;**6**(2):94-98. DOI: 10.7861/futurehosp.6-2-94

[60] Cohen I. Informed Consent and Medical Artificial Intelligence: What to Tell the Patient? Georgetown Law Journal. 2020;**108**:1425-1469. DOI: 10.2139/ssrn.3529576

[61] Academy of Royal Medical Colleges; Artificial intelligence in healthcare. Available from: https://www.aomrc.org.uk/wp-content/uploads/2019/01/artificial_intelligence_in_healthcare_0119.pdf

[62] Jones SM, Burleson B. The impact of situational variables on helpers' perceptions of comforting messages: An attributional analysis. Communication Research. 1997;**24**(5):530-555. DOI: 10.1177/009365097024005004

[63] Smith KA, Masthoff J. Can a Virtual Agent provide good Emotional Support? 10.14236/ewic/HCI2018.13

[64] Guzman AL, Lewis S. Artificial intelligence and communication: A Human–Machine Communication research agenda. New Media & Society. 2020;**22**(1):70-86. DOI: 10.1177/1461444819858691

[65] Wang W, Siau K. Living with Artificial Intelligence—Developing a Theory on Trust in Health Chatbots. In: Proceedings of the Sixteenth Annual Pre-ICIS Workshop on HCI Research in MIS. San Francisco, CA; 2018

[66] Bilquise G, Ibrahim S, Shaala K. Emotionally Intelligent Chatbots:

A Systemic Literature Review. DOI: 10.1115/2022/9601630. CORPUS id: 252552808

[67] Intelligent Healing for Mental Health. 2022 . Available from: https://www.twill.health/mental-health

[68] Meng J, Dai YN. Emotional support from AI Chatbots: Should a supportive partner self-disclose or not? Journal of Computer-Mediated Communication. 2021;**26**(4):207-222. DOI: 10.1093/jcmc/zmab005

[69] Diederich S, Brendel AB, Morana S, et al. On the design of and interaction with conversational agents: An organising and assessing review of human computer interaction research. Journal of the Association for Information Systems. 2022;**23**(1):96-138

[70] Sullivan Y, Nyawa S, Wamba SF. Combating Loneliness with Artificial Intelligence: An AI-Based Emotional Support Model URI: 2023. Available from: https://hdl.handle.net/10125/103173 978-0-9981331-6-4

[71] Picard RW. Affective Computing; MIT Media laboratory perceptual computing section technical report 321. 1995

[72] Aonghusa PM, Michie S. Artificial intelligence and behavioural science through the looking glass. Annals of Behavioral Medicine. 2020;**54**:942-947. DOI: 10.1093/abm/kaaa095

[73] Graham S, Depp C, Lee EE, Nebeker C, Tu X, Kim HC, et al. Artificial intelligence for mental health and mental illnesses: An overview. Current Psychiatry Report. 2019;**21**(11):116. DOI: 10.1007/s11920-019-1094-0

[74] Shaheen MY. AI in Healthcare: Medical and socio-economic benefits and challenges. 2021. Available at SSRN: https://ssrn.com/abstract=3932277 or DOI: 10.2139/ssrn.3932277

[75] Chakraborty N, Mishra Y, Bhattacharya R, et al. Artificial Intelligence: The road ahead for the accessibility of persons with Disability. Materials Today: Proceedings. 2021. DOI: 10.1016/j.matpr.2021.07.374. Available from: https://www.sciencedirect.com/science/article/pii/S2214785321052330

[76] Smith P, Smith L. Artificial intelligence and disability: Too much promise, yet too little substance? AI and Ethics. 2021;**1**:81-86. DOI: 10.1007/s43681-020-00004-5

[77] Wall DP, Dally R, Luyster R, et al. Use of artificial intelligence to shorten the behavioural diagnosis of autism. Plos One. 2021;**7**(8):e43855. DOI: 10.1371/journal.pone.0043855

[78] Chaddad A, Li J, Lu Q, et al. Can autism be diagnosed with artificial intelligence? A narrative review. Diagnostics. 2021;**11**:2032. DOI: 10.3390/diagnostics11112032

[79] McCoy LG, Nagaraju S, Morgado F, et al. What do medical students actually need to know about artificial intelligence? NPJ Digital Medicine. 2020;**2020**:86. DOI: 10.1038/s41746-020-0294-7

[80] Park SH, Do K-H, Kim S, et al. What should medical students know about artificial intelligence in medicine? Journal of Educational Evaluation Health Professor. 2019;**16**:18. DOI: 10.3352/jeehp.2019.16.18

[81] Masters K. Artificial intelligence in medical education. Medical Teacher. 2019;**41**(9):976-980. DOI: 10.1080/0142159X.2019.1595557

[82] Kennedy TJT, Glenn R, et al. Point-of-care assessment of medical trainee competence for independent clinical work. Academic Medicine. 2008;**83**(10):S89-S92. DOI: 10.1097/ACM.0b013e318183c8b7

[83] Santos DPS, Giese D, Brodehl S, et al. Medical students' attitude towards artificial intelligence: A multicentre survey. European Radiology. 2019;**29**:1640-1646. DOI: 10.1007/s00330-018-5601-1

[84] Gong B, Nugent JP, Guest W, et al. Influence of Artificial Intelligence on Canadian Medical Students' Preference for Radiology Specialty: A National Survey Study. Academic Radiology. 2018;**26**:566-577. DOI: 10.1016/j.acra.2018.10.007

[85] Asan O, Bayrak AE, Choudhury A. Artificial intelligence and human trust in healthcare: Focus on clinicians. Journal of Medicine Internet Research. 2020;**22**(6):e15154. DOI. 10.2196/15154

[86] LaRosa E, Danks D. Impacts on trust of healthcare AI. In: Proceedings of the 2018 AAAI/ACM Conference on AI, Ethics, and Society (AIES '18). New York, NY, USA: Association for Computing Machinery; 2018. pp. 210-215. DOI: 10.1145/3278721.3278771

[87] Kelly CJ, Karthikesalingam A, Suleyman M, et al. Key challenges for delivering clinical impact with artificial intelligence. BMC Medicine. 2019;**17**:195. DOI: 10.1186/s12916-019-1426-2

[88] Challen R, Denny J, Pitt M, et al. Artificial intelligence, bias, and clinical safety. BMJ Quality & Safety. 2019;**28**:231-237

[89] Duggal N: Advantages and disadvantages of artificial intelligence. 2023. Available from: https://www.simplilearn.com/advantages-and-disadvantages-of-artificial-intelligence-article

[90] Reinhart RJ. Available from: https://news.gallup.com/poll/228194/public-split-basic-income-workers-replaced-robots.aspx

Chapter 5

Artificial Intelligence Starts the Big Bang of Modern Medicine and Surgery

Tania María Blanchar Martinez and Fernando Pio de la Hoz Restrepo

Abstract

Objective. To identify the areas of application and uses of artificial intelligence and expert systems in medicine, surgical procedures, and surgical specialties, classifying the degree of agreement in articles published between 2010 and 2019. Materials and Methods. The methodology consists of a relational database model and an entity-relationship model. To determine the quality of each article, the classification by degrees of agreement between "highly concordant", "relatively concordant" or "not concordant" was created on our initiative. Results. A total of 146 articles were found, of which only 28 were highly concordant with the subject of interest. Conclusions. Artificial intelligence is the new research science that is revolutionizing the way of intervention in the different disciplines of the area of medicine.

Keywords: application of artificial intelligence, expert systems medicine, surgical specialties, and surgical procedures, science, technology

1. Introduction

The pure sciences, such as mathematics and physics, have been fundamental in evolution and human survival; the great researchers in these areas were the first Nobel Prize winners in the history of world discoveries. Discoveries that have undoubtedly marked a line in time, in the postulations of the different theories of physics have led to technological advances in different areas of science, whose origin has been observational and experimental from the beginning [1].

At this point in history, the different questions, predictions, and estimates related to the behavior of a certain event or circumstance began to take shape, which was references to other research areas, especially in the medical sciences, for the study of diseases, from the causative agents to the damage caused to health [1].

These pure sciences gave rise to computational sciences, which were the gateway to research focused on artificial intelligence. Shortly after the Second World War, around 1950, when the first article on artificial intelligence was published in the philosophical journal MIND Computing Machinery and Intelligence, Alan Turing was the first mathematician and researcher who applied his knowledge in developing a computational machine that could perform mathematical analysis. And at the same time, he wondered if this same computational machine could have the ability to think like a human being [2, 3].

The first works developed with artificial intelligence were focused on mathematical sciences, statistical analysis, and on an event that marked history during the Second World War: algorithms to decode the Nazis' attack plan towards the allied countries against the government of Adolf Hitler, and whose intervention saved thousands of soldiers and civilians from each of these countries. On this occasion, artificial intelligence was used for the common good, to stop the machiavellian attacks from a sick and ambitious mind that took more than 20 million people [2, 3].

However, parallel to these feats uncertainty also grows to arise from the historical background of advances in the pure sciences. Such as the discovery of uranium and nuclear weapons, for human survival purposes, the discovery of dynamite to accelerate construction and firearms, for human defense. All of these have been questioned for their use in world wars, where human annihilation has prevailed, the most famous of all, the atomic bomb [2, 3].

Today we are thinking of artificial intelligence for the benefit of health, just health, which allows the approach from genetic and environmental risk factors and social and institutional determinants of the population. However, arises the concern as to whether the use of artificial intelligence is only of interest to ensure the survival of human beings from many diseases of the XXI century and its evolution, or whether we are approaching our annihilation [2–4].

The survival of the human race has been constantly threatened since ancient times by different outbreaks, epidemics, and pandemics of different infectious agents such as bacteria and viruses, an example of this, is the bubonic plague or black plague that wiped out 50% of the European population, and currently, the Covid-19, that had a demographic, social, economic and social impact. This has brought the world population to its knees and has made us understand that we are not indestructible, in fact, we are very vulnerable, and we must take into account nature's limits, the environment that surrounds us, and that exceeding them has led us to commit recklessness that has led to the annihilation of the human race [5].

The question we ask ourselves now is if we have learned the lesson from previous experiences, which have put human survival at risk. Or whether in this case, artificial intelligence will focus only on preserving human life and the environment around us improving our quality of life, or otherwise, we will be conquered again by the ambition for power, expansion, and wanting to be superior to others when we should be working together for our well-being.

The big bang of artificial intelligence focused on medicine and surgical procedures has already begun, the latest industrial revolution, a technological avalanche focused on the solution of more timely health interventions, reflecting real-time decision making, and influencing the health of different specific populations.

Likewise, it is urgent to regulate the uses and applications of artificial intelligence with laws and norms, imposing limits that guarantee the use of this technology only to preserve the human race, not replace it, much less annihilate it.

All countries, whether developed or developing, without exception, must sign international agreements and treaties in which they commit to use it only for the common good.

Being prudent in the development of these technologies and sharing this knowledge among sister countries that we are, without a doubt, would allow an unprecedented advance in science in general.

We must be very alert, and be able to impose limits on ourselves so that we do not engage in unethical behavior that puts the human race at risk.

We are in a historical moment, where technological advances have allowed the survival of the human race, it is important to mention that all the technology used for the creation in record time of vaccines against the covid-19 disease, which has taken so many lives worldwide.

In this way, we must unite our knowledge and efforts from all research fields, and educational institutions, such as universities worldwide, are the guarantors of imposing the limits of the different research approaches, thus favoring the good use of artificial intelligence applications.

If the academy is the one that produces the generation of knowledge for research purposes, and to solve problems, which in this case is focused on the solution of health problems, then it should impose the limits of uses on human beings and their environment.

Each research group, in their different areas, from different universities, should be able to build their methods focus on this discipline, to generate high-level knowledge, which can be translated into different computational languages, with the only purpose of making decisions in real-time.

Currently, the areas of development of artificial intelligence are focused on: Machine learning (machine learning, deep learning, unsupervised, supervised), driven by Massive Data (massive exploitation of data, identifying relationships between them, detecting patterns, making inferences, and learning through probabilistic mathematical models), natural language processing (content extraction, classification, translation, text generators), expert systems (knowledge and rule-based systems, diagnostics), computer vision (exploring the recognition and understanding of images and videos), robotics (advanced laparoscopic surgery such as Da Vinci, the Sojourner, Spirit, Opportunity, and Curiosity robots for space research) and speech recognition [6–8].

The applications, however, are focused on language analysis and understanding, information retrieval, information extraction, answer searches, automatic summaries, automatic translation, automatic document classification, speech recognition, chatbot, child content control, document and opinion detection, and anti-spam filters. Spam, voice assistants, Siri as Apple assistant, Cortana, Alexa, and Bixby all these applications use natural language techniques [6–8].

Search engines and entertainment and communications platforms such as Google Search, Google Maps, Netflix, and social networks such as Facebook, Pinterest, Twitter, Instagram, and Google Photos [6–8].

The challenge in the health areas is not only to create information systems with artificial intelligence, big data, and data mining with sophisticated algorithms for information management; making decisions in real-time is the key to intervening quickly in health problems [6–8].

2. Methodology

Descriptive methodology, with a systematic literature search in four phases, of potentially relevant articles published about artificial intelligence and expert systems applied in the areas of medicine and surgical procedures.

2.1 First phase (research question)

This phase will specify the structured research question, the population to be studied, the what, the when, the where, and the delimitation of the review time, which in this case is 10 years, and the context of interest, whose key event is the application of artificial intelligence in medicine, specialties, and surgical procedures.

In which areas of medicine, surgical specialties, and surgical procedures have artificial intelligence and expert systems been applied from 2010 to 2019?

How well do published articles on artificial intelligence and expert systems applied in the area of medicine, surgical specialties, and surgical procedures from 2010 to 2019 match?

In how many of these articles on artificial intelligence and expert systems applied in the area of medicine, surgical specialties, and surgical procedures were there decision-making from 2010 to 2019?

2.2 Second phase (selection and localization of databases - relational database model - entity-relationship model of the databases)

The location and selection of databases will be done, where the search for articles with the subject of interest will be carried out.

We will use a relational database model and an entity-relationship model to guarantee the referential entity of which the databases and the articles are part.

The Relational Model Relationship refers to the entities and their respective relationships with the other entities; therefore, it allows referential integrity to take place [9].

The Entity-Relationship Model consists of representing descriptively1 and through a diagram the information system, formalizing all the storage structure of the database (**Figure 1**) [9].

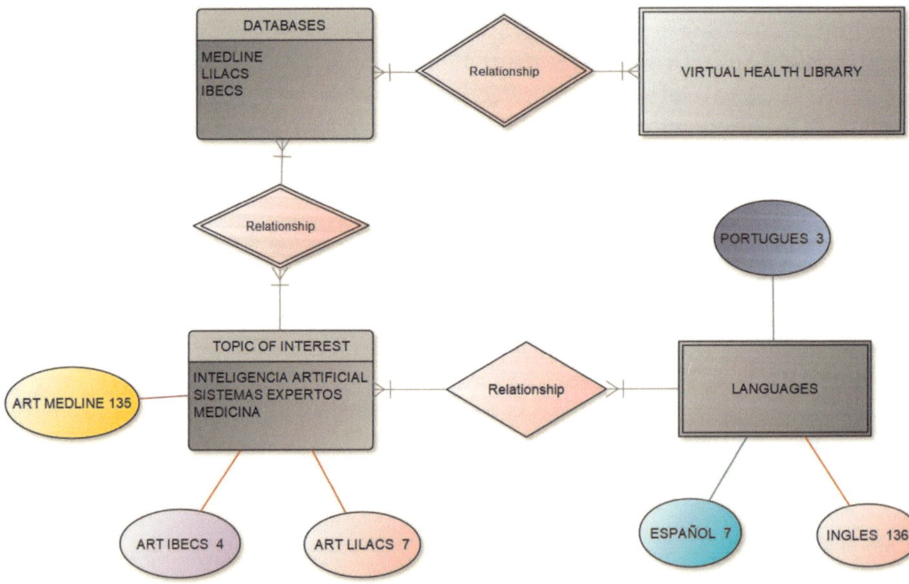

Figure 1.
Model entity general relationship model of the systematic review of the literature on a particular topic. Source: Taken and adapted from the book Relational Database Programming.

Inclusion and exclusion criteria will be applied to guarantee the following good selection of articles.

2.2.1 Inclusion criteria

The inclusion criteria will take into account the central theme, which is artificial intelligence and expert systems applied in medicine and surgical procedures, in English, Portuguese, and Spanish; other criteria will be electronic publications in the virtual health library from 2010 to 2019.

2.2.2 Exclusion criteria

The exclusion criteria included the Virtual Health Library database.

2.3 Third phase (selection of the articles in the languages of interest)

The list of eligible articles will be drawn up, and the concordance with the established objectives should be evaluated to avoid invalidating the results of the systematic reviews.

This list of eligible articles will be organized in a matrix with a degree of concordance; it will be identified qualitatively and quantitatively by identifying the titles and abstracts (**Figure 2**).

Very concordant = The title of the article and the research question have a clear relationship with the topic of artificial intelligence, expert systems, and description of uses.

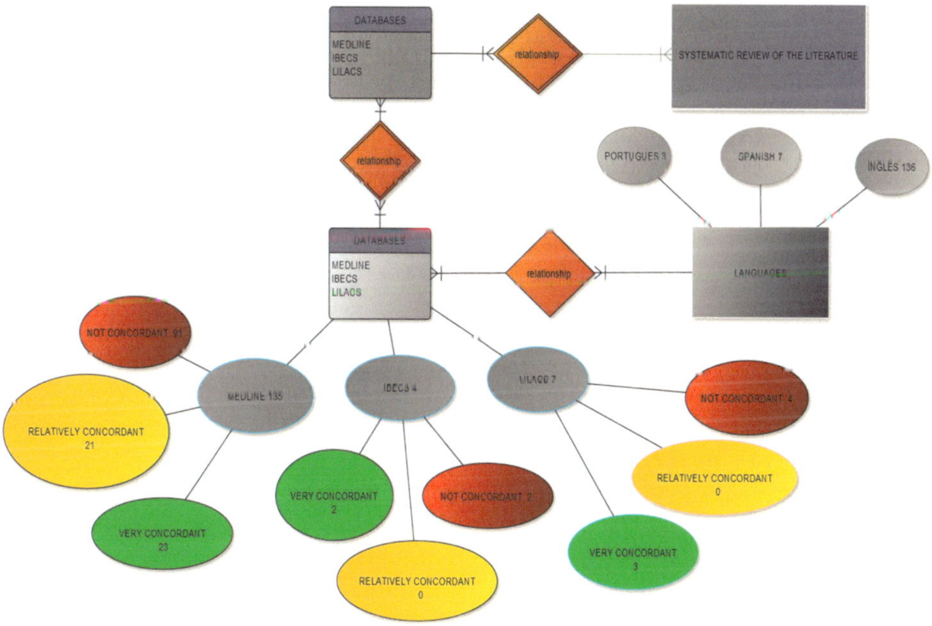

Figure 2.
Entity-relationship model of selected article databases. Source: Taken and adapted from the book Relational Database Programming.

Relatively concordant = The title of the article and the research question are partially related to the subject of artificial intelligence, expert systems, and description of uses.

not concordant = The title of the article is not related to the research question, subject of Artificial intelligence, expert systems, and uses.

2.4 Fourth phase (inspection, observation, and content extraction)

Inspection, observation, and extraction of the content of each of the articles relevant to the systematic review of the literature.

Each of the selected contents will also be organized in a matrix according to the degree of concordance.

Very concordant = The content of the article must be related to the subject of interest artificial intelligence, expert systems, objectives, and description of uses.

Relatively concordant = The content of the article must be partially related to the subject of interest artificial intelligence, expert systems, objectives, and description of uses.

Not concordant = The content of the article is not related to the subject of Artificial intelligence, expert systems, objectives, and description of uses.

3. Results

During the systematic reviews performed in the virtual health library database with the keywords artificial intelligence and surgical procedures, a total number of 100 articles were found. 65 from which did not match the keywords, 63 from which were from the MEDLINE database, and two from the LILACS database; 19 were relatively concordant, all from the MEDLINE database, and only 16 were highly concordant with the topic of interest, according to the MEDLINE database (see **Table 1**).

About the Systematic Reviews carried out with the keywords Artificial Intelligence and Medical Specialties, a total number of 39 articles were found, from which 29 were not concordant, eight were very concordant with the subject of interest, and only two were relatively concordant (**Table 2**).

Artificial intelligence in surgical procedures		Languages	Very concordant	Relatively consistent	Not concordant	Total
Medline	98	English (97) / Spanish (1)	16	19	63	98
Lilacs	2	Portuguese /Ingles	0	0	2	2
Total	100					100
Source: Own elaboration.						

Table 1.
Systematic review of artificial intelligence in surgical Procedures.Colombia,2019.

Artificial intelligence and medical specialties		Languages	Very concordant	Relatively consistent	Not concordant	Total
Medline	35	**English (35)**	7	2	26	35
Ibecs	1	English	0	0	1	1
Lilacs	3	Portuguese (2) Spanish 1	1	0	2	3
Total	39					39

Source: Own elaboration.

Table 2.
Systematic review of artificial intelligence and medical specialties. Colombia, 2019.

Artificial intelligence and expert systems in medicine		Languages	Very concordant	Relatively consistent	Not concordant	TOTAL
Medline	2	English	0	0	2	2
		Spanish (2)	2	0	1	3
Ibecs	3	English (1)				
Lilacs	2	English (2)	2	0	0	2
Total	7					7

Source: Own elaboration.

Table 3.
Systematic reviews of artificial intelligence and expert Systems in Medicine. Colombia, 2019.

In the Systematic Review with the keywords Artificial Intelligence and Expert Systems in Medicine, seven articles were found, from which four were highly concordant and three were not concordant (**Table 3**).

4. Final evaluation of the articles of the systematic review virtual health library

A total of 146 articles were evaluated, of which 97 were not concordant, 28 were highly concordant and 21 were relatively concordant.

The red non-concordance refers to the fact that the article does not make any reference to the stated objectives and the subject of interest, to the research question, or to the uses.

The highly concordant articles, identified with the green color, are directly related to the subject of interest, the stated objectives, the research question, and the uses.

In the case of the relatively concordant category, identified with the yellow color, they have partially related to the subject matter and the research question, but not to the objectives or uses (see **Table 4**).

During the Virtual Health Library Systematic Review, 135 articles from the MEDLINE database, seven articles from the LILACS database, and four from the IBECS database were analyzed.

Degrees of agreement	Total items
Very concordant	28
Relatively consistent	21
Not concordant	97
Total	**146**

Source: Own elaboration.

Table 4.
Compliance follow-up matrix resulting from the evaluation of systematic review articles. Colombia, 2019.

Twenty-eight highly concordant articles were identified, whose analysis consisted of organizing them by areas of artificial intelligence; to be able to visualize the approaches that are currently being applied in medicine, surgical procedures, and medical specialties. This analysis produced the following findings from the evidence found by area of artificial intelligence:

5. Automatic reasoning or machine learning

Based on contexts of repeating patterns or parameters, it groups and analyzes them and then identifies the behavior or tendency of a certain event or circumstance to suggest different predictions. It is also a specialized tool in extracting stored information to answer questions and draw conclusions to detect patterns, draw conclusions to detect patterns, of certain epidemiological behaviors.

In this area of artificial intelligence, applications were recognized in Education research: digital health: intersections between scientific research and its mediatization. Medical education: opportunities for collaborative work towards artificial intelligence tools in medical education, improvement of pedagogical techniques for learning. Dermatology: diagnosis by dermatoscopy (sonification), laboratory, and prospective observational study. Public health: comparison of the performance of machine learning algorithms in predictive analytics in public health and medicine, predictive and probabilistic models for estimating the risk of health events or diseases. Occupational health: human activity recognitions based on feature selection in the smart home using a backpropagation algorithm. Deep machine learning for workflow recognition during surgery. Occupational medicine: artificial intelligence in occupational medicine. Pneumology: prediction of asthma exacerbations, and chronic disease changes, using algorithms and predictive models of Bayesian classifiers and support vector machines with artificial intelligence Internal medicine: mobile application of intensive insulin therapy based on artificial intelligence techniques. Anesthesiology: artificial intelligence system for endotracheal intubation. Pediatric surgery: preoperative prediction of surgical morbidity in children: comparison of five statistical models, logistic regression models. General surgery: development of an intelligent surgical training system for thoracentesis. Laparoscopic surgery: Analysis and counting of the uses of the multifunctional or modular tool in mixed procedures of cholecystectomies and Nissen judicature to reduce operating room time and decrease patient risk, by means of a video using fuzzy logic techniques, to analyze the types of instruments used, the duration of each use and the function of each instrument. Diagnostics. fuzzy naive Bayesian model for medical diagnostic decision support, medical applications as a diagnostic aid in medicine, SOFTEL-MINSAP experience, and segmentation methods based on machine learning algorithms for large-scale magnetic resonance imaging. Technological focus on diagnostic aids for cancerous lesions using learning algorithms. Anatomical diagnosis: stable segmentation based on atlas mapped prior (stamp) machine learning for large-scale multicenter MRI data. Diagnostic Microbiological Metabolic Profiling: predicting colonic polyps with machine learning based on urinary metabolomics. Cardiology: machine learning system to improve heart failure patient care, predicting heart attacks four hours in advance in patients with a history of heart disease with a tendency to myocardial infarction, and improving prediction times for cardiologists. This system was fed with clinical data from each patient, incorporating clinical parameters to make the prediction. Physiotherapy: a computerized behavioral system for home.

physiotherapy exercises using an RGBD camera. Research: artificial intelligence applied to evidence-based surgery. Rheumatology. identifies new pathways associated with demineralization in a viral model of multiple sclerosis, prediction of HIV-associated neurocognitive disorder from three genetic features of the gp 120 glyco-protein envelope, and Molecular biology prediction of interactions between HIV-1 and human proteins by information integration. Genetics prediction of virus mutations by statistical relational learning, Microbiology Genetics virus detection by statistical gene expression analysis, and classification of therapy resistance based on longitudinal biomarker profiles [10–25].

6. Big data and machine learning

The combination of big data and machine learning has enabled data processing and analysis to have a greater opportunity to participate in decision-making in a timely manner. There are many areas of healthcare in which such combinations of algorithmic functions have shown positive results for intervention in this case of chronic diseases and their respective treatments. Among these applications, the following stand out: Intensive care medicine: artificial intelligence in the intensive care unit using big data and machine learning in intensive care medicine. Improved specificity of networked distributed physiological alarms based on a simple deterministic reactive intelligent agent in the intensive care environment, Programmed databases to analyze clinical questions of patient diseases and treatments, and intervention protocols to generate new lines of research [26–28].

7. Computer vision

Explores the recognition and understanding of images and videos, The tool is able to perceive each of these. Recognized in Neurology: neuro GPS: automated neuron localization for brain circuits using the L1 minimization model, automated neuron localizations through biophysical models, concerning the morphology of the neural axoma, through a Neurog method, to localize neurons in various parts of the brain Oncology: detection of cancer cells to design a tool with precise optics for rectal colon biopsy. Diagnostic Endoscopy: the potential of artificial intelligence-assisted colonoscopy using an endocystocope with video optical biopsy, making use of an ultra-magnified endoscope [3, 29, 30].

8. Expert systems

Designed to solve complex problems by making decisions based on a knowledge base and rules for applying that knowledge. Recognized in Surgery: reduction of operating room time and reduction of patient risk through the use of modular surgical instrumentation with artificial intelligence. Internal Medicine: Improved specificity of networked distributed physiological alarms based on a simple deterministic reactive intelligent agent in the intensive care setting [31, 32].

9. Deep learning

Attempts to mimic the functioning of the human nervous system, using what is known as neural networks or layers of the processing unit (artificial neurons) that specialize in identifying characteristics or patterns determined in objects or unstructured data sets, without the need for prior training with a set of structured or labeled data. Neural networks: in Neurology, clinical applications of neural networks in sleep apnea-hypopnea syndrome were recognized, and *backpropagation* (BP) algorithms were also programmed. The BP algorithm is used to train the feed-forward neural network for human activity recognition in intelligent home environments in conjunction with probabilistic algorithms: the Naïve Bayes (NB) classifier and the Hidden Markov Model (HMM), neural networks for diabetes control using a multipanel graphic interface, neurological disease estimation [31, 33].

10. Automatic reasoning, expert systems, logistic regression

In these specialized areas of artificial intelligence, they have focused their algorithm progradation in the medical area of infectious diseases; machine learning has specialized in the realization of algorithms for statistical inferences, optimizing problems of analysis and interpretation of results from research studies, and the application of models for representations and evaluations of statistical data using techniques to predict response to antiretroviral therapy. Expert systems in organizing through knowledge based on rules and categories focused on diagnostics to solve decision making, and regression logistics in performing decision making based on a continuous variable, taking values and predicting the outcome for decision making [34, 35].

11. Analysis of artificial intelligence applications by tendency of use in medical areas

The trend of artificial intelligence in healthcare marks a meeting point between the pure sciences and the medical sciences.

The most pronounced trend is machine learning. In this application area, the medical specialties in which the greatest applications were developed were in the diagnostic area with the use of advanced optics, on a large scale for the observation of cancer cells in different parts of the body. Additionally in combination with Big Data and automatic reasoning in internal medicine, have intervened in important areas such as chronic non-communicable diseases, rheumatology, pulmonology, cardiology, and diabetes diseases for intensive insulin therapy. Additionally, the most intervened surgical specialties or surgery are pediatric surgeries, ophthalmologic surgeries, and general surgery.

The second trend is identified as Computer Vision, focused on image and video recognition with ultra-magnified large-scale optics and also identification with precise biopsy of colon cancer cells and finally, detection of cancer cells, and anatomical identification of neuron parts.

The third trend focused on expert systems, where genetics and genetic microbiology are identified in studies of viral mutations and DNA sequencing. Additionally, knowledge is based on diagnostic rules for early detection of cancer in its early stages and deep learning with the application of neural networks, estimation, and neurological diseases.

There are also applications combined with machine learning and big data for the use of physiological alarms structured in a network with intelligent agents, and evidence-based medicine through questions and answers of diseases and treatments, generating new research lines. Other combinations were machine learning, expert systems, and logistic regression used in antiretroviral treatment predictions.

12. Graphical representation simulation modified endemic index of the development trend of artificial intelligence by specialized medical areas

With this graphical representation, the behavior of the areas of development of artificial intelligence in medicine by medical specialty can be established, and the future behavior of each area can be monitored and, why not, predicted.

The results were organized in a traffic light fashion, with green being the most trending AI development behavior, yellow the second most trending development behavior and red the least trending.

In the green-colored success zone, the artificial intelligence area of Machine learning or Machine Learning is identified, it is the most developed area in medicine and health. This is because it was the first to be developed and put into practice, additionally because it has a lot of theoretical information. After all, it has been widely used in the financial and business area for predictions and analysis of economic behavior, financial profitability, and others. Nowadays it is used in the area of medical sciences and health.

Therefore, in this area of artificial intelligence, it is where great decisions have been made in the economic area and also in the health area, due to the large number of applications developed.

The majority of scientific publications in the area of artificial intelligence were found in this area of success, and the language in which most of them were published was English.

In the security zone, marked in yellow, Computer Vision is identified. This area was the second zone in which artificial intelligence applications were developed, focused on diagnostic methods with large-scale optics and in the English language.

In the red alarm zone, deep learning and expert systems were identified, where applications of neural networks were found, these being the most complex to develop, requiring a lot of expertise and focused on the central nervous system; however, expert systems are also complex, given the rule-based systems in which they are structured, they can be a good area of application that could be focused on molecular biology and DNA sequencing.

Finally, in this area, the smallest number of artificial intelligence applications were developed, since it is the least explored due to its degree of complexity, also in English (**Figure 3**).

In the three zones of the traffic-light simulation, developed countries were involved, with a notorious difference in participation compared to developing countries.

Investments in education focused on technological areas have allowed for significant progress in the different academic and research sectors.

The advantage that developed countries have over developing countries is related to budget allocations and investments in the education and technological innovation area.

Therefore, they are the pioneers in presenting the different advances in areas related to information systems, research, health, economics, pedagogical and educational strategies, robotics, and other areas (**Figure 4**).

The following graph shows the development trend of artificial intelligence by area and medical specialty. The most developed area of artificial intelligence was machine learning, being located in the zone of success since it was applied in several medical specialties; to name, including medical education, and specialized surgeries such as ophthalmology, general surgery, and pediatrics. However, much progress has been

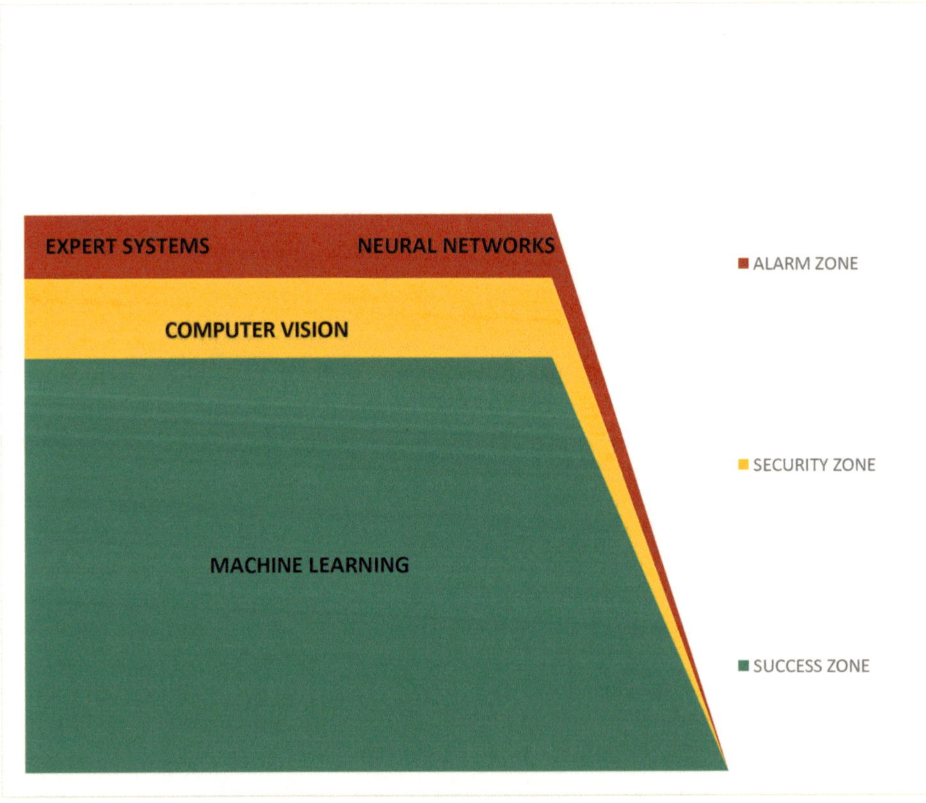

Figure 3.
Simulation graphical representation modified endemic index of areas of development of artificial intelligence applications according to trend.

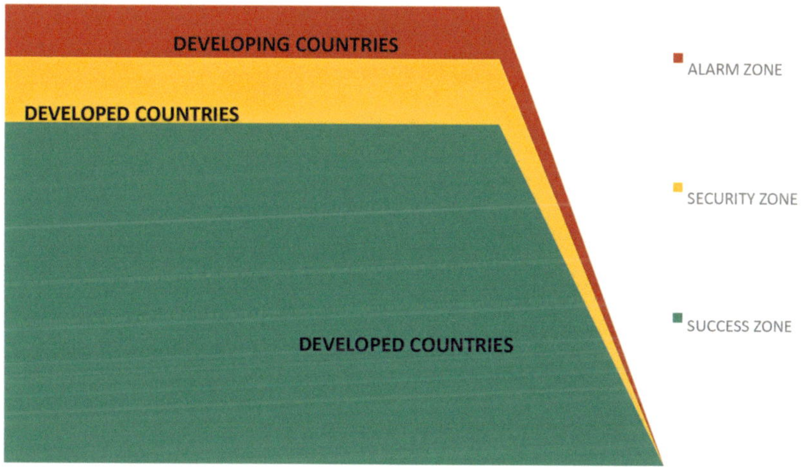

Figure 4.
The trend of artificial intelligence in developed countries VS developing countries.

made in diagnostic areas through the use of advanced and large-scale optics in oncology (**Figure 5**).

During the review of the content of each of the articles, located in the three simulated areas of the endemic channel, it was found that, in each of the medical specialties, where the different areas of artificial intelligence were developed and strategically applied, clinical decisions were made that allowed timely intervention in real-time, according to the needs required in each of them (**Figure 6**).

In all these areas, decisions were made after applying each of these in the different areas of medicine and health. It allowed for generating an impact in the intervention of chronic and transmissible diseases and treatments for each one of them.

13. Limitations

Many of the languages were also limiting for the review of the articles.

14. Discussion

There are many technological applications being made focused on the area of medicine, but not all of them are structured under artificial intelligence and expert systems. This led to evaluate current healthcare technologies in terms of artificial intelligence and expert systems.

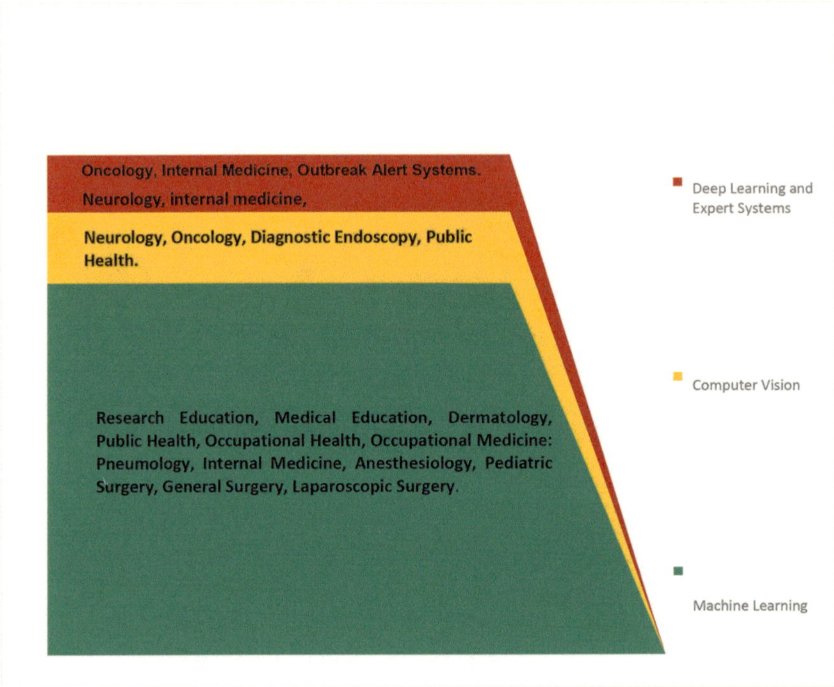

Figure 5.
Development of artificial intelligence application by medical specialty.

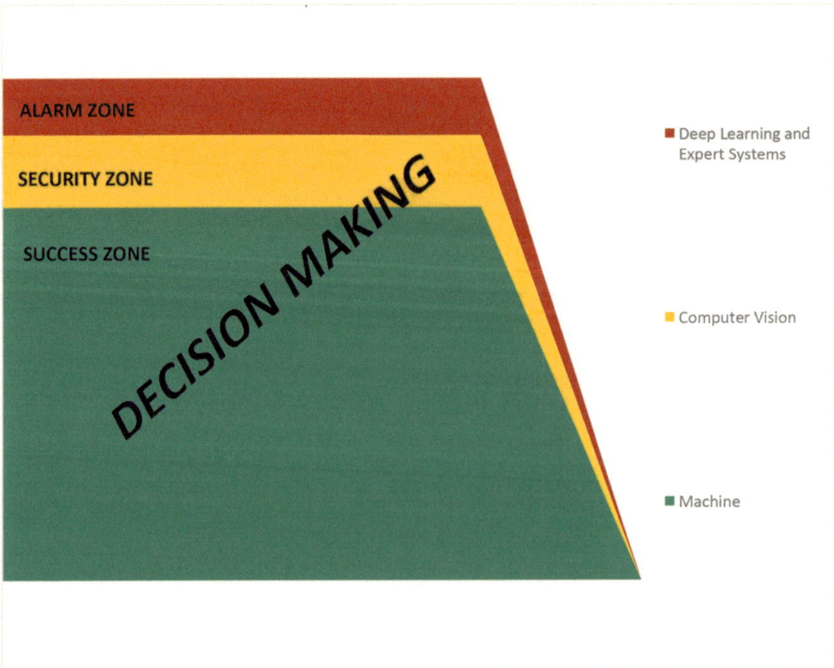

Figure 6.
Decision making by artificial intelligence specialty.

Important findings were obtained with respect to the interventions that have been applied in the clinical part.

Among the most relevant findings, it was recognized that the areas of artificial intelligence where different medical applications were developed were automatic reasoning, computer vision, expert systems, and deep learning with neural networks.

The articles identified as highly concordant were in English, whose applications were implemented in developed countries. This demonstrates the great void of projects and studies on technologies in developing countries, where there is little economic investment in technology and research.

In addition, the epidemiological studies that apply to each of the areas of artificial intelligence were identified, represented by observational, descriptive, analytical, predictive, and experimental studies.

When comparing this article with another research conducted on artificial intelligence in communicable diseases, we can observe that the total number of articles found according to the degree of agreement was 70, compared to 146 in this study; 16 studies were highly concordant compared to 28 in this research. The trend by areas of artificial intelligence focused mainly on automatic reasoning, computer vision, expert systems, and neural networks; in this study, the same result was obtained according to the approach.

In both studies, it could be observed that the area of neural networks is the least developed, the most published and very concordant studies were in the English language in developed countries and in the Medline database, which demonstrates the economic, educational, and research investment that these countries have made in comparison with developing countries.

In addition, it reflects the transformation and technological advances that these countries have made in different areas. The areas of health where there was greater development were public health and epidemiology in infectious diseases, unlike this study, which was in the area of internal medicine.

On the other hand, it made it possible to identify which clinical issues have been evaluated and do not require further research, as well as which texts or topics do not require further research. It also allowed professionals to keep up to date on current trending topics.

We were able to assess the consistency of studies and explore the main sources of variability in studies with apparently beneficial results. Different predictive models of morbidity were identified.

The quality assessment of the body of evidence obtained was performed by two reviewers or peers independently, and the differences in the results of the evaluation of each aspect were discussed until a consensus was reached. The differences between the peers between each of the filters were minimal.

15. Conclusion

It is interesting to observe how medical and technological sciences have been harmonized with the only purpose of finding solutions to daily problems in the care of patients and in search of improving their health condition.

The results of this systematic review of the literature will serve to have a qualitative and quantitative balance of these medical interventions, allowing to an evaluation of their benefits.

Decisions on the forms of medical intervention should be based on the evaluation of the balance between the benefit and the risks or harm they generate; this evaluation will make it possible to obtain relevant and valid information that will allow the search for different forms of intervention.

The search strategy was based on a relational model and an entity-relationship model, in addition to a model for evaluating the thematic quality of the articles found, which made it possible to establish strategies to minimize biases and avoid making systematic errors when selecting or evaluating the relevant literature.

On this occasion, a systematic review of the literature was carried out, not based on clinical or experimental studies, but focused on reviewing and evaluating health technologies, specifically artificial intelligence and expert systems applied to medicine, medical specialties, and surgical procedures.

The contribution that artificial intelligence is making to medical science, research, and the population's health has been fundamental in the advance of public health interventions and in the approach to diseases. However, it is a cause for concern since technology is advancing faster than the regulatory, ethical, and legal framework; and to what extent these new technologies can benefit or harm humanity.

Conflicts of interest

There are no conflicts of interest.

Author details

Tania María Blanchar Martinez[1*] and Fernando Pio de la Hoz Restrepo[2]

1 Public Health Department, Epidemiology and Health Evaluation Research Group, University National, Colombian College of Surgical Instrumentation, University Juan N Corpas, University del Cesar, Bogotá, Colombia

2 Department of Public Health, School of Medicine, Research Group on Infectious Diseases, Epidemiology and Evaluation in Public Health, National University of Colombia, University of London, Bogotá, Colombia

*Address all correspondence to: tmblanchar@gmail.com

References

[1] Hawking SW. A Very Short History of Time. First ed. Drakontos Pockets. Barcelona: Booket; 2006. p. 2

[2] Turing AM. I.—Computing machinery and intelligence. Mind. 1950; **LIX**(236):433-460, Published 01 October. DOI: 10.1093/mind/LIX. 236.433

[3] Rusells NP. Inteligencia artificial, un enfoque moderno. Madrid: Prentice Hall Hispanoamericana S.A; 1996

[4] Lasala P. Introduction to Artificial Intelligence and Expert Systems. 1st ed. Calleja: Prensas Universitarias; 1994

[5] Rius GC. La peste a lo largo de la historia. Servicio de Epidemiología. Agència de Salut Pública de Barcelona. Barcelona. CIBER Epidemiología y Salud Pública (CIBERESP), Madrid. Review Enfermedades Emergency. 2019;**18**(3): 119-127

[6] Zamarripa Franco RA. Curso virtual. Introducción a la Inteligencia Artificial. México: Red de Universidades de Anáhuac; 2020 [acceso 2/11/2019] Disponible en: https://www.edx.org/es/school/anahuacx

[7] Wilkins N. Inteligencia Artificial: Una Guía Completa sobre la IA, el Aprendizaje Automático, el Internet de las Cosas, la Robótica, el Aprendizaje Profundo, el Análisis Predictivo y el Aprendizaje Reforzado. Estados Unidos de América: Bravex Publications; 2020

[8] Lee KF. Superpotencias de la inteligencia artificial: China, Silicon Valley y el nuevo orden mundial. Barcelona, España: Grupo planeta. Deusto s. a ediciones; 2020

[9] Martinez López F, Gallegos RA. Relational database programming. Bogotá: Editions de la U; 2017

[10] Lermen, from Falco Brasileiro. Digital Health: Intersections between Scientific Research and its Mediatization. 2019. Available from: https://pesquisa.bvsalud.org/portal/resource/es/biblio-1005610.

[11] Walker BN, Rehg JM, Kalra A, Winters RM, Drews P, Dascalu J, et al. Dermoscopy diagnosis of cancerous lesions utilizing dual deep learning algorithms via visual and audio (sonification) outputs laboratory and prospective observational studies. eBioMedicine. 2019;**40**:176-183. Available from: https://pesquisa.bvsalud.org/portal/resource/es/mdl-30674442

[12] Santos, Hellen Jeremias dos, Comparison of machine learning algorithms performance in predictive analyzes in public health and medicine. São Paulo; s.n; 2018. 187 p. Available from: https://pesquisa.bvsalud.org/portal/resource/es/biblio-970061.

[13] Finkelstein J, Wood J. Predicting asthma exacerbations using artificial intelligence. Studies in Health Technology and Informatics. 2013;**190**. 56. Available from: https://pesquisa.bvsalud.org/portal/resource/es/mdl-23823374

[14] Carlson J, Das, S, De la Torre F, Frisch A, Guyette F, Hodgins J, et al. A Novel Artificial Intelligence System for Endotracheal Intubation. 20(5): 667-71. Available from: https://pesquisa.bvsalud.org/portal/resource/es/mdl-26986814.

[15] Cooper JN, Wei L, Fernandez SA, Minneci PC, Deans KJ. Pre-operative Prediction of Surgical Morbidity in

Children: Comparison of Five Statistical Models. 2015. Available from: https://pesquisa.bvsalud.org/portal/resource/es/mdl-26986814.

[16] Núñez Reiz A, Martínez Sagasti F, Álvarez González M, Blesa Malpica A, Martín Benítez JC, et al. Organizing Committee of the Madrid 2017 critical care Datathon big data and machine learning in critical care: Opportunities for collaborative research. Intensive Medicine Madrid improved edition. 2019;**4**:52-57. Available from: https://pesquisa.bvsalud.org/portal/resource/es/ibc-181530

[17] De la Cruz FL, Fernández Rodríguez R, González RM. Towards artificial intelligence tools in medical education. Preliminary approach. Revista cubana de inform medicine. 2018;**10**(1):68-75. Available from: https://pesquisa.bvsalud.org/portal/resource/es/biblio-960451

[18] Cabrera Hernández M, Paderni López M, Hita Torres R, Delgado Ramos A, Tardío López M, Derivet Thaureaux D. Medical applications as an aid to diagnosis in medicine. SOFTEL-MINSAP Experience Revista cubana de inform medicine. 2012;**4**(2):199-212. Available from: https://pesquisa.bvsalud.org/portal/resource/es/lil-739202

[19] Guidi G, Pettenati MC, Melillo P, Iadanza E. A machine learning system to improve heart failure patient assistance. IEEE Journal of Biomedical and Health Informatics. 2014;**18**(6):1750-1756. Available from: https://pesquisa.bvsalud.org/portal/resource/es/mdl-25029521

[20] Ilktan A, Yusuf A. A computerized recognition system for home-based physiotherapy exercises using an RGBD camera. IEEE Transactions on Neural Systems and Rehabilitation Engineering. 2014;**22**(6):1160-1171. Available from: https://pesquisa.bvsalud.org/portal/resource/es/mdl-2486003

[21] Paddy N. Machine and deep learning for workflow recognition during surgery. Minimally Invasive Therapy & Allied Technologies. 2019;**28**(2):82-90. Available from: https://pesquisa.bvsalud.org/portal/resource/es/mdl-3084926

[22] Jordi NL. Artificial intelligence applied to evidence-based surgery/Inteligencia artificial aplicada a la cirugía basada en la evidencia. CirEsp. 2019;**97**(2):6364. Available from: https://pesquisa.bvsalud.org/portal/resource/es/mdl-30744823

[23] Nakawala H, Ferrigno G, De Momi E. Development of an intelligent surgical training system for thoracentesis. Artificial Intelligence in Medicine. 2018;**84**:50-63. [Nov-13-2019] Available from: https://pesquisa.bvsalud.org/portal/resource/es/mdl-29169646

[24] Kim EY, Magnotta VA, Liu D, Johnson HJ. Stable atlas-based mapped prior (STAMP) machine-learning segmentation for multicenter large-scale MRI data. Magnetic Resonance Imaging. 2014;**32**(7):832-844. Available from: https://pesquisa.bvsalud.org/portal/resource/es/mdl-24818817

[25] Eisner R, Greiner R, Tso V, Wang H, Fedorak RN. A machine-learned predictor of colonic polyps based on urinary metabolomics. BioMed Research International. 2013;**2013**:303982. Available from: https://pesquisa.bvsalud.org/portal/resource/es/mdl-24307992

[26] Lovejoy C, Buch V, Maruthappu M. Artificial intelligence in the intensive care unit. Critical Care. 2019;**23**(1):7. Available from: https://pesquisa.bvsalud.org/portal/resource/es/mdl-30630492

[27] Yu KH, Beam AL, Kohane IS. Artificial intelligence in healthcare.

Nature Biomedical Engineering. 2018; **2**(10):719-731. Available from: https://pesquisa.bvsalud.org/portal/resource/es/mdl-29169646

[28] Blum JM, Kruger GH, Sanders KL, Gutierrez J, Rosenberg AL. Specificity improvement for network distributed physiologic alarms based on a simple deterministic reactive intelligent agent in the critical care environment. L. Journal of Clinical Monitoring and Computing. 2009;**23**(1):21-30. Available from: https://pesquisa.bvsalud.org/portal/resource/es/mdl-19169835

[29] Mori Y, Kudo S, Mori K. Potential of artificial intelligence-assisted colonoscopy using an endocytose (with video). Digestive Endoscopy. 2018;**30** (Suppl. 1):52-53. Available from: https://pesquisa.bvsalud.org/portal/resource/es/mdl-29658647.pop

[30] Quan T, Zheng T, Yang Z, Ding W, Li S, Li J, et al. Sci NeuroGPS: Automated localization of neurons for brain circuits using L1 minimization model. Reports. 2013;**3**:1414. Available from: https://pesquisa.bvsalud.org/portal/resource/es/mdl-23546385

[31] Miller DJ, Nelson CA, Oleynikov D. Shortened OR time and decreased patient risk through the use of a modular surgical instrument with artificial intelligence. Surgical Endoscopy. 2009; **23**(5):1099-1105. Available from: https://pesquisa.bvsalud.org/portal/resource/es/mdl-19184205

[32] Campo F, Hornero R, Marcos JV, Álvarez D, Zamarrón C. Clinical applications of neural networks in sleep apnea-hypopnea hypopnea syndrome. Sleepwake Sleep. 2013;**25**(1):34-43. Available in: IBECS (bvsalud.org). https://pesquisa.bsalud.org/portal/resource/es/ibc-111436

[33] Fang H, He L, Si H, Liu P, Xie X. Human activity recognition based on feature selection in a smart home using back-propagation algorithm. ISA Transactions. 2014;**53**(5):1629-1638. Available from: https://pesquisa.bvsalud.org/portal/resource/es/mdl-25016308

[34] Curran K, Nichols E, Xie E, Harper R. An intensive insulin therapy mobile phone application built on artificial intelligence techniques. Journal of Diabetes Science and Technology. 2010;**4**(1):209-220. Available from: https://pesquisa.bvsalud.org/portal/resource/es/mdl-20167186

[35] Alpaydın E. Introduction to Machine Learning. London, England: The MIT Press; 2010

Section 3

Focus on Clinical Applications of Artificial Intelligence and Machine Learning

Chapter 6

Human-Machine Collaboration in AI-Assisted Surgery: Balancing Autonomy and Expertise

Gabriel Szydlo Shein, Ronit Brodie and Yoav Mintz

Abstract

Artificial Intelligence is already being actively utilized in some fields of medicine. Its entrance into the surgical realm is inevitable, sure to become an integral tool for surgeons in their operating rooms and in providing perioperative care. As the technology matures and AI-collaborative systems become more widely available to assist in surgery, the need to find a balance between machine autonomy and surgeon expertise will become clearer. This chapter reviews the factors that need to be held in consideration to find this equilibrium. It examines the question from the perspective of the surgeon and the machine individually, their current and future collaborations, as well as the obstacles that lie ahead.

Keywords: surgery, artificial intelligence, computer assisted surgery, robotic surgery, surgical technology

1. Introduction

Artificial Intelligence (AI) is an exponentially growing field that has already impacted many industries. Although the foundations of AI were laid out by Alan Turing as early as the Second World War, recent advances in machine learning and deep learning have bolstered the field, making it one of the most exciting areas of research and development in today's technology landscape. AI focuses on developing systems to perform tasks that would normally require human intelligence, including activities such as problem solving, pattern recognition, decision making, and even creativity. In recent years, as AI popularity has increased, its impact on various elements of the medical industry have become more visible, a harbinger to the future integration of AI technology into the surgeon's daily toolbox.

As this technology continues to mature, and integrates into surgical practice, the questions surrounding its role in the operating room will become more complex. While the primary question of "what can AI do for surgeons?" might soon have an obvious answer, it will open the door to the more nuanced inquiry of "how will surgeons adopt this technology and how can we mark the boundaries of what we should permit AI to do in the operating room?"

We herein discuss all the necessary information for the surgical community to understand the issues at hand surrounding AI, and we lay the framework to assist in making appropriate choices when it comes to balancing Human-AI collaboration in the operating room (OR). The chapter is divided into three sections: The human perspective of the collaboration, the machine side of the collaboration, and the balance between Surgeon and Machine.

2. Methodology

A through literature search was conducted utilizing the online databases of PubMed, Google Scholar, ResearchGate as well as relevant websites. The search terms used were "artificial intelligence," "machine learning," "deep learning," "neural networks," "computer vision," "computer assisted surgery," "machine automation," "machine autonomy," "surgery automation," "surgery autonomy," "robotic surgery," "surgeon responsibility", "surgeon psychology", "surgical training," "technology adoption," and "levels of automation." Inclusion criteria were peer reviewed articles and book chapters published in the English language from 2018 to 2023. As this chapter includes a thorough examination of current technologies, product and company websites were also included that lead to further articles. Excluded articles included those that were not published in the English Language, that were not related to the subject and that were not available in full text.

Our search initially yielded 6887 articles. After excluding articles and removing duplicates, all abstracts were screened, resulting in 60 full text articles that met our inclusion criteria.

The snowball sampling technique was utilized to identify additional relevant articles by reviewing the reference lists of the included articles. This resulted in an additional 10 articles that met our inclusion criteria.

3. The human perspective of the collaboration

3.1 The surgeon's responsibility in the operating room

Surgeons are trained to make complex decisions under pressure and to act on those decisions with appropriate speed. This requires constant situation assessment and analysis, and reassessment and reanalysis [1]. When leading a multidisciplinary team, the surgeons are held responsible for their patient's welfare, safety and wellbeing. From the very beginning of a surgeon's professional life this personal responsibility for their patients' outcome is instilled in them, and is constantly reinforced throughout their career [2, 3]. The American College of Surgeons describes the surgical profession as one of responsibility and leadership, where the surgeon is ultimately in charge of every aspect of the patients' well-being, even if they are not directly involved [4, 5]. While some of these responsibilities might be obvious, others may perhaps be less obvious, as laid out in **Table 1** [6].

The tremendous weight of carrying all this responsibility often creates a psychological mindset where the delegation of responsibilities becomes a difficult task that must be managed with great assiduity. Surgeons learn via their training to "trust no one", to delegate tasks with caution, and to personally review all data [7]. This constant and obviously essential need for oversight raises the question - What does it

Responsibility of the surgeon to ensure patient safety	
Responsibility	**Description**
Preoperative preparation	Oversee proper preoperative preparation of the patient with standardized protocols. Achieving optimal preoperative preparation frequently requires consultation with other physicians from different disciplines; however, the responsibility for attaining this goal rests with the surgeon.
Informed consent	Obtain informed consent from the patient regarding the indication for surgery and surgical approach, with known risks.
Consultation with OR team	Consult with anesthesia and nursing teams to ensure patient safety. Oversee all appropriate components of the surgical time-out (Identification of patient, procedure, approach, etc.).
Safe and competent operation	Lead the surgical team in performing the operation safely and competently, mitigating the risks involved. Ensure anesthesia type is appropriate for the patient and procedure. Including planning the optimal anesthesia and postoperative analgesic method with the anesthesia team.
Specimen labeling and management	Overseeing specimen collection, labeling, and management with completion of the pathology requisition.
Disclose operative findings	Disclose operative findings and the expected postoperative course to the patient.
Postoperative care	Personal participation and direction of the postoperative care, including the management of postoperative complications. If some aspects of the postoperative care may be best delegated to others, the surgeon must maintain an essential coordinating role.
Follow up	Ensure appropriate long-term follow-up for evaluation and management of possible extenuating problems associated with or resulting from the patient's surgical care.

Table 1.
Responsibilities of the surgeon as the treating physician.

take for surgeons to feel comfortable delegating responsibility? When do surgeons feel at ease when relinquishing part of this control? And subsequently, what does it take for the surgical profession to adopt new technologies that take part of this burden of responsibility away from the surgeon?

3.2 The surgeon as an innovator and the process of adopting new technology

Although surgical training is based on apprenticeship, where the student learns from the master and replicates the master's actions exactly, the advancement of surgical capabilities has always relied heavily on the innovation and adoption of new technologies. Throughout history, the desire to help their patients has motivated surgeons worldwide to be creative in finding new solutions to their problems [8]. The evolution and adoption of change within the actual surgical practice, however, is rather complicated. Some surgeons are constantly innovating by customizing therapies and procedures to meet the uniqueness of each patient, while most continue to follow the path that was laid out by their mentors, often reluctant to adopt new technologies. As such, the integration of novel technologies or procedures into a surgeon's daily practice is influenced by many factors, including the possible benefit the innovation provides to the patient, the patient's demand for it, the learning curve required for skill acquisition by the surgeon, and the amount of disruption it would create within their practice [9]. Take for example, laparoscopic cholecystectomy; it took only four years from its introduction, to become the gold standard for gallbladder removal, as this procedure had obvious and very tangible benefits for the patients compared to open cholecystectomy, and the amount of disruption to the surgical practice was low. In contrast, laparoscopic simple nephrectomy attained only a mere 20% acceptance rate by surgeons thirteen years after its introduction – most likely due to the lack of perceived benefit of changing the standard of care by the surgeons [10]. The question then arises, how does one promote and move forward a new concept so that it can be adopted?

The process by which a cohort adopts a new concept (idea, technology, procedure, etc.,) can be studied and understood with the Technology Adoption Curve (TAC). TAC is a sociological model that divides individuals into five types of people with different desires and demands, and explains what it takes for each of these groups to adopt an innovation. These five groups are the innovators, the early adopters, the early majority, the late majority, and the laggards (**Figure 1**) [11].

The TAC model, used to describe adoption in the general population can be extrapolated and applied to the adoption of technology by surgeons [12].

Innovator surgeons are enthusiastic about new technologies and are willing to take the risk of failure. They are willing to test a new procedure even if it is in experimental stages. *Early adopters* are the trendsetters, they are also comfortable with risk, but they want to form a solid opinion of the technology before they vocally support it. These surgeons are comfortable trying a novel procedure that has enough published literature to be regarded as safe.

Surgeons in the *early majority* are interested in innovation but want definitive proof of effectiveness. The benefits of a procedure are more important to them than

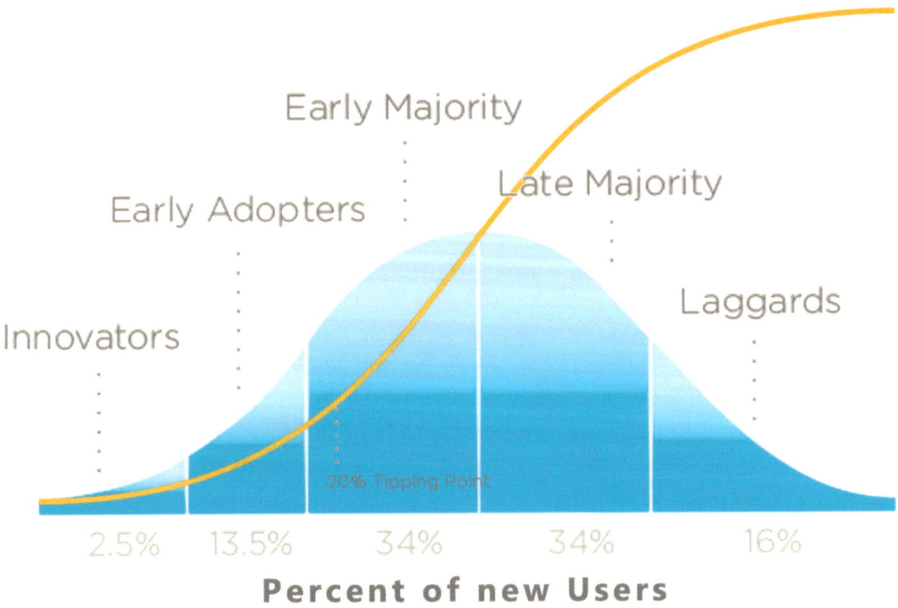

Figure 1.
Technology adoption curve. Bell-curve represents the variation of adoption, and S-curve represent the accumulated adoption over time.

Technology adoption curve	Stages of surgical innovation
Innovators	Development
Early Adopters	Exploration
Early Majority	Assessment
Late Majority	Long Term Implementation
Laggards	

Table 2.
Stages of surgical innovation according to Barkun et al. and how they compare to the TAC model.

the novelty. The *late majority* are averse to risk, as such, they need to be convinced that the new procedure is worth their time. While *Laggards* are skeptical and wary of change, making them reluctant to change, preferring to continue with what is familiar to them.

In an effort to better relate the model to evidence-based practices like surgery, Barkun et al. proposed some adaptations, allowing for critical appraisal and assessment of the technology. In their model every stage would require peer review, thereby promoting a more scientific approach to the application of new technology in surgery (**Table 2**) [13].

On average, for a new concept to be considered adopted, 20% of people must have already begun to use the technology [9], in other words, some but not all people in the *early majority* group of the TAC. For this to happen with AI in the OR, the benefit of the technology must be proven beyond the proof-of-concept stage. Once the technology has been proven to be safe and beneficial then it will be easier to convince more individuals to try it, thereby promoting wider spread acceptance, adoption and eventually integration into daily practice.

4. The machine side of the collaboration

4.1 The basics of artificial intelligence

Artificial intelligence (AI) is defined as the simulation of human intelligence in machines programmed to think and learn like humans. The aim of AI is to create machines with the ability to perceive their environment, reason with it and act in such a way that would normally require human intelligence or to process data whose scale exceeds what humans can analyze [14]. In other words, to create systems that have a certain degree of autonomy [15]. Within the framework of autonomy in AI there is a hierarchy, comprised of three main tiers:

4.1.1 Artificial narrow intelligence

Systems designed to perform a specific task or solve a specific problem. As such, they have a narrow range of parameters allowing them to simulate human behaviors in specific contexts such as face or speech recognition and processing, voice assistance, or autonomous driving. They are "intelligent" only within the specific task they are programmed to do.

4.1.2 Artificial general intelligence

Systems designed to perform any intellectual task that a human can [16]. Apart from mimicking human intelligence, these systems have the ability to learn and adapt. Additionally, they can think, learn, understand, and act in a way that is indistinguishable from that of a human being in any situation.

4.1.3 Artificial superintelligence

A system designed to surpass human intelligence in every aspect with the ability to improve its own capabilities rapidly [17]. This system is designed to have consciousness and be sentient [18], surpassing humans in every way: science, analysis, medicine, sports, as well as emotions and relationships.

While the tiers of AI are each fascinating in their own way, currently the only type of AI that exists is Artificial Narrow Intelligence. The remaining tiers are merely theoretical and philosophical concepts, as such have yet to be achieved, and are beyond the scope of this chapter.

To further understand how AI works, it is important to discuss the concepts of Machine Learning, Artificial Neural Networks, and Deep Learning. These terms are used to describe the techniques that organize the basis of AI systems and are important to understand how AI is achieved. These terms refer to different techniques used to train machines on data, each one building upon the prior one in order to reach more complex results [19–21].

- Machine Learning (ML) is the process by which an AI system can automatically improve with experience; this process allows a system to learn from data without being explicitly programmed. Machine learning algorithms can analyze large amounts of information to identify patterns and make predictions or decisions based on that analysis.

- Artificial Neural Network (ANN) is a type of machine learning algorithm based on a collection of connected units called "neurons" that loosely model neurons in the biological brain. Each connection can transmit a signal to other "neurons" which in turn receive the signal, process it and forward a new signal to other neurons connected to it. A neuron can only transmit its processed signal if it crosses a certain threshold, a process similar to the depolarization of biological neurons, hence the term neural network.

- Deep Learning (DL) is a type of neural network that is designed to learn and make decisions based on multiple hidden layers of interconnected neurons. Deep learning algorithms are capable of learning and representing complex relationships in multiple datasets automatically (**Figure 2**).

Now that the techniques that serve as the basis of AI have been clarified, it is important to understand how they are applied to create actual usable systems that can perform a task. These basic applications of AI include Natural Language Processing, Computer Vision, and Expert Systems, which leverage Machine Learning, Artificial Neural Networks and Deep Learning to solve specific problems [22–24].

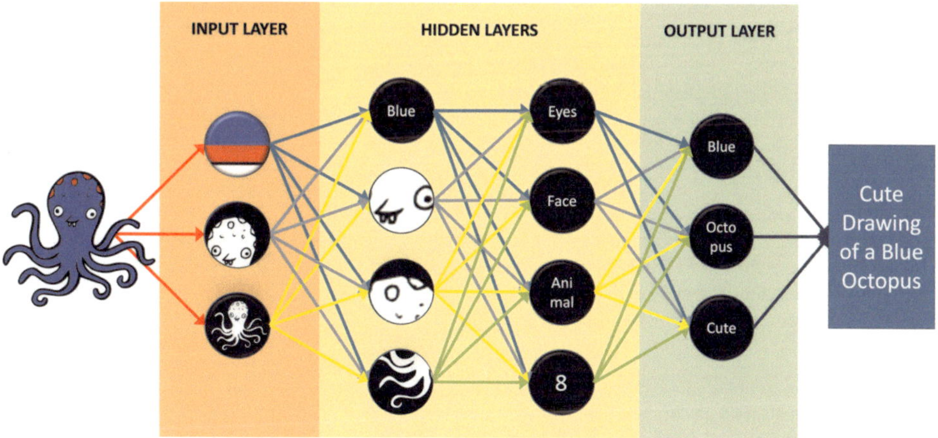

Figure 2.
Deep learning example of an artificial neural network where an image is pushed through several algorithms in hidden layers. Once all layers are processed the outcome can be reached, in this case a definition of the image.

- Natural Language Processing (NLP) is the ability of AI systems to understand, process, and interpret human language.

- Computer Vision (CV) is the ability of AI systems to interpret and understand visual data, such as images and videos.

- Expert Systems (ES) is the ability of AI systems to emulate the decision-making capacity of a human expert.

For the purpose of simplification one can say that there are different techniques to train artificial intelligence (ML, ANN and DL) which each perform specific tasks (CV, NLP, ES) in order to solve a specific problem (**Figure 3**).

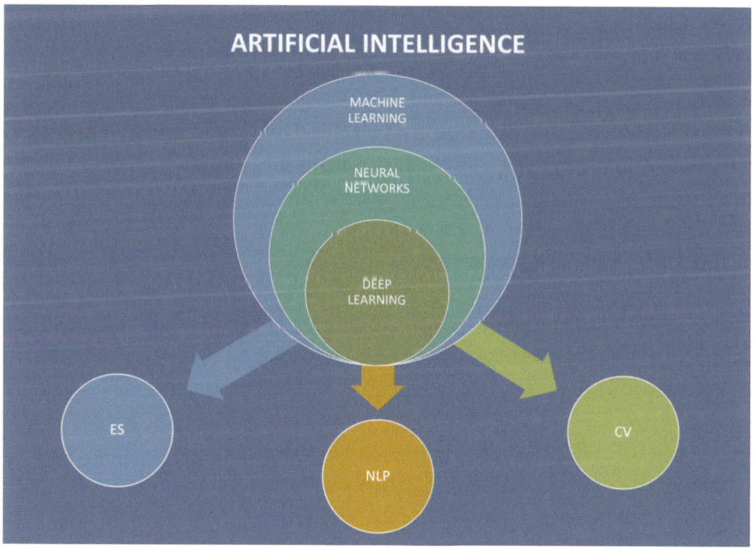

Figure 3.
Relationship between basic concepts of artificial intelligence.

Principle	Analogy	Real world	Medical world
Machine Learning	Teaching a child to recognize an object by showing it pictures of the object, without telling the child what it is.	Netflix, Inc. uses machine learning to recommend personalized content to each user [25].	Owkin, Inc. [26], a company that uses machine learning to improve drug discovery and clinical trial design.
Neural network	The human brain processes and interprets information from the senses to make decisions and control the body.	AlphaZero™ by Deepmind, Ltd. is a chess engine which after 24 hours of training defeated world-champion chess programs [27].	PhysIQ, Inc. is a company using neural networks to continuously monitor at-risk patients remotely and alert their physicians in real time [28].
Deep learning	A student who starts learning basic concepts in class and continues to self-teach building-up to more complex ideas.	Tesla, Inc. uses deep learning algorithms to constantly improve their cars' self-driving system [29].	AIdoc, Ltd. [30] is a company that uses deep learning algorithms for image analysis to detect and prioritize acute abnormalities in radiology.
Natural language processing	A translator between people who speak different languages.	Alexa™ by Amazon, Inc. is a virtual assistant that can understand, process and respond to language prompts [31].	The UNITE algorithm developed at Harvard University can automatically assign ICD codes based on clinical notes without human supervision [32].
Computer Vision	A child that can see any picture of a dog and know it's a dog.	Google Lens ™ [33] can process an image and offer actions depending on what it sees.	DeePathology, Ltd. has created an algorithm that can autonomously detect *H. Pylori* in pathology slides [34].
Expert Systems	A firm that has a lawyer on retainer to answer any question at any time.	AITax, Ltd. has an AI system that can automatically check and file user taxes [35].	Merative™ (formerly IBM Watson Health) [36], is a clinical decision-support system for the diagnosis and treatment planning.

Table 3.
AI basic concepts with examples used in the real world and in the medical world today.

Most of the cutting-edge AI systems available today use a variety of these algorithms in tandem to accomplish their tasks. **Table 3** presents examples of technologies that use specific AI algorithms for each concept discussed above.

4.2 AI in medicine and its current applications

Today AI is already being utilized in medicine, and thus far, its applications have shown promising results as demonstrated by improved patient outcomes, optimized clinical workflows, and accelerated research. To date, there are 521 AI-Enabled medical devices approved by the FDA [37], with the overwhelming majority of these products being in the field of radiology used to process images for all pathologies, excluding cancer [38]. Other AI applications currently available are used in the fields of anesthesiology, cardiology, gastroenterology, general and plastic surgery, hematology, microbiology, neurology, obstetrics and gynecology, ophthalmology, orthopedics, pathology and urology. Given the broad spectrum of applications within varying fields of medicine, one understands that AI utilization is not only based on type but also on what its end goal is. Generally, AI technologies in medicine can be classified by the end goal they achieve; these include everything from screening and diagnosis, to triage and clinical trial management. Multiple applications are currently being utilized and under further development, including:

Computer-Aided Detection (CADe) technology is being developed to aid in marking/localizing regions that may reveal specific abnormalities. Its goal is to elevate the sensitivity of screening tests. Curemetrix, Inc. product cmAssist™, for example, has shown a substantial and statistically significant improvement in radiologists' accuracy and sensitivity for detection of breast cancers that were originally missed [39].

Computer-Aided Diagnosis (CADx) is being developed to help characterize or assess diseases, disease type, severity, stage, and progression. An example of the application of this technology is GI Genius™; an Intelligent Endoscopy Module by Medtronic, plc. That can analyze a colonoscopy in real-time and estimate the possible histology of colorectal polyps [40].

Computer-Aided Triage (CADt) aids in prioritizing time sensitive patient detection. VIZ™LVO is a software by Viz.ai, Inc. that detects large vessel occlusion strokes in brain CT scans and directly alerts the relevant specialists in a median time of 5 minutes and 45 seconds, as opposed to 1 hour which is the standard of care today, significantly shortening the time to diagnosis and treatment [41].

Computer-Aided Prognosis (CAP) can provide personalized predictions about a patient's disease progression. The EU-funded CLARIFY Project (Cancer Long Survivor Artificial Intelligence Follow-Up) is working in harnessing big data and AI to provide accurate and personalized estimates of a cancer patient's risk for complications, including rehospitalization, cancer recurrence, treatment response, treatment toxicity, and mortality [42].

Clinical Decision Support Systems (CDSS) are being employed to aid healthcare providers in the diagnoses and treatment of patients in the most effective way possible. Babylon AI, by Babylon, Inc. for example, is a system that uses data to decide on, and provide information about the likely cause of people's symptoms. It can then suggest possible next steps, including treatment options. The system has demonstrated its ability to diagnose as well as or even better than physicians [43].

Remote Patient Monitoring (RPM) systems are being used to monitor patients, and Virtual Rehabilitation is being developed to help patients recover from illnesses and injuries. Systems like CardiacSense Ltd. Medical Watch continuously monitor heart rate and blood pressure, process the data and update the physician in real time. This noninvasive monitoring system allows the physician to change treatment according to data that would not have been available otherwise [44].

Health Information Technology (HIT) is being employed to improve disease prevention and population health. Medial EarlySign, Ltd. mines data from electronic medical records for early detection of patients with high risk of colorectal cancer. Patients determined to have a high risk by the system are flagged and consequently scheduled for colonoscopy. This system has achieved early detection of an additional 7.5% of colorectal cancers that would otherwise have been caught in more advanced stages [45].

Clinical Trials Management Systems (CTMS) are being developed to help streamline all aspects of clinical trials including preclinical drug discovery, clinical study protocol optimization, trial participant management, as well as data collection and management. These types of systems enable researchers to improve study design by utilizing the guidance in choosing the best study design, determination of number of patients needed for each study arm, optimizing candidate selection, as well as tracking and analyzing large amounts of data. CTMS are helping researchers create stronger and more efficient trials [46].

As demonstrated by the above systems, the implementation of these types of AI has significantly and measurably improved the field of medicine. As the benefit of AI continues to be appreciated, via the understanding as to how it aids in providing better and more efficient care to patients, more professionals will begin to utilize it. With improved acceptance, the previously discussed adoption model that Barkun et al. [13] proposed will continue to shift towards long term implementation.

4.3 Potential benefits of AI in surgery

Improved patient care has historically been linked to technological advancements. Laparoscopic cameras have evolved from simple VHS quality to HD and 4 K cameras and even 3D vision with Near Infra-Red capabilities that allow the surgeon to see beyond the naked eye. Laparoscopic instruments evolved from simple straight and rigid instrumentation to articulating and flexible tools, providing a limitless range of motion. Standardization and precision-surgery have infiltrated the OR in the form of staplers for the creation of anastomosis, advanced energy tools for cutting and coagulation, and robotic assisted surgery that combines all of the above technologies together to enhance human precision. Most recently, AI has started to appear in the surgical field, albeit in the perioperative setting. These systems are helping surgeons with decision making processes both pre- and post-operatively by predicting complications and managing different aspects of patient variables [47]. Nevertheless, AI has yet to penetrate the walls of the OR.

The disparity between the advancement of AI in surgery and other fields in medicine is probably because most applicable AI technologies today are focused on vision and reporting, i.e. diagnosis and big data analysis. Surgery at its core is about both vision and action, which presents a much more complex challenge. This challenge, however, has not stopped research efforts in the field of Computer Assisted Surgery. A PubMed query revealed that in 2022, there were more than 5200 publications discussing AI in surgery, and according to The Growth Opportunities in Artificial Intelligence and Analytics in Surgery study, by 2024 the AI market for surgery will reach $225.4 million [48].

Prototypes, proof of concept and pilot studies are being developed around the world, focusing mainly on improving patient safety and refining workflows in the OR [49]. There are already published reports of AI projects in Expert Systems, Computer Vision, image classification, as well as data acquisition and management that show promising results. Studies have reported success of Computer Vision systems for recognition of surgical tools, surgical phases and anatomic landmarks.

Research on videos of laparoscopic cholecystectomy, for example, has reported success of tool recognition such as graspers, hooks and dissectors; other studies have been successful in phase recognition during laparoscopic cholecystectomy. The tested systems have demonstrated the ability of understanding and reporting when the surgeon is dissecting the cystic duct, separating the gallbladder from the hepatic bed or removing it from the body. More advanced systems have demonstrated the ability to recognize and mark the critical view of safety [50, 51].

While these research efforts are certainly demonstrating promising results, the application of AI within the operating room itself remains in its infancy.

5. The balance between human and machine

When trying to find an adequate balance between human and machine collaboration in the OR the subject of autonomy is a natural starting point. Surgical teams today are comprised of highly specialized professionals that need to work in perfect synchrony for surgical procedures to run smoothly. The surgeon, as the leader, must find balance between managing everything going on with a high degree of control, whilst still allowing for the autonomy and independence of each team member. Most surgeons are authoritative leaders within these teams, meaning that they retain control while still empowering the freedom of self-management where each member can be engaged, motivated and focused on their personal tasks at hand [52]. Although the surgeon is ultimately responsible, he or she will not intervene in a nurse's needle or instrument counts, or check whether the anesthesia machine is properly working. Surgeons authorize themselves to relinquish this direct control because via a strong culture, values and guidelines they ultimately continue to provide the critical oversight and supervision for effective risk-management [52].

Besides team management, the surgeon may be liable for equipment malfunctions, therefore there is a certain underlying hesitancy in giving autonomy to machines. A 2013 systematic review of surgical technology and operating room safety failures found that up to 24% of errors within the OR are due to equipment malfunction [53]. This has not, however, stopped us from relinquishing control in certain parts of the surgery and delegating it to tools which we cannot always fully control. Advanced hemostatic devices like Ligasure™ for example, automatically adjusts and discontinues the delivery of energy based on its own calculations without any surgeon input. Similarly, the Signia™ Stapling System has Adaptive Firing™ technology that automatically and autonomously makes adjustments depending on the tissue conditions it senses [54, 55]. So, while there is hesitancy from the surgeon side for adopting new autonomous devices, if the surgeon is able to see the benefits as with the Ligasure™ and Signia™ systems, these types of tools can in fact break the barrier of more advanced machines into daily OR practice.

5.1 Machine autonomy in other fields and how they can relate to the OR

Whether we are aware of it or not, AI is already affecting the world and making our everyday lives easier. It is there every time we search for something online. It automatically recognizes us in pictures we take, it recommends new music, food or products we will like. AI helps us hear what is written and read what is spoken. It protects us from credit card fraud and helps us make smarter investments. At home it manages our thermostat and decides when and where to vacuum clean the floors.

Moreover, machines are already responsible for millions of human lives on a daily basis, albeit indirectly. The oldest and most famous example is probably the autopilot in airplanes; multiple studies have shown that in 95% of commercial flights, pilots spend less than 440 seconds manually flying the plane [56, 57]. Other examples include the automation of emergency medical service dispatchers and the automation of trains and metros, where nearly a quarter of the world's metro systems have at least one fully automated line in operation [58–60].

The advancements of automation in settings where human lives are at stake have pushed society to further debate the autonomy versus control issue. Depending on the field, different scales have been proposed to define levels of automation and autonomy. These scales have been important as they help define the capabilities and limitations of a system's autonomous features and establishing expectations around the operator's behavior and responsibilities. In addition, they have helped build trust and reduce anxiety around autonomous machines, while ensuring that legal and ethical concerns are considered as technologies continue to develop.

The most prominent autonomy scales revolve around the automotive and aviation industries. The main difference between the two is that the automotive scale encompasses all the systems in a car as a single unit and the vehicle is labeled depending on its capability as a whole [61]. While in the aviation scale, each system in an airplane receives a level of automation independent from other available autonomous systems on the same plane [62]. It is important to note that the scales defining the levels of autonomy in cars, trains, and planes all have basic similarities which are adapted to each specific industry. These adaptations are dependent on the level of complexity of each industry, and the training of the average operator. All the scales, across the various industries begin at level 0 where there is no automation at all, gradually increasing to level 5 (or the maximum of 4 in trains [63]) where there is full machine autonomy without the need for human input at all.

In the field of surgery, the question of how to define the levels of autonomy in systems within the OR has already begun, and although surgical systems are not yet as advanced as other industries', it is important to have a standardized language when referencing this subject. Yang GZ et al.'s proposal for defining the levels of autonomy for medical robotics [64] has been extremely effective in catalyzing the debate of defining the levels of autonomy in surgery. This scale is loosely based on the automotive levels of autonomy as it grades a robotic system as a whole depending on all of its capabilities.

The scale is composed of 6 levels (0–5) as follows:

- Level 0: No autonomy. This includes currently available robots which are master-slave systems that follow the surgeon's movements.
- Level 1: Robot assistance. The robot provides some mechanical assistance, while the human has continuous and full control of the system.
- Level 2: Task autonomy. The robot can autonomously perform specific tasks when asked by the surgeon.
- Level 3: Conditional autonomy. A system suggests and then performs a number of tasks when approved by the surgeon.
- Level 4: High autonomy. The robot can make medical decisions while being supervised by the surgeon.
- Level 5: Full autonomy. The robot can perform an entire surgery without the need for a human surgeon.

Others have built upon this scale, using similar classification methods for surgical robot autonomy [65, 66]. Current technology in robotic surgery is only at Level 0, but when the objectives of the research projects described above are met, we might reach level 1 and 2.

As surgeons, our experience in the OR environment is more comparable to flying a sophisticated airplane than driving a car. A surgeon's professional responsibility is similar to that of a pilot, as such the expected capabilities from autonomous systems in the OR might be similar to those in an airplane's cockpit, where each system has their own level of autonomy, independent from other available systems. Therefore, it may be more beneficial to expand the robotic surgery scale, creating a more comprehensive autonomy scale in surgery encompassing all the types of technology used within the OR. To this end one must first understand the flow of a surgical procedure. Every surgery is built on a series of different phases, each of which are divided into tasks based on specific steps (**Figure 4**). A surgeon's job in the OR is to perform a series of steps in order to complete tasks in different phases of a procedure. After fulfilling all steps within each task and phase, the surgery is said to have been completed.

The following scale (**Table 4**), adapted from the levels of automation in aviation, may be used to address the role of automation and autonomy in surgery as it

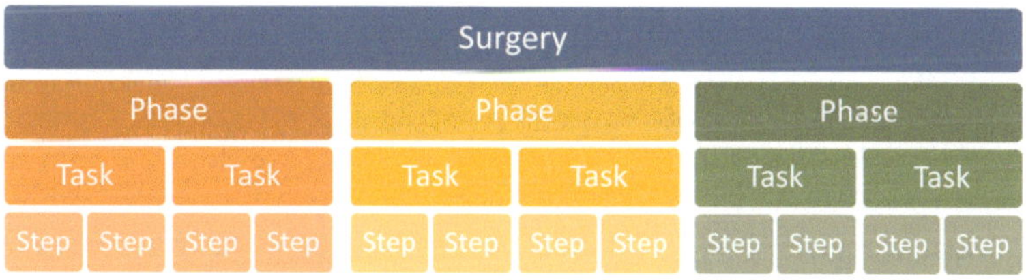

Figure 4.
Divisions of a surgery. The tasks and phases can be done in tandem or can be partially achieved and completed following completion of another task.

Level	Description	Supervision
0: Complete Human autonomy	• The surgeon performs all steps of in every task.	The surgeon is in complete control
1: Task Assistance	• The system executes a specific step of a task.	The surgeon is in complete control.
2: Task Automation	• The surgeon delegates execution of multiple steps of a task to one or more systems.	The surgeon monitors performance of the system during the execution of the specific steps. The system requires active permission from the surgeon to advance to next step.
3: Phase Automation	• The surgeon delegates most steps of multiple tasks to the system • The surgeon performs a limited set of actions in support of the tasks.	The surgeon monitors performance of the system and responds if intervention is requested/required by the system. The system reviews its own work in order to advance to the next step.
4: Full Autonomy	• The surgeon delegates execution of all steps of a task in any phase to the system. • The system can manage most steps of the task under most conditions.	The surgeon actively supervises the system and has full authority over the system.
5: Complete system autonomy	• Execution of all steps of a task in all phases is done by an automated system. • The system can manage all steps of the task under complicated conditions.	The surgeon passively monitors performance of the system.

Table 4.
Levels of automation in surgery.

encompasses every type of technology. It proposes a description of each level of automation, taking into consideration the division of a surgery into phases, tasks and steps.

5.2 The P.A.D. taxonomy—A novel scale for automation and autonomy in the OR

Every surgical procedure is completed based on a series of perceptions, actions and decisions made by the surgeon. These three different duties are important aspects of surgery and must be included in the conversation regarding AI and its application in surgery (**Table 5**).

Perception refers to the recognition of variables in the surgical environment. Surgeons do this instinctively using their senses. Systems sense using sensors like cameras with computer vision, heat detectors, impedance measurements, etc., to convert data from a physical environment into a computational system. As an example, basic bipolar devices transfer a fixed amount of energy through the target tissue for as long as it is activated by the surgeon regardless of the state of the tissue. While using the basic bipolar it is important for the surgeon to use their own senses to see that the tissue appears to have undergone coagulation in order to stop applying energy and prevent inadvertent injury. Over-activation after the tissue has already been coagulated will create a different path of energy transfer that could damage nearby tissues. Advanced bipolar devices, in contrast, sense the tissues impedance, regulating

	System		
	Perception	**Action**	**Decision**
Level 0: Complete Human autonomy			
Level 1: Task Assistance	The system has the ability of basic sensing.	The system performs a step in a specific task.	The system may give basic warnings
Level 2: Task Automation	The system has the ability of general phase, tool and anatomy recognition.	The System performs multiple steps of a task within a phase.	The system understands current step and reacts accordingly.
Level 3: Phase Automation	The system recognizes most phases, tools, and anatomical variables. The system can detect abnormal events.	System can perform most tasks within a phase.	The system understands current task, can predict next actions and react accordingly.
Level 4: Full Autonomy	The system can identify every aspect of a procedure under most conditions.	The system can perform all tasks of every phase in a procedure under most conditions.	The system has full understanding of current phase under most conditions. It plans and reacts accordingly.
Level 5: Complete Autonomy	The system recognizes every aspect and abnormal event of a procedure under any condition.	The system can perform all tasks of every phase of a procedure under any condition.	The system has full understanding of every aspect of the procedure and its variables. It plans and reacts according to any event under any condition.

Table 5.
The PAD (perception, action, decision) scale for surgical autonomy.

the amount of energy dispensed, and automatically discontinuing the activation when the tissue is coagulated.

Action refers to the maneuvers performed in order to execute a task. Surgeons perform actions depending on their perception of a specific scenario. Basic tools and systems can perform actions without having the ability to sense. Advanced systems have the ability to perform an action depending on what they sense. The advanced bipolar device, for example, acts to continue energy or stop it according to its own perception (sensing).

Decision refers to the capability of reaching a conclusion after considering different variables. Advanced systems can give real-time feedback to the surgeon during a procedure, either passively in the form of alerts, warnings and suggestions, or actively in the form of whole system halts, or action restrictions. For example, an advanced laparoscopic stapler can sense the cartridge type inserted to the device as well as the distance and physical resistance between its two jaws. When the stapler is ready to fire, if these variables exceed the stapler's ability, it makes the decision not to fire.

With this taxonomy, one can describe easily the level of AI autonomy by combining each section into a shortened form. As such, the current standard of care is at P1A1D2, because although AI is not yet commercially available, we do have tools like advanced devices that perform certain actions autonomously. Applying the scale to these commercially available devices, we can say that advanced bipolar devices are a Level 1 automated systems as they measure the impedance of a tissue to automatically decide when a cycle is completed. A procedure using this device would therefore be characterized as a P1A1D1 procedure. Smart staplers such as the Signia™ would also be a Level 1 system and a surgeon using it would also be performing a P1A1D2 procedure. As current technologies are further developed with the evolution of AI into more clinical applications, procedures at the level of P2A1D3 may in fact be in our near future.

It is important to note that according to these Levels of Autonomy in Surgery, the responsibility still always falls upon the surgeon, independently of the amount of control and relative autonomy that the system has. The natural path of the debate in the field will bring surgeons (and healthcare professionals in general) to reach a consensus on the amount of control we are willing to give up for the whether it should be ethical and legal for a surgeon to actually relinquish control and autonomy to the point where the burden of responsibility should not be placed on them.

5.3 Will AI replace surgeons?

As with any industry, the perceived threat of AI taking control and pushing away human involvement holds true in medicine. Although at the peak of the hype of AI in radiology and pathology many experts predicted that humans would soon be replaced by machines in these fields, they quickly revised their opinions, with the realization that rather than replacement, the technology had arrived to augment their field's possibilities [67]. This is true in the surgical field as well, and as part of the adoption of AI, surgeons will have to adapt training methods to include these new systems. Not as a way of replacing, but as a way of augmenting the surgeon's capabilities. As such, it is imperative that surgeons understand the capabilities and limitations of the technology, that they know how to use it and problem solve with it, with enough exposure during their training to feel comfortable adding it to their bag of armament. More importantly, as the technology advances it remains imperative that the surgeons retain the ability to perform a surgery with all the necessary tasks safely, even without the use of automated systems. This is particularly important when faced with ensuring safety of patients: Imagine the problematic hypothetical scenario of surgeon who is unable to perform a cholecystectomy due to lack of the ability to recognize the triangle of safety because they rely solely on AI. Conversely, imagine the exciting scenario where a surgeon who is trained to recognize the triangle of safety can utilize AI tools to augment its visualization in a patient with complex anatomy, bringing an added benefit to the patient and the surgeon themselves.

Fundamentally, it is possible to continue to build on the basis of the surgeon's knowledge while maintaining control and delegating specific tasks to AI in order to augment their capabilities, not replace them. As long as the human understands the capabilities and limitations of an AI system as laid out above, the loss of control is thereby mitigated.

It cannot be stressed enough that medicine is a profession of empathy. As physicians we consider more than just the patient's diagnosis in order to propose an appropriate treatment and management. Surgeons must weigh the patient's prognosis, social support system, risks involved in surgery, and patient expectations in order to propose the best treatment. Moreover, during surgery we make an immeasurable amount of decisions and subsequent actions based on the unique patient laying on our table. We cannot say that AI has the ability to consider a patient's environment, desires and expectations, nor can we say that it is machine-proof, but the potential for an AI system with the ability to make such decisions with empathy remains only a theoretical concept for now.

6. Conclusion

The goal of this chapter was to present the factors that both humans and machines face in the evolution of surgery, as well as the balance needed to have a fruitful collaboration. As the field of artificial intelligence has been catapulted into the medical field with many new innovations, the transformation of the medical field is inevitable. The question of how AI technology will affect the surgical profession has become pivotal, as the technology continues to grow, finding new ways to benefit surgeons and patients alike. AI should be viewed not as a threat, rather as another tool in the surgeon's armament for augmenting their skills, further benefiting the patients. The challenge facing AI integration into the operating room are not simple, but as presented herein, we already have some AI available at our fingertips. In the chapter we proposed a novel taxonomy scale encompassing every type of technology that could one day be used in the OR in a comprehensive manner. The PAD taxonomy for Surgical Autonomy may help to bring more awareness to surgeons. With a simple method for stratification of AI, surgeons may begin to feel more confident and be more willing to adopt newer options by understanding what they are utilizing.

Questions remain with regards to the legality and ethics of AI in surgery, specifically with regards to autonomy and task delegation, which may take time to understand and develop. As with any innovation, it is imperative to continue discussions within the surgical community to find the ideal way of collaboration between surgeons and advanced AI systems, to ensure a beneficial partnership.

Author details

Gabriel Szydlo Shein*, Ronit Brodie and Yoav Mintz
Department of General Surgery, Hadassah Hebrew University Medical Center, Jerusalem, Israel

*Address all correspondence to: gabriels@hadassah.org.il

References

[1] Riskin DJ, Longaker MT, Gertner M, Krummel TM. Innovation in surgery: A historical perspective. Annals of Surgery. 2006;**244**(5):686-693. DOI: 10.1097/01.sla.0000242706.91771.ce

[2] Responsible surgery [Internet]. AAO-HNSF Bulletin. 2016. Available from: https://bulletin.entnet.org/home/article/21246793/responsible-surgery [Accessed: February, 2023].

[3] Randle RW, Ahle SL, Elfenbein DM, Hildreth AN, Lee CY, Greenberg JA, et al. Surgical trainees' sense of responsibility for patient outcomes: A multi-institutional appraisal. Journal of Surgical Research. 2020;**255**:58-65

[4] What is the job description for surgeons? [Internet]. ACS. Available from: https://www.facs.org/for-medical-professionals/education/online-guide-to-choosing-a-surgical-residency/guide-to-choosing-a-surgical-residency-for-medical-students/faqs/job-description/ [Accessed: February, 2023]

[5] Principles Underlying Perioperative Responsibility [Internet]. ACS. Available from: https://www.facs.org/about-acs/statements/principles-underlying-perioperative-responsibility/ [Accessed: February, 2023].

[6] Patient Safety in the Operating Room: Team Care [Internet]. ACS. Available from: https://www.facs.org/about-acs/statements/patient-safety-in-the-operating-room/ [Accessed: February, 2023].

[7] Lee TC, Reyna C, Shah SA, Lewis JD. The road to academic surgical leadership: Characteristics and experiences of surgical chairpersons. Surgery. 2020;**168**(4):707-713. DOI: 10.1016/j.surg.2020.05.022

[8] Gauderer MW. Creativity and the surgeon. Journal of Pediatric Surgery. 2009;**44**(1):13-20. DOI: 10.1016/j.jpedsurg.2008.10.006

[9] Wilson CB. Adoption of new surgical technology. BMJ. 2006;**332**(7533):112-114. DOI: 10.1136/bmj.332.7533.112

[10] Miller DC, Wei JT, Dunn RL, Hollenbeck BK. Trends in the diffusion of laparoscopic nephrectomy. Journal of the American Medical Association. 2006; **295**(21):2476

[11] Adapted from: A graph of Everett Rogers Technology Adoption Lifecycle model. Distributed under the GNU Free Documentation License. Available from: https://commons.wikimedia.org/wiki/File:DiffusionOfInnovation.png

[12] Barrenho E, Miraldo M, Propper C, Walsh B. The importance of surgeons and their peers in adoption and diffusion of innovation: An observational study of laparoscopic colectomy adoption and diffusion in England. Social Science & Medicine. 2021;**272**:113715. DOI: 10.1016/j.socscimed.2021.113715

[13] Barkun JS, Aronson JK, Feldman LS, Maddern GJ, Strasberg SM, Balliol Collaboration, et al. Evaluation and stages of surgical innovations. Lancet. 2009;**374**:1089-1096. DOI: 10.1016/S0140-6736(09)61083-7

[14] What Is Artificial Intelligence (AI)? [Internet]. Google Cloud. Available from: https://cloud.google.com/learn/what-is-artificial-intelligence [Accessed: February, 2023].

[15] Chen J, Sun J, Wang G. From unmanned systems to autonomous intelligent systems. Engineering. 2022; **12**:16-19. DOI: 10.1016/j.eng.2021.10.007

[16] Shevlin H, Vold K, Crosby M, Halina M. The limits of machine intelligence: Despite progress in machine intelligence, artificial general intelligence is still a major challenge. EMBO Reports. 2019;**20**(10):e49177. DOI: 10.15252/embr.201949177

[17] Saghiri AM, Vahidipour SM, Jabbarpour MR, Sookhak M, Forestiero A. A survey of artificial intelligence challenges: Analyzing the definitions, relationships, and evolutions. Applied Sciences. 2022;**12**(8):4054. DOI: 10.3390/app12084054

[18] Buttazzo G. Artificial consciousness: Hazardous questions (and answers). Artificial Intelligence in Medicine. 2008;**44**(2):139-146. DOI: 10.1016/j.artmed.2008.07.004

[19] Mitchell TM. Machine Learning. New York: McGraw-Hill; 1997. p. 414

[20] What are neural networks? [Internet]. IBM. Available from: https://www.ibm.com/topics/neural-networks [Accessed: February, 2023].

[21] Deng L, Yu D. Deep learning: Methods and applications. Foundations Trends Signal Processing. 2014;**7**(3–4):197-387. DOI: 10.1561/2000000039

[22] What is Natural Language Processing? [Internet]. IBM. Available from: https://www.ibm.com/topics/natural-language-processing [Accessed: February, 2023].

[23] Huang T. Computer vision: Evolution and promise. 19TH CERN School of Computing. 1996:21-25. DOI: 10.5170/CERN-1996-008.21

[24] Jackson P. Introduction to Expert Systems. Harlow, England: Addison-Wesley; 1999

[25] How Netflix's Recommendations System Works [Internet]. Netflix Help Center. Available from: https://help.netflix.com/en/node/100639 [Accessed: February, 2023].

[26] Find the right treatment for every patient [Internet]. Owkin. Available from: https://owkin.com/ [Accessed: February, 2023].

[27] AlphaZero: Shedding new light on chess, shogi, and Go [Internet]. Deepmind. Available from: https://www.deepmind.com/blog/alphazero-shedding-new-light-on-chess-shogi-and-go [Accessed: February, 2023].

[28] PhysIQ [Internet]. PhysIQ. Available from: https://www.physiq.com/ [Accessed: February, 2023].

[29] Autopilot [Internet]. Tesla Autopilot. Available from: https://www.tesla.com/autopilot [Accessed: February, 2023].

[30] Healthcare AI. [Internet]. Aidoc. Available from: https://www.aidoc.com/ [Accessed: February, 2023].

[31] Conversational AI/Natural language processing [Internet]. Amazon Science. Available from: https://www.amazon.science/research-areas/conversational-ai-natural-language-processing [Accessed: February, 2023].

[32] Sonabend A, Cai W, Ahuja Y, Ananthakrishnan A, Xia Z, Yu S, et al. Automated ICD coding via unsupervised knowledge integration (UNITE). International Journal of Medical Informatics. 2020;**139**:104135. DOI: 10.1016/j.ijmedinf.2020.104135

[33] Google Lense [Internet]. Google. 2022. Available from: https://lens.google/howlensworks/ [Accessed: 2023].

[34] Klein S, Gildenblat J, Ihle MA, Merkelbach-Bruse S, Noh KW, Peifer M, et al. Deep learning for sensitive detection of helicobacter pylori in gastric biopsies. BMC Gastroenterology. 2020; **20**(1):417. DOI: 10.1186/s12876-020-01494-7

[35] The AiTax Corporation [Internet]. AiTax. Available from: https://www.aitax.com/ [Accessed: February, 2023].

[36] Clinical Decision Support [Internet]. IBM Watson. Available from: https://www.ibm.com/watson-health/solutions/clinical-decision-support [Accessed: February, 2023].

[37] Artificial Intelligence and machine learning (AI/ml)-enabled medical Devices [Internet]. U.S. Food and Drug Administration. FDA; Available from: https://www.fda.gov/medical-devices/software-medical-device-samd/artificial-intelligence-and-machine-learning-aiml-enabled-medical-devices [Accessed: February, 2023].

[38] US Food and Drug Administration. Computer-assisted detection devices applied to radiology images and radiology device data—Premarket notification [510 (k)] submissions. Available from: https://www.fda.gov/regulatory-information/search-fda-guidance-documents/computer-assisted-detection-devices-applied-radiology-images-and-radiology-device-data-premarket

[39] Watanabe AT, Lim V, Vu HX, Chim R, Weise E, Liu J, et al. Improved cancer detection using artificial intelligence: A retrospective evaluation of missed cancers on mammography. Journal of Digital Imaging. 2019;**32**:625-637. DOI: 10.1007/s10278-019-00192-5

[40] Hassan C, Balsamo G, Lorenzetti R, Zullo A, Antonelli G. Artificial intelligence allows leaving-in-situ colorectal polyps. Clinical Gastroenterology and Hepatology. 2022; **20**(11):2505-2513. DOI: 10.1016/j.cgh.2022.04.045

[41] Golan D, Shalitin O, Sudry N, Mates J. AI-powered stroke triage system performance in the wild. Journal of Experimental Stroke & Translational Medicine. 2020;**12**:3

[42] Torrente M, Sousa PA, Hernández R, Blanco M, Calvo V, Collazo A, et al. An artificial intelligence-based tool for data analysis and prognosis in cancer patients: Results from the Clarify study. Cancers. 2022;**14**(16):4041. DOI: 10.3390/cancers14164041

[43] Richens JG, Lee CM, Johri S. Improving the accuracy of medical diagnosis with causal machine learning. Nature Communication. 2020;**11**(1): 3923. DOI: 10.1038/s41467-020-17419-7

[44] Chorin E, Hochstadt A, Schwartz AL, Matz G, Viskin S, Rosso R. Continuous heart rate monitoring for automatic detection of life-threatening arrhythmias with novel bio-sensing technology. Frontiers in Cardiovascular Medicine. 2021;**8**:707621. DOI: 10.3389/fcvm.2021.707621

[45] Hornbrook MC, Goshen R, Choman E, O'Keeffe-Rosetti M, Kinar Y, Liles EG, et al. Early colorectal cancer detected by machine learning model using gender, age, and complete blood count data. Digestive Diseases and Sciences. 2017;**62**: 2719-2727. DOI: 10.1007/s10620-017-4722-8

[46] Weissler EH, Naumann T, Andersson T, Ranganath R, Elemento O, Luo Y, et al. The role of machine learning in clinical research: Transforming the future of evidence generation. Trials. 2021;**22**(1):1-5. DOI: 10.1186/s13063-021-05571-4

[47] Loftus TJ, Tighe PJ, Filiberto AC, Efron PA, Brakenridge SC, Mohr AM, et al. Artificial intelligence and surgical decision-making. JAMA Surgery. 2020, 2020;**155**(2):2. DOI: 10.1001/jamasurg.2019.4917

[48] Kite-Powell J. Artificial Intelligence Set To Dominate Operating Rooms By 2024 [Internet]. Forbes 2020. Available from: https://www.forbes.com/sites/jenniferhicks/2020/06/25/artificial-intelligence-set-to-dominate-operating-rooms-by-2024/ [Accessed: February, 2023].

[49] Mintz Y, Brodie R. Introduction to artificial intelligence in medicine. Minimally Invasive Therapy & Allied Technologies. 2019;**28**(2):73-81. DOI: 10.1080/13645706.2019.1575882

[50] Padoy N. Machine and deep learning for workflow recognition during surgery. Minimally Invasive Therapy & Allied Technologies. 2019;**28**(2):82-90. DOI: 10.1080/13645706.2019.1584116

[51] Mascagni P, Alapatt D, Sestini L, Altieri MS, Madani A, Watanabe Y, et al. Computer vision in surgery: From potential to clinical value. npj Digital Medicine. 2022;**5**(1):163. DOI: 10.1038/s41746-022-00707-5

[52] Gilbert G. The paradox of managing autonomy and control: An exploratory study. South African Journal of Business Management. 2013;**44**(1):1-4. DOI: 10.4102/sajbm.v44i1.144

[53] Weerakkody RA, Cheshire NJ, Riga C, Lear R, Hamady MS, Moorthy K, et al. Surgical technology and operating-room safety failures: A systematic review of quantitative studies. BMJ Quality & Safety. 2013;**22**(9):710-718. DOI: 10.1136/bmjqs-2012-001778

[54] LigaSure technology [Internet]. Medtronic. Available from: https://www.medtronic.com/covidien/en-us/products/vessel-sealing/ligasure-technology.html [Accessed: February 20, 2023].

[55] Signia stapling system [Internet]. Covidien. Available from: https://www.medtronic.com/covidien/en-us/products/surgical-stapling/signia-stapling-system.html [Accessed: February 20, 2023].

[56] Cummings ML, Stimpson A, Clamann M. Functional Requirements for Onboard Intelligent Automation in Single Pilot Operations. AIAA Infotech@ Aerospace; 2016. p. 1652. DOI: 10.2514/6.2016-1652

[57] Barry D. How long do pilots really spend on autopilot? [Internet]. Cranfield. Available from: https://saiblog.cranfield.ac.uk/blog/how-long-do-pilots-really-spend-on-autopilot [Accessed: February, 2023].

[58] Uitp SB. World Report on Metro Automation 2018. Observatory of Automated Metros Brussels. Belgium; 2020

[59] The world's leading intelligent safety platform. RapidSOS; Available from: https://rapidsos.com/ [Accessed: February, 2023].

[60] Predict prevent crime [Internet]. PredPol. 2018. Available from: https://www.predpol.com/ [Accessed: February, 2023]

[61] Taxonomy and Definitions for Terms Related to Driving Automation Systems for On-Road Motor Vehicles. SAE International. Available from: https://www.sae.org/standards/content/j3016_202104/

[62] Anderson E, Fannin T, Nelson B. Levels of aviation autonomy. In: 2018 IEEE/AIAA 37th Digital Avionics Systems Conference (DASC). London,

England: IEEE; 2018 Sep 23. pp. 1-8. DOI: 10.1109/DASC.2018.8569280

[63] IEC–International Electrotechnical Commission. Railway applications–Urban guided transport management and command/control systems. Available from: https://webstore.iec.ch/publication/6777

[64] Yang GZ, Cambias J, Cleary K, Daimler E, Drake J, Dupont PE, et al. Medical robotics—Regulatory, ethical, and legal considerations for increasing levels of autonomy. Science Robotics. 2017;**2**(4):eaam8638. DOI: 10.1126/scirobotics.aam8638

[65] Battaglia E, Boehm J, Zheng Y, Jamieson AR, Gahan J, Fey AM. Rethinking autonomous surgery: Focusing on enhancement over autonomy. European Urology Focus. 2021;**7**(4):696-705. DOI: 10.1016/j.euf.2021.06.009

[66] Attanasio A, Scaglioni B, De Momi E, Fiorini P, Valdastri P. Autonomy in surgical robotics. Annual Review of Control, Robotics, and Autonomous Systems. 2021;**4**:651-679. DOI: 10.1146/annurev-control-062420-090543

[67] Langlotz CP. Will artificial intelligence replace radiologists? Radiology. Artificial Intelligence. 2019;**1**(3):e190058. DOI: 10.1148/ryai.2019190058

Chapter 7

Application of Computer-Assisted Surgery System Based on Artificial Intelligence in Pediatric Precise Oncological Surgery

Wenli Xiu, Xiwei Hao, Nan Xia, Yongjian Chen, Haitao Niu and Qian Dong

Abstract

Pediatric oncological surgery is difficult and challenging, especially in children with malignant solid tumors. Compared with adults, children have immature organs, thin blood vessels, and poor surgical tolerance. Moreover, pediatric malignant solid tumors are often huge, complex in location, fast-growing, and highly malignant. With artificial intelligence and machine learning breaking through many bottlenecks, computer-assisted precision medicine has also taken a quantum leap forward. Ten years ago, Professor Dong's group invented the Computer-assisted Surgery System (Hisense CAS). Now, this three-dimensional (3D) visualization technology based on artificial intelligence has been used for pediatric precise oncological surgery and has been upgraded to version 5.0. Hisense CAS was developed based on enhanced pediatric CT data, so it has advantages in displaying pediatric solid tumors. CAS can display the adjacent relationships of the tumor with the surrounding tissues (especially the compressed blood vessels) in a 3D, dynamic, and complete manner through rapid and accurate 3D reconstruction of organs, tumors, and blood vessels. Then, precise preoperative evaluations and surgical planning can be carried out. This chapter focuses on individualized computer-assisted surgical planning and progress in common and complex pediatric tumors (such as malignant liver tumors, retroperitoneal tumors, and mediastinal tumors) and introduces experience in improving the resectability of tumors and reducing surgical complications.

Keywords: tumor, surgery, pediatric, computer-assisted, precise surgery

1. Introduction

With decreasing mortality from infectious diseases and increasing cure rates for congenital malformations, pediatric tumors have become an important disease factor endangering the health of children, and their incidence continues to rise [1, 2]. Surgical resection is the most effective and important treatment for the eradication of pediatric solid tumors, especially malignant solid tumors. However, pediatric tumors are often diverse, complex in location, and large in size compared to tumors in the young body. Malignant tumors are highly malignant and grow rapidly. Moreover, compared with that of adults, the organ structure of pediatric patients is slender and has poor tolerance, thus the space for surgical treatment is limited. Therefore, there is a greater need for high-technology tools that help perform precise and meticulous surgical procedures [3].

Technological innovation and interdisciplinary integration have brought surgery to a brand new stage, namely, the era of precision surgery. Precision surgery is a whole process of surgery-centered surgical practices, covering all stages from disease assessment, clinical decision-making, surgical planning, and surgical resection to perioperative management. Computer-assisted surgery (CAS), a typical representative of medical-industrial integration, is a new technology based on artificial intelligence and machine learning that can process and learn large amounts of medical data and information at high speed and then provide technical support to surgeons through a virtual surgical environment to assist in the realization of precision surgery [4].

2. Methodology

This chapter provides a retrospective summary of the key technologies of our self-developed computer-assisted surgery system "Hisense CAS" and analyses its practical application in pediatric oncological surgery, providing individualized computer-assisted surgical planning for common and complex pediatric tumors (such as malignant tumors of the liver, retroperitoneal tumors, and mediastinal tumors) to improve tumor resectability and reduce surgery-related complications [5, 6].

3. Computer-assisted surgery

CAS is a new surgical concept that refers to the use of computer technology for presurgical planning and to guide or assist surgical procedures. CAS is generally considered to include (i) creation of virtual images of patients; (ii) analysis and in-depth processing of patient images; (iii) diagnosis, presurgical planning, and simulation of surgical steps; (iv) surgical navigation; and (v) robotic surgery. With its development and use in the medical field, CAS has helped realize precision surgery.

3.1 Digital three-dimensional reconstruction and simulation surgery

The technical basis of digital three-dimensional (3D) reconstruction is to convert two-dimensional (2D) cross-sectional images such as CT or MRI into 3D visual images using computer algorithms to provide the operator with more intuitive stereoscopic images for diagnosis and preoperative evaluation. Through the virtual reality surgeries available through modern computer technology, a virtual surgery model for specific individualized surgical modality evaluations can be established. The surgeon can input the conceived surgical plan into the computer, combine it with the presurgical medical images, and form a three-dimensional image after processing by the software system to understand in detail the specific location, involvement range, and adjacent relationships of the tumor, especially the involvement of blood vessels. Medical image data and virtual surgery systems are also used to reasonably customize individualized surgical plans to reduce surgical injury, avoid damage to surrounding tissues, improve the precision of lesion localization, and increase the success rate of surgery [7].

3.2 Research and development of CAS based on artificial intelligence

The Hisense Computer-assisted Surgery System (Hisense CAS) was developed by Prof. Dong's group in 2013. This system can perform medical image preprocessing with CT imaging DICOM data, especially low-quality data that can be enhanced in high definition before preprocessing. The medical images labeled with features such as greyscale and texture features are then subjected to deep machine learning by U-Net on a large number of standard DICOM files. Thus, automatic and accurate segmentation of new input data is achieved. The segmentation results are processed by filtering, CT interlayer adaptive correspondence point interpolation, morphology, pattern recognition, and other algorithms, and a self-learning topological model is established to model and track the vessel shape in the three phases (arterial phase, venous phase, and balance phase) of imaging. Then, the matching cubes and ray cast algorithms are used for color rendering, and finally, the 3D alignment algorithm is used to stereoscopically align the three-phase data to accurately obtain enhanced 3D images visualizing the target organs, lesions, and blood vessels. This system can precisely observe the relationships of the lesion with blood vessels and organs in 3D, calculate the volume of the organs, lesions, and blood supply area of each blood vessel branch, perform virtual surgical resection, and determine the best surgical resection line.

With the progression of clinical needs, artificial intelligence technology, and machine learning based on big data, Hisense CAS has been updated to version 5.0. The improved algorithm enables less manual operation and a 25–30% reduction in 3D reconstruction time, and the whole process takes approximately 20 minutes. Hisense CAS can reconstruct more than 4 levels of vessels and distinguish tumors and vessels with 0.5 cm spacing. The Dice value of solid tissues can reach more than 95%, and that of ducts can reach more than 90%. Hisense CAS can also display the overall 3D anatomical relationship and pipeline variations in a semitransparent and interactive way, calculate the distance between any two points and the angle of travel of any blood vessel, the range of innervation or drainage, and the volume of organs and tumors, and provide other information that cannot be obtained from traditional 2D images. In addition, a cloud-based 3D visualization platform for precision surgery based on B/S architecture was constructed to realize the data interactions between the PC terminal browser and CAS and to store, manage and share 2D and 3D image data (**Figure 1**) [8, 9].

3.3 Gesture control intelligent display module (Hisense SID)

Real-time surgical navigation is used to accurately correspond the preoperative image with intraoperative organ anatomy, and through instruments or signal transmission, real-time feedback to the image is provided to reconstruct the model, enable clear positioning, and achieve precision surgery. The 3D image gesture control intelligent display module (Hisense SID) developed by Prof. Dong's group, based on somatosensory interaction, motion capture, and other technologies, can quickly and precisely realize human-computer interactions through simple gesture operations within a specific range to ensure intraoperative sterility. The operator can rotate,

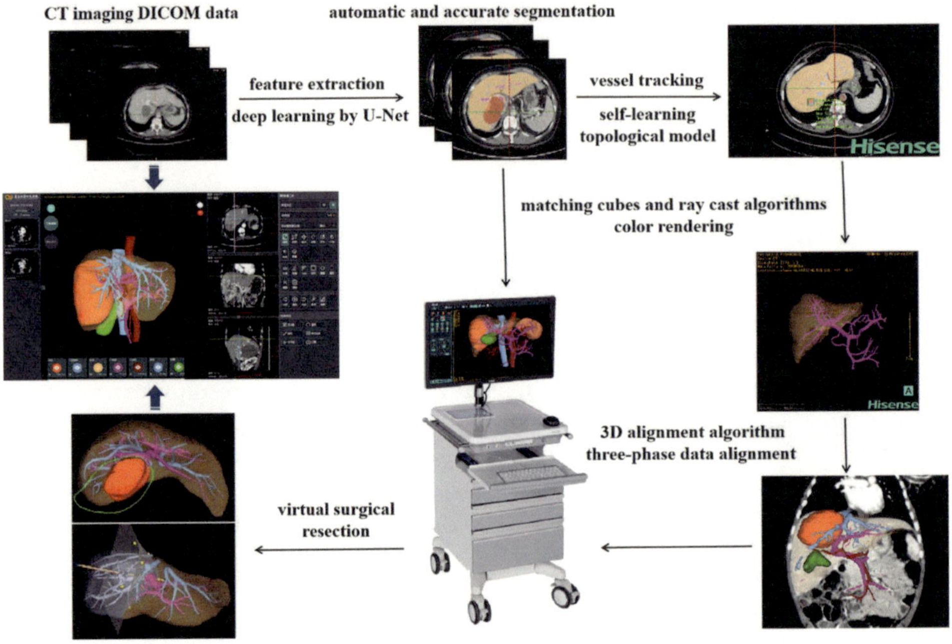

Figure 1.
Hisense computer-assisted surgery system based on artificial intelligence.

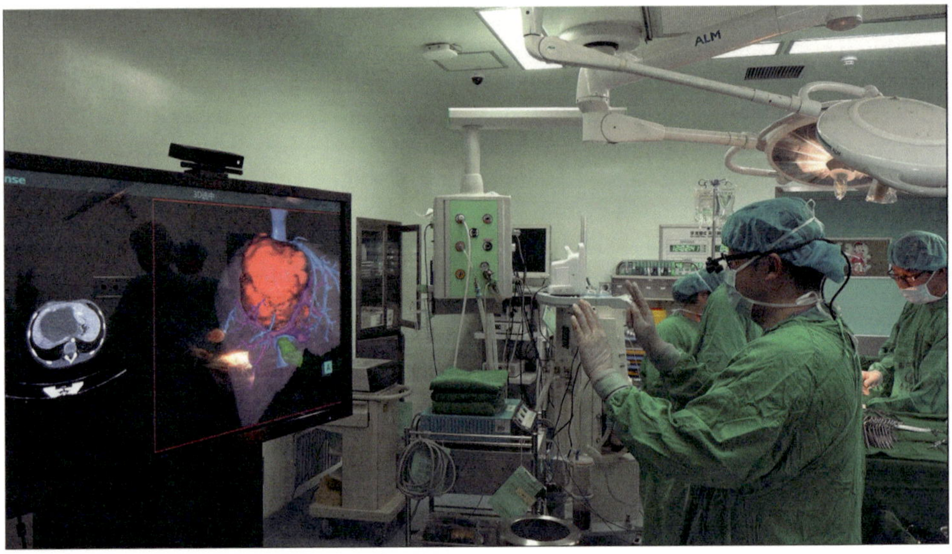

Figure 2.
Real-time surgical navigation through Hisense SID gesture intelligent control.

zoom in and zoom out on the digital 3D image through different gesture control commands to view the required details. In addition, the system provides intelligent tracking of specific operators, thus eliminating interference from surrounding personnel, reducing misuse, and improving recognition rates (**Figure 2**) [10].

4. Application of CAS in pediatric precise oncological surgery

According to a survey by the International Society of Pediatric Oncology, the incidence of pediatric tumors has increased at a rate of 2.8% each year over the past 10 years, and pediatric malignant solid tumors have become a major cause of illness and death in children. Primary surgical resection or surgical resection after other treatments is still recognized as the current first choice for the treatment of pediatric malignant solid tumors and is the only means to achieve a radical cure for malignant tumors. However, the necessity of pursuing radical surgery in children and the special characteristics of pediatric tumors put forward higher requirements for pediatric precision surgery.

4.1 Pediatric liver tumor

The anatomical structure of the liver is complex, and internal vascular and biliary tract variants are common, especially in the hepatic vein. The structure of the intrahepatic vascular system in pediatric patients is very delicate, and the organ is small in size and poorly tolerant to surgical trauma. Moreover, pediatric liver tumors are often huge, complex, fast-growing, and highly malignant. Tumors often squeeze and deform the surrounding blood vessels, and the compression or invasion of the adjacent liver area is difficult to identify. Large tumors involving the hepatic porta and tumors originating from the hepatic porta are still difficult to treat surgically. In addition, pediatric liver volume changes greatly with age and weight, so individualized liver anatomy and volume analyses are very important [11].

Hepatoblastoma (HB) is the most common primary malignant tumor of the liver in children. Its incidence rate is the highest among infants and children under 5 years old, with an annual incidence of approximately 1.5 cases per 1 million. The increasing incidence year by year and disparities between races have attracted widespread attention. With the combination of surgery and chemotherapy, especially neoadjuvant chemotherapy, the prognosis of children with HB has improved significantly, with survival rates increasing from 30% to approximately 80% [12, 13]. However, surgical resection is still an important and indispensable treatment for HB, and whether the tumor can be completely removed with a sufficient liver remnant volume is the key factor affecting the prognosis of such children [14].

All current collaborative trial groups used PRETEXT/POSTTEXT to assess the surgical resectability of HB before surgery. This staging is based on 2D cross sectional images and is performed on the basis of Couinaud's liver segmentation by determining the number of consecutive tumor-free liver sections. In practice, this approach is of limited help to the surgeon, and the assessment of staging and surgical resectability by window level selection and artificial measurements is severely limited by anatomical basis, image interpretation experience, and surgical experience. Only a very rough estimate of the expected surgical procedure difficulty can be made. In addition, although Couinaud's segmentation is very classical and practical, it is limited by the small number of dissection cases available when the classification was established and some differences between the isolated and living liver. PRETEXT also provides a detailed and cumbersome description of vascular variants, but as definitions, their clinical application is limited [15].

From the point of view of surgical resection, regardless of the strategy and staging, what must be assessed is vascular involvement, which was also defined by

PRETEXT as the annotation factors V and P [13]. In clinical practice, the extent of tumor involvement in major vessels is difficult to assess due to the limitations of 2D images and the deformation variability of the liver vascular system. Another key consideration for surgical resection is the future liver remnant (FLR). An adequate postoperative FLR volume is important, as a small FLR volume can lead to acute liver failure or even death. For HB, guidelines emphasize anatomic hepatic resection, which allows for more normal liver tissue located >1 cm outside the tumor to be removed. Non-anatomic hepatic resection for advanced HB is often considered, such as extended major hepatectomies, mid-liver lobectomy, or segmental resections, which require more precise assessments of FLR [16].

3D imaging technology based on CT images is able to display the positional relationships of the liver, tumor, and all internal ductal structures in a comprehensive and simultaneous manner to achieve accurate evaluations of distances in three-dimensional space, which has obvious advantages in vessels with compression deformation or individual anatomical variations. The ability to track the route of each vessel and determine the drainage segment of each vein is important for determining individualized liver segmental anatomy [15, 17]. In addition, this technology allows for continuous assessments of preoperative chemotherapy and postoperative liver regeneration, which is of greater value in selecting the optimal timing of surgical resection and assessing postoperative liver recovery. Hisense CAS was developed based on enhanced pediatric CT data, so it has more advantages in displaying pediatric liver tumors, especially huge tumors compressing the hepatic porta. Hisense CAS can clearly show the relationships between the tumor and blood vessels and improve the resectability of liver tumors.

Two typical cases of patients with HB who underwent surgical planning with Hisense CAS are shown below. **Figure 3** demonstrates a 4-year-old boy with a large

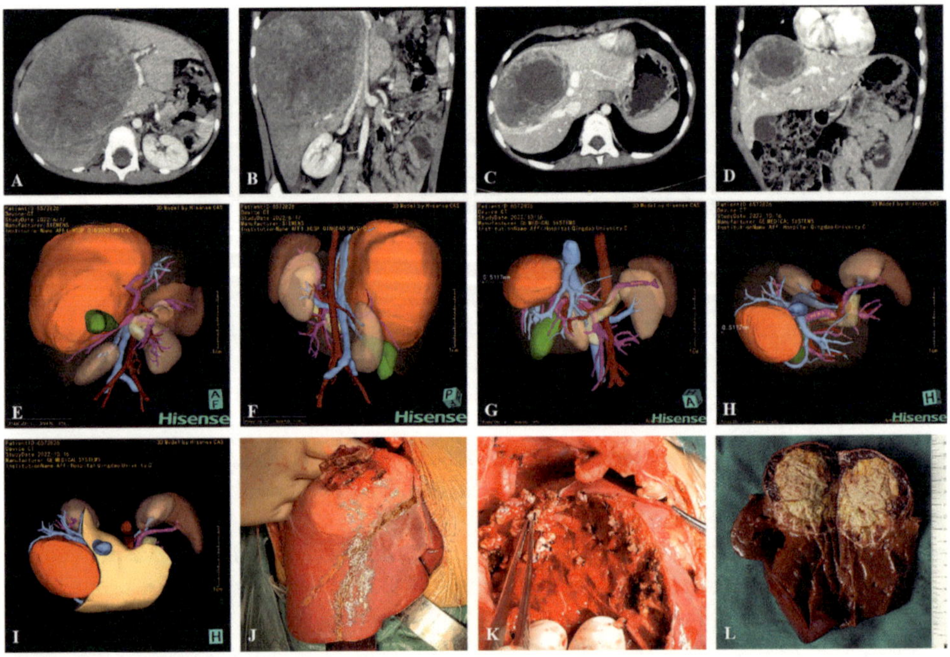

Figure 3.
Computer-assisted resection of the liver tumor with hepatic vein variation.

liver tumor. Enhanced CT allowed for an approximate analysis of the tumor size and the adjacent relationships (**Figure 3A–D**). 3D imaging based on CT could show the location of the liver, the tumor, and all internal ductal structures in relation to each other in a comprehensive, whole, and simultaneous manner. When vascular involvement was evaluated after 5 cycles of neoadjuvant chemotherapy, it was found that the left hepatic vein cointersected with the middle hepatic vein and merged into the inferior vena cava. The tumor margin was only 0.5117 mm from the cointersection (**Figure 3E–H**). Preoperative simulation of right hemicolectomy showed that the residual liver volume was sufficient. The surgery was performed according to the preoperative plan, and the cointersection and the middle hepatic vein were successfully preserved (**Figure 3I–L**).

Figure 4 shows another 3-month-old girl with a massive tumor volume (459.1 ml) when her liver-occupying lesion was detected. The tumor was compressing and invading important blood vessels of the liver, and an aspiration biopsy confirmed HB. Neoadjuvant chemotherapy was the only option other than liver transplantation (**Figure 4A** and **B**). The tumor remained unresectable based on the evaluation performed after 4 cycles of neoadjuvant chemotherapy (**Figure 4C** and **D**). The re-evaluation after 5 cycles of neoadjuvant chemotherapy showed no significant change in tumor volume, from 35.7 ml to 35.0 ml, and the tumor was still too close to the important blood vessels of the liver and could not be operated on (**Figure 4E** and **F**). The re-evaluation after 6 cycles of neoadjuvant chemotherapy showed that the tumor was slightly reduced in size, from 35.0 ml to 25.9 ml, and the tumor was in contact with blood vessels, so surgical resection was considered (**Figure 4G** and **H**). Intraoperative 3D images assisted the surgery. The operation was successful, the

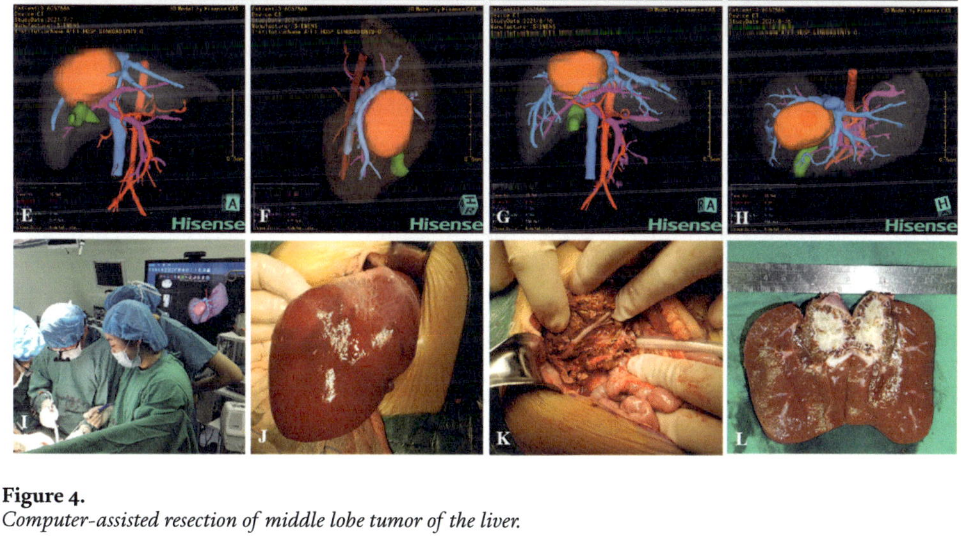

Figure 4.
Computer-assisted resection of middle lobe tumor of the liver.

tumor was completely removed, and the middle hepatic vein and portal vein were successfully preserved (**Figure 4I–L**).

4.2 Pediatric retroperitoneal tumor

Retroperitoneal tumors (RTs) are insidious in origin, lack specific clinical manifestations, and have multiple pathological types. Due to their special anatomical location, these tumors are often found to involve large blood vessels and adjacent organs. The incidence of RTs is low, accounting for approximately 0.07%–0.20% of systemic tumors [18]. However, its malignant degree and recurrence rate are high, so complete surgical resection is the most effective treatment and affects the prognosis [19, 20]. Therefore, it is particularly important to accurately evaluate the anatomical relationships of RTs.

At present, the preoperative evaluation of RTs mainly relies on ultrasound, CT, and MRI. Among them, CT is fast, with high resolution and clear images, and can objectively reflect the compression and displacement of tumors with the surrounding organs and large blood vessels, and it has good reference value [21]. However, CT can only provide simple 2D images, and surgeons can generally judge the tumor's size, location, and adjacent relationships by reading consecutive 2D images. However, this lacks objective accuracy and does not facilitate preoperative communication with colleagues and family members. In addition, more importantly, CT images can only show blood vessels along a specific cross-section and cannot fully display the course and wall shape of the curved blood vessels or show large compressed vessels such as the abdominal aorta, inferior vena cava, portal vein, mesenteric arteries, and iliac vessels in detail.

The application and development of digital medical technology overcame the disadvantages of CT. 3D reconstruction of CT images has made it possible to display the relationships of the tumor with surrounding adjacent organs and blood vessels in a three-dimensional, dynamic, and visualized manner. Hisense CAS can also build a 3D model, which can be rotated, scaled, and combined in any way to clearly show the size and shape of the tumor and the anatomical relationships and invasion situation between the tumor and the organs and blood vessels, especially the shape of the vasculature, thus reducing the subjective error of reading the original CT images to assess the size and degree of tumor invasion and making the preoperative assessment more realistic and reliable.

Pediatric RTs are mostly neuroblastic tumors, including neuroblastoma (NB) and ganglioneuroblastoma (GNB), which are malignant tumors, and ganglioneuroma (GN), which is a benign tumor. All three types originate from primitive neural crest cells in the neuroectoderm but are difficult to distinguish and can be mutually transformed [22]. NB is one of the most common malignant solid tumors in children and has no specific symptoms or signs. Its CT manifestations are as follows: mostly lobulated; poorly defined; often with coarse, patchy calcifications within the tumor; infiltrative growth across the midline; and high rate of involvement of the surrounding vital tissues and organs. Pediatric RTs are often found in stages III and IV and enveloping and infiltrating large retroperitoneal vessels, and up to 45% of abdominal neuroblastomas have invasion into the renal pedicle. Often the preoperative differential diagnosis between pediatric RTs and nephroblastoma becomes difficult due to excessive invasion of the kidney. This makes it difficult to resect NB. Despite chemotherapy, there are still quite a number of cases with only biopsy or partial resection, and radical surgery without a tumor at the surgical margin under the microscope is actually impossible. However, complete surgical resection of NB is the basis for further treatment, improves the confidence of both physicians and patients in treatment, and is associated with prognosis [23]. Hisense CAS assists in the anatomical analysis of important retroperitoneal vessels to improve surgical resectability and reduce the incidence of surgical complications such as vascular injury and kidney damage.

GN is generally insensitive to chemotherapy, and radical surgical resection is the first choice to confirm the diagnosis and cure. The CT manifestations are often a well-defined, regular-shaped mass, with mostly speckled calcifications in the tumor. The tumor mainly pushes and compresses the surrounding vessels and can grow along the peri-organ space and encircle the blood vessels. Despite the vessels being encircled, the vessels are generally not invaded, and the shape of the vasculature is natural and straight, with few occlusions or stenoses. To avoid sampling errors in aspiration biopsy, to relieve the symptoms of tumor compression already present, and to reduce the possibility of malignant transformation, surgical resection of suspected GN or GNB can be performed. In giant GN/GNB of retroperitoneal origin, the base of the tumor is often the mesenteric root, and involvement of the abdominal aorta, inferior vena cava, and mesenteric arteries is often the main reason for complete resection of the tumor [24]. Hisense CAS aids in the complete resection of the tumor to reduce recurrence and protects important vessels to avoid complications such as bleeding, intestinal obstruction, and intestinal necrosis.

Figure 5 shows a typical case of a 4-year-old child with an RT. Enhanced CT of the abdomen showed a huge mass-like mixed-density lesion in the abdominal cavity with a maximum cross-section of approximately 123 mm × 85 mm. The radiologists considered the mass to be a tumor (NB?), and there was a very thick blood vessel inside the tumor (**Figure 5A–C**). To clarify the diagnosis and decide on the next treatment, ultrasound-guided abdominal mass aspiration biopsy was performed. The pathologists first considered the mass to be a GN. Thus, surgical resection was the best option for this type of benign tumor. For precise preoperative evaluation, 3D reconstruction was performed using CAS. The reconstructed image clearly showed that the tumor was located in the retroperitoneum, and the mass had a volume of 676.7 ml. The mass was extremely close to the abdominal aorta. The superior mesenteric vein was pushed forwards, and the inferior mesenteric artery passed through the tumor (**Figure 5D–F**). The intraoperative exploration was completely consistent with the preoperative three-dimensional evaluation, and the tumor had a relatively complete fibrous capsule. The superior mesenteric vein was pushed to the front of the tumor. The tumor was close to the abdominal aorta, and the inferior mesenteric artery penetrated the tumor. After splitting the tumor with a CUSA knife, the inferior mesenteric artery that was encased by the tumor could be seen. Arterial pulsation was seen in the exposed inferior mesenteric artery, and the distal sigmoid colon and rectum were ruddy. The tumor section was yellowish-white with a straight and intact vascular sheath, and the postoperative tumor weight was 820 g (**Figure 5G–L**). The tumor was finally diagnosed as a GNB.

4.3 Pediatric mediastinal tumor

Most mediastinal tumors have an insidious onset and lack specific clinical manifestations, and most of them have no clinical symptoms in the early stage. However, because there are many important organs and structures in the mediastinum, such as the heart, superior vena cava, trachea, and esophagus, the thorax, which has a bony structure, is not as elastic as the abdomen. Because they have less space for

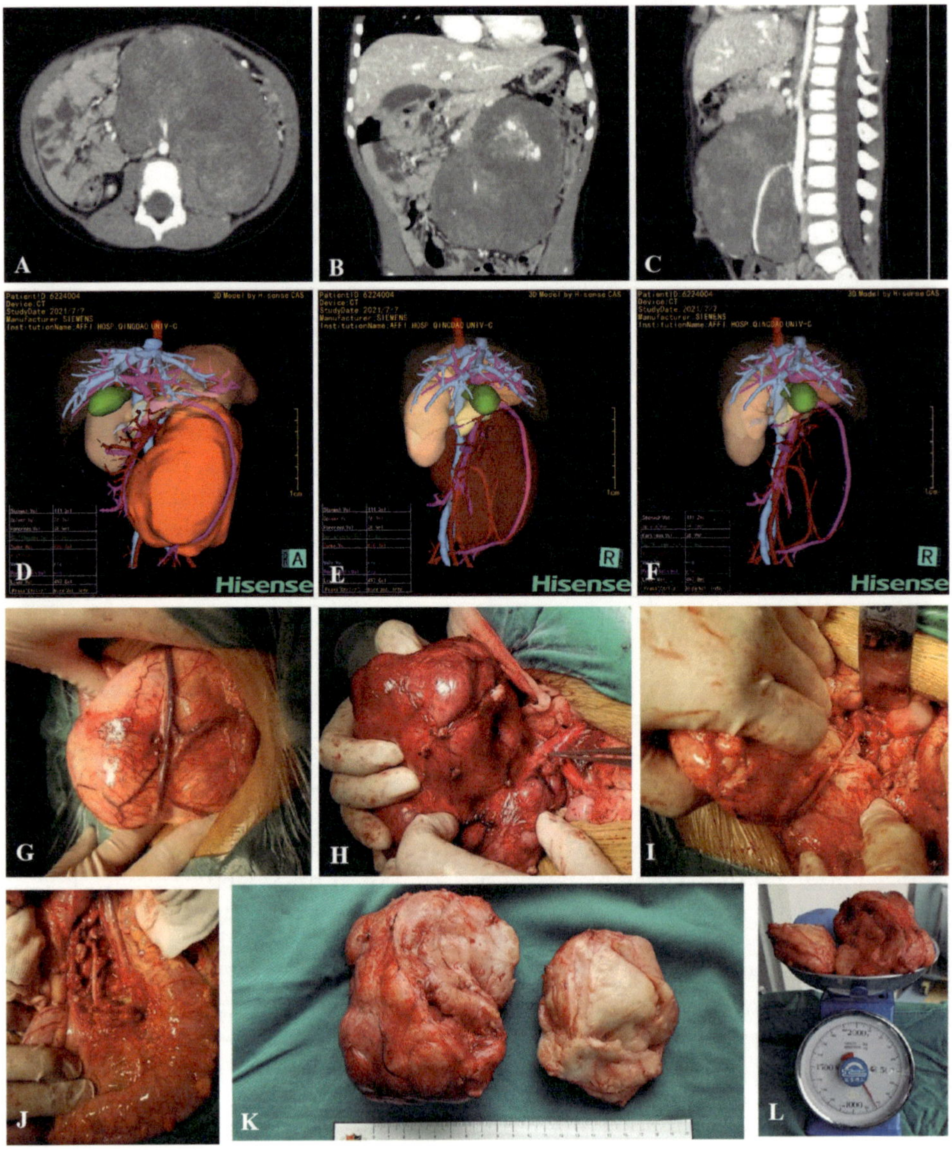

Figure 5.
Computer-assisted resection of retroperitoneal tumor (With the permission of the author).

cushioning, mediastinal masses are prone to compressing important organs and the corresponding symptoms, namely, mediastinal mass syndrome (MMS) [25]. Compared with that in adults, the thoracic cavity in children is relatively smaller in size, and therefore, its complex anatomic-spatial relationships and dense vascular-neural structures have brought more challenges for surgical treatment [26].

Mediastinal tissues are of complex origin, and a variety of benign or malignant primary tumors can occur. Neuroblastic tumors are the most common mediastinal tumors in children. In principle, once a mediastinal mass is found, it should be actively treated. Tumors with clear borders and small volumes can be considered for radical surgery. For malignant tumors with high surgical risk, biopsy should be considered, followed by a combination of chemotherapy, surgery, radiotherapy, and immunotherapy. The difficulty of surgery lies in separating the tumor from the arteries, thoracic vertebrae, chest wall, and lung lobes. In children, the mediastinum is small, and the tissues are delicate. Thus, it is easy to inadvertently damage blood vessels and nerves during surgery, resulting in massive hemorrhage or vascular injury or even death. Therefore, accurate preoperative positioning is particularly important [27]. In addition, it has been reported that the blood vessels supplying mediastinal tumors are highly variable and may come from intercostal arteries, coronary arteries, the thyroglossal trunk, internal thoracic arteries, bronchial arteries, etc. Mediastinal tumors usually have an abundant blood supply from multiple arteries, and surgical resection may lead to severe blood loss.

Compared with 2D CT images, 3D reconstructed images can better visualize the adjacent relationships of important mediastinal tissues, whether the tumor invades the blood vessels, and the variations of the blood vessels so that surgeons can clarify the anatomical relationships. Hisense CAS aids in the precise localization of mediastinal tumors and the accurate assessment of important and variant vessels to reduce damage to vital organs and vessels [6, 17].

Figure 6 shows a three-year-old girl with a mediastinal tumor. Enhanced CT of the thorax suggested that the tumor was located in the left posterior part

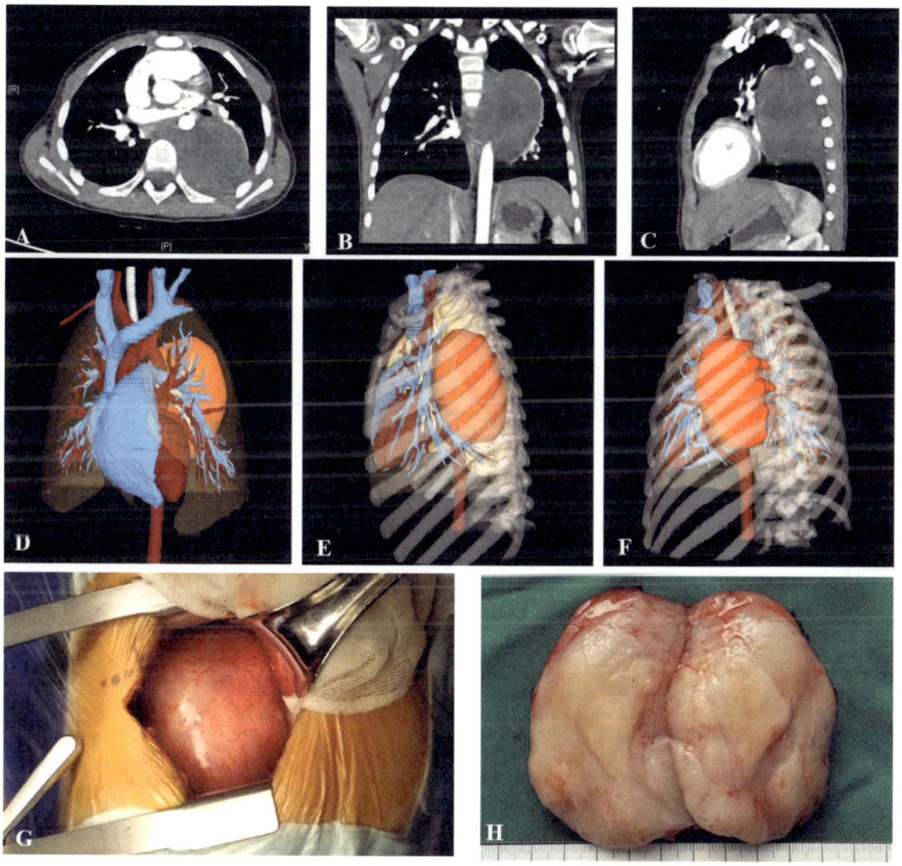

Figure 6.
Computer-assisted resection of mediastinal tumor.

of the heart and T4-T9 left the paravertebral region, measuring approximately 61.15 mm × 42.00 mm. The tumor pushed the adjacent lung tissue, and part of the tumor extended to the spinal canal (**Figure 6A–C**). 3D reconstruction suggested that the tumor originated from the posterior mediastinum and was closely adhered to the thoracic aorta and thoracic vertebra. The three supply vessels of the tumor came from the branches of the thoracic aorta, and part of the tumor protruded into the intervertebral foramen (**Figure 6D–F**). Intraoperatively, the anatomical relationship of the tumor was approximately the same as the preoperative three-dimensional reconstruction results. The tumor was very densely adherent to the thoracic vertebrae and rib space, and part of the periosteum and rib space were excised to gradually remove the tumor completely (**Figure 6G** and **H**). The postoperative pathological diagnosis was a GNB.

In summary, artificial intelligence technology has made significant breakthroughs and clinical applications in the field of precision surgery. Computer-assisted medical technology combines the interdisciplinary disciplines of imaging, medical image processing, and computer science, focusing on the development of assisted clinical treatment and surgical planning and simulation systems, and has become a frontier in the development of modern medical technology. Computer-assisted pediatric precise surgery improves tumor resection rates and surgical safety in a comprehensive and objective manner using artificial intelligence. In the future, individualized 3D-based precision surgery may be a new direction for surgical research.

Author details

Wenli Xiu[1,2], Xiwei Hao[1], Nan Xia[2], Yongjian Chen[2], Haitao Niu[2,3] and Qian Dong[2]*

1 Department of Pediatric Surgery, The Affiliated Hospital of Qingdao University, Qingdao, China

2 Shandong Provincial Key Laboratory of Digital Medicine and Computer-Assisted Surgery, Shandong College Collaborative Innovation Center of Digital Medicine Clinical Treatment and Nutrition Health, Qingdao University, Qingdao, China

3 Department of Urology, The Affiliated Hospital of Qingdao University, Qingdao, China

*Address all correspondence to: 13608968352@163.com

References

[1] Steliarova-Foucher E, MM F, Colombet M, et al. Changing geographical patterns and trends in cancer incidence in children and adolescents in Europe, 1991-2010 (Automated Childhood Cancer Information System): A population-based study. The Lancet Oncology. 2018;**19**(9):1159-1169

[2] Ni X, Li Z, Li X, et al. Socioeconomic inequalities in cancer incidence and access to health services among children and adolescents in China: A cross-sectional study. Lancet. 2022;**400**(10357):1020-1032

[3] Fuchs J. The role of minimally invasive surgery in pediatric solid tumors. Pediatric Surgery International. 2015;**31**(3):213-228

[4] Kenngott HG, Wagner M, Nickel F, et al. Computer-assisted abdominal surgery: New technologies. Langenbeck's Archives of Surgery. 2015;**400**(3):273-281

[5] Su L, Zhou XJ, Dong Q, et al. Application value of computer assisted surgery system in precision surgeries for pediatric complex liver tumors. International Journal of Clinical and Experimental Medicine. 2015;**8**(10):18406-18412

[6] Liu Y, Xia N, Duan Y, et al. Application of computer-assisted surgery in pediatric mediastinal tumor surgery. International Journal of Medical Robotics. 2022;**2022**:e2489

[7] Fang C, An J, Bruno A, et al. Consensus recommendations of three-dimensional visualization for diagnosis and management of liver diseases. Hepatology International. 2020;**14**(4):437-453

[8] Liu J, Xiu W, Duan G, et al. Application of 3D simulation software in chemotherapy and hepatoblastoma surgery in children. Frontier in Surgery. 2022;**9**:908381

[9] Xiu W, Liu J, Li T, et al. Application value of computer-assisted surgery system in pediatric hepatic hemangioma. Pediatric Surgery International. 2021;**37**(11):1575-1583

[10] Zhu CZ, Dong BZ, Dong Q. Imaging evaluation of liver tumors in pediatric patients. Liver Research and Clinical Management. 2018:57-72

[11] Yang X, Wang H, Dong B, et al. Standard liver volume-predicting formulae derived from Normal liver volume in children under 18 years of age. Frontiers in Pediatrics. 2021;**9**:629645

[12] Katzenstein HM, Langham MR, Malogolowkin MH, et al. Minimal adjuvant chemotherapy for children with hepatoblastoma resected at diagnosis (AHEP0731): A Children's Oncology Group, multicentre, phase 3 trial. The Lancet Oncology. 2019;**20**(5):719-727

[13] Meyers RL, Maibach R, Hiyama E, et al. Risk-stratified staging in paediatric hepatoblastoma: A unified analysis from the Children's Hepatic tumors International Collaboration. The Lancet Oncology. 2017;**18**(1):122-131

[14] Ziogas IA, Benedetti DJ, Wu WK, et al. Management of hepatoblastoma in the United States: Can we do better? Surgery. 2021;**170**(2):579-586

[15] Towbin AJ, Meyers RL, Woodley H, et al. 2017 PRETEXT: Radiologic staging system for primary hepatic malignancies of childhood revised for the Paediatric Hepatic International Tumour Trial

(PHITT). Pediatric Radiology. 2018;**48**(4):536-554

[16] Fuchs J, Cavdar S, Blumenstock G, Ebinger M, Schäfer JF, Sipos B, et al. POST-TEXT III and IV Hepatoblastoma: Extended hepatic resection avoids liver transplantation in selected cases. Annals of Surgery. 2017;**266**(2):318-323

[17] Lamadé W, Glombitza G, Fischer L, Chiu P, Cárdenas CE Sr, Thorn M, et al. The impact of 3-dimensional reconstructions on operation planning in liver surgery. Archives of Surgery. 2000;**135**(11):1256-1261

[18] Serio G, Tenchini P, Nifosi F, et al. Surgical strategy in primary retroperitoneal tumours. The British Journal of Surgery. 1989;**76**(4):385-389

[19] Pierie JP, Betensky RA, Choudry U, et al. Outcomes in a series of 103 retroperitoneal sarcomas. European Journal of Surgical Oncology. 2006;**32**(10):1235-1241

[20] An JY, Heo JS, Noh JH, et al. Primary malignant retroperitoneal tumors: Analysis of a single institutional experience. European Journal of Surgical Oncology. 2007;**33**(3):376-382

[21] Neville A. Herts B.CT characteristics of primary retroperitoneal neoplasms. Critical Reviews in Computed Tomography. 2004;**45**(4):247-270

[22] Cohn SL, Pearson ADJ, London WB, et al. The international Neuroblastoma Risk Group (INRG) classification system: An INRG Task Force report. Journal of Clinical Oncology. 2009;**27**(2):289-297

[23] la Quaglia MP. Surgical management of neuroblastoma. Seminars in Pediatric Surgery. 2001;**10**(3):132-139

[24] Alexander N, Sullivan K, Shaikh F, et al. Characteristics and management of ganglioneuroma and ganglioneuroblastoma-intermixed in children and adolescents. Pediatric Blood & Cancer. 2018;**65**:e26964

[25] Shi X, Liu X, Dong X, et al. Trends, symptoms, and outcomes of resec-table giant mediastinal tumors. Frontiers in Oncology. 2022;**12**:820720

[26] Chen CH, Wu KH, Chao YH, Weng DF, Chang JS, Lin CH. Clinical manifestation of pediatric mediastinal tumors, a single center experience. Medicine (Baltim). 2019;**98**(32):e16732

[27] Liu FY, Wang MQ, Duan F, et al. Combined embolization and surgical resection of a giant mediastinal tumor. The Thoracic and Cardiovascular Surgeon. 2014;**62**(3):265-269

Chapter 8

Application and Prospect of Telesurgery: The Role of Artificial Intelligence

Haitao Niu

Abstract

Remote surgery refers to a new surgical mode in which doctors operate on patients with the help of surgical robots, network technology, and virtual reality technology. These robots are located far away from patients. The remote surgical robot system integrates key technologies such as robot, communication technology, remote control technology, space mapping algorithm, and fault tolerance analysis. Apply a variety of emerging networking modes such as 5G, optical fiber private network, fusion network technology, and deterministic network to realize the motion of the subordinate surgical robot and the vision of the main knife, and ensure stable signal transmission and safe remote operation. The development and application of remote surgical robots has become a new trend, which helps to break the barriers of unbalanced regional medical resource allocation, promote the rational allocation of high-quality medical resources, and solve the telemedicine problems in special areas and special circumstances. The development prospect is broad. In the future, relying on the 5G network technology with high speed, low power consumption, and low latency, remote surgery can operate more efficiently and stably, and the surgical robot will also develop toward a more portable and flexible direction, so as to better serve patients.

Keywords: telesurgery, artificial intelligence, 5G network, master/slave signal communication, network delay, outlook

1. Introduction

Telesurgery is an emerging model in which the physician and the patient are located in geographically distant locations and the physician performs surgery on the patient with the help of surgical robotics, network technology, and virtual reality. The idea of telesurgery was first proposed during wartime, with the aim of providing fast, high-quality surgical treatment to forward hospital trauma patients. However, the progress of related research was slow due to the limited level of robotics, network, and other technologies at that time. The uneven distribution of modern medical resources and the limited distribution of resources in special areas have led to many patients losing the best surgical opportunities, and the demand for telesurgery has increased in modern society. With the development of telecommunication technology and surgical robotics, the idea of telesurgery has gradually become a reality and has already benefited some patients. Artificial intelligence is a new technical science that delves into the development of theories, methods, core technologies, application software, and control systems for simulating the extension and expansion of the intelligence of the human brain. Its areas include robotics, image recognition, and expert systems. AI has important applications in many medical disciplines.

1.1 Method

We searched for literature on PubMed and the Internet using keywords such as "remote surgery," "artificial intelligence," "digital twin technology," "quantum communication," and "5G network," and summarized the retrieved literature.

2. History and current status of telesurgery development

2.1 History of the development of telesurgery abroad

As a country with advanced medical care, the United States has conducted early research in the field of telemedicine, and basic research such as teleconsultation in multiple hospitals and televideo medical education has been conducted before entering into formal research on telesurgery. Since the 1990s, telemedicine for surgical procedures has developed rapidly, and a large number of research results have been reported. The first real-time teleconsultation for telesurgery was reported in 1992 in which a standard telephone network was used to transfer pathology slides between surgical procedures and to give real-time pathology diagnosis by a remote pathologist, but only 37% of the 35 cases received diagnostic help due to the limited network technology and medical level at that time [1]. In the same year, Satava et al. used the SRI remote operating system to directly control the movement of the mechanical needle tip to perform part of the operation and developed the famous da Vinci robot based on this operating system [2], which was the beginning of telesurgical robotics and the turning point of telesurgery.

In the 1990s, based on the continuous exploration of telesurgery, some foreign countries have mastered the key of technology in telesurgery, from the initial remote simple operation to the basic formation of telesurgery system, and began to try the real meaning of independent telesurgery. In 2001, the first real telesurgery was completed, namely the famous "Charles Lindbergh surgery" [3]. The patient was a 68-year-old woman with gallbladder stones in Strasbourg, France, and the surgeon was operating 7000 km away in New York, USA. A special dedicated network was applied to transfer signals between the surgeries, and the data transmission was stable during the surgery, with smooth transmission of operational and imaging signals and low network latency maintained. This is a milestone in telesurgery, and it validates the feasibility of telesurgery technology.

2.2 History of telesurgery development in China

Medical resources in China are unevenly distributed. Highly qualified surgeons and advanced medical equipment are basically distributed in large- and medium-sized cities, while rural and remote areas are significantly lagging behind, and there are obvious geographical differences. Many patients in need of surgery are unable to receive timely and high-quality surgical treatment, which seriously threatens their lives and health safety. Therefore, there is a need for the development of telesurgery in China. Although the research on telesurgery in China started late, it is developing rapidly.

In the early twenty first century, the Naval General Hospital used a remote surgical robot system to perform stereotactic biopsy surgery for brain tumor patients, completing the first off-site brain surgery in China. Beijing Jishuitan Hospital applied the master-slave robotic surgery system to perform remote orthopedic assisted surgery operations. Although the two surgeries were completed successfully, the telesurgery system in the study only played the role of auxiliary positioning and image transmission.

The application of 4G network communication has promoted the development of telesurgery in China, and its network stability is better than that of satellite communication. In 2015, the domestic "Myriad S" surgical robot completed remote wireless animal experiments at an interval of about 170 km with the help of 10 Mb/s bandwidth commercial network. Although the whole experiment was relatively successful, the narrow bandwidth and high latency of the 4G network still limit the extension of the clinical application of telesurgery.

2.3 The status of telesurgery abroad

In 2003, Anvari M's team set up a telesurgery system between a teaching hospital and a rural hospital 400 km apart in Hamilton. This study led to the completion of 21 telesurgeries in 2005, successfully establishing the world's first tele-robotic system to serve rural communities.

In 2014, a study by Xu et al. showed that a time delay below 200 ms is ideal for remote surgery, but up to 300 ms does not affect the successful completion of the procedure. A higher network latency would affect the safety and accuracy of the procedure, or even make it impossible for the operator to perform the operation. This conclusion has also been used as a criterion for network selection in many domestic and international remote studies [4].

Since the beginning of 2019, many foreign studies have started to use 5G networks for remote surgery. And satisfactory surgical results have been obtained. Lacy's team applies 5G network to remote surgical coaching of young physicians in off-site locations [5]. In February 2019, a Spanish medical team used 5G network to remotely perform an intestinal tumor resection. This is the world's first human remote surgery done using 5G network.

2.4 The current status of telesurgery in China

The commercialization of 5G network is a sign that China's telesurgery has entered modernization, and its low latency, high bandwidth, and high mobility meet the demand for real time, high efficiency and stability of remote surgery, advancing the research boom of domestic telesurgery. In December 2018, the People's Liberation Army General Hospital applied a domestic self-developed surgical robot to successfully complete 5G telesurgery animal experiments in Fuzhou. The physician remotely controlled the robotic arm and the lens arm to remove part of the pig liver, and the intraoperative high-definition 3D image and sound transmission were in real time and stable. The robotic arm operated flexibly with good master-slave consistency, and the one-way average time delay between the two ends was less than 150 ms. In September 2019, the National Institute of Hepatobiliary Surgery completed the world's first multi-point collaborative 5G remote multidisciplinary animal experiment with stable network latency, smooth surgical operation, and stable intraoperative animal vital signs. The surgical experiment allowed two physicians located in Beijing and Suzhou to perform gastrointestinal resection and liver resection on the experimental animals through remote control of the robotic arm. This experiment broke the traditional mode of single-point consultation and surgery between doctors and patients, and provided patients with multidisciplinary remote consultation and treatment options, realizing multidisciplinary cooperation in telesurgery.

Chinese telesurgery is developing rapidly with the help of 5G networks. And it has transformed from a single-center, few-sample exploration model to a multi-center, large-sample clinical research model. Since September 2020, Prof. Niu Haitao's team at the Affiliated Hospital of Qingdao University has conducted a large sample, multicenter remote robot-assisted urological surgery study based on animal experiments and simulated time-delay experiments. More than 50 cases of telesurgery have been completed, further confirming the safety and feasibility of telesurgery [6].

In February 2023, Prof. Niu Haitao's team completed the first case of quantum telesurgery in China. The implementation of telesurgery with the help of quantum communication technology means that the development of telesurgery has entered a brand new stage, which greatly expands the spatial scope for physicians to perform complex surgeries and creates more convenient conditions for people in remote areas to enjoy high-quality medical services.

In order to ensure the high requirements of network for telesurgery, more and more new network technologies are applied to the network line. The multi-link aggregation transmission technology is a more mature and widely used network technology in telesurgery. Multi-link aggregation technology ensures data transmission capability for remote surgery. It adds a virtual layer on top of the traditional link layer, which implements the distribution of data frames that are distributed to each link through a rotation algorithm, successfully aggregating the transmission bandwidth of multiple physical links, thus achieving the effect of high-speed transmission with bandwidth overlay on the same terminal. Multi-link transmission and single-link transmission can coexist, and either multi-link transmission or single-link transmission can be selected according to the actual needs of the application. As an auxiliary technology of the networking scheme, it can guarantee the future development of telesurgery after the 5G network mode is popularized and has great development potential.

3. Application of digital twin technology based on artificial intelligence in remote surgery

The application of artificial intelligence in remote surgery is a new emerging technology, also known as remote intelligent surgery or robot-assisted remote surgery. Its core is to combine robotic surgery systems with Internet technology, allowing surgeons to perform surgery remotely *via* the network. This technology can help patients in areas with limited medical resources to receive better medical services.

In this technology, artificial intelligence can identify human tissues and organs during surgery and provide accurate location and size information through deep learning and image recognition technology. In addition, based on patient medical data and surgical history, artificial intelligence can provide personalized surgical plans and treatment recommendations to surgeons. Moreover, artificial intelligence can also perform automatic control and adjustment during surgery to ensure accuracy and safety. Combining digital twin technology derived from artificial intelligence with remote surgery greatly enhances the safety of the surgical process.

Digital twin is a digital representation of real-world entities or systems, creating virtual models of physical entities in a digital way that can describe the process of "symbiosis" between physical objects and their dynamic processes throughout their lifecycle. By simulating the behavior of physical entities in a real environment with interactive feedback between virtual and real worlds, data fusion analysis, and iterative decision optimization, and digital twin can add or expand new capabilities to physical entities and serve as a bridge and link between the physical and digital worlds. Currently, the concept and technology of robotic digital twin are also entering the medical and health fields from the industrial sector. The potential applications of digital twin include patient health monitoring, personalized medication, medical equipment, hospital operation management, etc. These characteristics are expected to play an important role in overcoming the limitations of remote surgery technology and expanding its application scenarios.

3.1 Establishment of artificial intelligence digital twin models in remote robot-assisted surgery interactive processes

In remote robot-assisted surgery, stereoscopic image processing and remote transmission are the main factors causing delays, making it difficult for doctors to obtain real-time information about the current movement of instruments within the body cavity. Therefore, using artificial intelligence technology, real-time monitoring of the surgical process can be achieved through 3D images and laser scanning, helping doctors to more accurately locate and handle problems during surgery. Artificial intelligence can also apply digital twin technology to the surgical process and perform twinning of the expected movements of instruments in real time at the doctor's end. By establishing a digital representation of the entity model's geometric dimensions, physical relationships, and motion behaviors in multiple dimensions and expressing the entity's characteristics using mesh simplification and entity rendering methods, a twinning model of instrument movement can be constructed. This twinning surgical instrument can interact with the main operating hand operated by the doctor in real time to reflect the ideal posture of the instrument under the current instructions of the doctor.

3.2 Dynamic fusion of digital twin model and real surgical scene

The interactive process observed by doctors during remote surgery is a delayed scene, while the digital twin environment can accurately reflect the real-time position and posture of surgical instruments being operated by the doctor. By integrating these two, comprehensive remote operation information can be provided to ensure operational safety and avoid damage to intra-abdominal organs. Since both are time-varying scenes, a virtual scene perspective coordinate system is first constructed based on the endoscopic camera coordinate system. Then, artificial intelligence techniques such as deep learning and image morphology are used to accurately segment the real instrument pole, determine the control points and the scaling relationship between the twin and real scenes, and reverse correct the coordinate system deviation introduced by the camera and disparity. Based on the control point registration, virtual and real image fusion is achieved to accurately present the twin instrument model under the real endoscopic image.

3.3 Representation of motion correlation between real surgical instruments and their digital twin models

The motion of the digital twin surgical instrument and the real surgical instrument is homologous but not synchronous, and the motion deviation of the two needs to be extracted to ensure remote operation safety. In the abovementioned fused environment of real and twin scenes, intelligent algorithms are used to establish the expression of the twin and real instruments in the image coordinate system based on the principle of projective geometry, and the spatial deviation between them is described by pixel difference. Based on this, the transparency of the twin instrument is controlled by the deviation, with smaller deviations resulting in greater transparency and larger deviations resulting in greater visibility. Without interfering with the doctor, the delay of the remote instrument is visually displayed to the doctor.

3.4 Virtual fixture and safety force feedback strategy for virtual-real fusion

A virtual fixture is constructed by introducing a gravitational potential field, with the reference point of the real instrument's end point in the image as the zero point of the potential energy, and the distance between this reference point and the twin instrument's end point used to represent the potential energy size. Dead zone and extreme value processing are performed on this potential energy to ensure model stability. Based on this, the potential energy generated by the virtual-real fusion is fed back to the primary operator as impedance force within the extreme value range. When the twin model's potential energy reaches the safety threshold, the system automatically generates feedback force to resist the driving force of the primary hand and waits for delayed motion to follow. If the feedback exceeds the limit value, the master-slave operation pause command is executed, and the remote robot motion is stopped within one network transmission and robot execution cycle (less than 40 ms).

Remote surgical operation delay is currently a critical factor affecting the success of remote surgeries and patient safety. To address the core challenge of operation delay in robot-assisted remote surgeries, remote surgeons combine artificial intelligence and digital twin technology. The AI system analyzes and deeply learns the basic principles of expressing delay based on the remote surgeon's ideal operation behavior in virtual space and the observed real operation behavior. It achieves quantitative expression in both visual and tactile dimensions, making delay a visible and tangible physical quantity. Based on this, the surgeon's operation process is intervened to provide safe and reliable guarantees for remote operations.

4. Remote surgical robot equipment and technology

4.1 Remote surgical robot system architecture

Remote surgical robot is a complex of multidisciplinary and high-tech means. It is composed of two parts: the doctor's operation end and the operation end. It has two modes of traditional local surgical function and remote surgical function. The emergence of remote surgical robot is of great significance. It is completely different from the traditional surgical concept. Through the remote surgical robot system, surgeons can carry out surgical treatment for patients in different geographical locations [7, 8]. This is another milestone in the history of surgical development.

The remote surgical robot control system consists of five parts: the doctor console, the master communication control box, the patient console, the slave communication control box, and the three-dimensional endoscope camera system.

4.1.1 Doctor console

The doctor console is the control center of the surgical robot system and the interactive platform of the system at the doctor's end. The surgeon controls the surgical instruments and three-dimensional laparoscopy by operating the two mechanical arms on the doctor's console. The motion scaling function is added to the remote surgery robot system, which maps the motion of the doctor's mechanical arm to the motion of the patient's mechanical arm after reducing it to a certain proportion, minimizing the unconscious motion of the doctor's hand, and improving the operation quality of the remote surgery.

In addition, the doctor console in the remote surgical robot system also includes the main communication control box, which is composed of industrial computer, display, controller, image processor, keyboard, etc. At the main operation end of remote surgery, the communication control box at the main end is connected with the doctor's console. At the same time, all signals are collected and transmitted to the remote patient end, and the transmission signals and three-dimensional images from the remote patient end are received to the doctor's console.

4.1.2 Patient console

The patient console is the executive part of the remote surgical robot system to implement minimally invasive surgery. Its main structure is to provide support for two patient manipulators and one image arm. In the process of remote surgery, the surgical assistant is also required to work next to the patient operating table in the sterile area, responsible for replacing the surgical instruments and three-dimensional laparoscopy, and assisting the chief surgeon to complete the operation. The operation of the remote surgical robot system must always be under the absolute control of the chief surgeon or surgical assistant and meet a certain priority relationship, that is, the surgical assistant next to the patient's console has the highest priority, and they can adjust the robot's motion at any time according to the actual situation of the operation.

Similarly, the patient console also includes the slave communication control box, which is composed of industrial computer, display, image processor, keyboard, etc. At the slave operation end of remote surgery, the slave communication control box is connected with the patient console for use, receives all signals from the remote master operation end, and simultaneously sends all signals and three-dimensional images to the remote master operation end.

4.1.3 3D endoscope camera system

The three-dimensional endoscope camera system collects the three-dimensional images in the body cavity area and then presents the image data on the three-dimensional display. During the operation, it is located outside the sterile area and can be operated by itinerant nurses, and various auxiliary surgical equipment can be placed. Three-dimensional laparoscopy is a high-resolution optical three-dimensional lens, which can magnify the surgical field by more than 10 times, and can obtain three-dimensional high-definition images of the surgical field, so that the surgeon can get a clearer understanding of the structure, reduce visual fatigue, and improve the accuracy of surgery.

4.1.4 Other equipment

The doctor's console, patient's console, and 3D endoscope camera system all need separate power supply. There is a backup battery on the patient console. In order to prevent emergencies, always connect the power supply to ensure that the backup battery is in full charge.

In the process of remote surgery, the patient's slave operation terminal and the doctor's console at the master operation terminal are connected through 5G network. The rest of the equipment is connected through the control signal line. Each time the remote surgery is performed, the labels at both ends of each cable need to be confirmed to ensure that the connection is correct.

4.2 Core technology and security processing mechanism of remote surgical robot

4.2.1 System architecture

The key to implement remote surgery is the development of remote surgery robot system. Traditional commercial surgical robots are mainly used in the same physical space. To build a remote surgical robot system, the key is to add a reliable remote communication system. Among them, the remote robot system includes the patient console, the doctor console, the attached endoscope system, and the surgical instrument unit. The remote communication system mainly provides a network channel for the transmission of multimodal signals at the master and slave ends of the robot.

4.2.2 Remote signal transmission mechanism

In order to ensure the smooth operation of remote surgery, doctors not only need to control the robotic arm at the patient end to perform surgery, but also need to constantly confirm the feedback information at the patient end. Therefore, the transmission of remote signals needs to have a high real-time two-way transmission mechanism. At present, the transmission hardware of the remote communication system is mainly based on the upper computer, and most of the transmission mechanisms adopt the robot control information transmission protocol based on UDP [9]. However, due to the low transmission reliability of UDP transmission protocol, developing a real-time and reliable transmission mechanism is one of the important research directions for the future development of remote surgical robots.

4.2.3 Video compression processing mechanism

The doctors of remote robot surgery can obtain a wider and clearer operation field through 3D laparoscopy, and how to obtain a high-resolution 3D laparoscopy image is one of the key technologies of robot remote surgery. Because the laparoscopic image is a 3D high-definition image, which requires high bandwidth and network real-time, an external high-speed data acquisition card needs to be used at the patient end for image acquisition and 3D compression processing, which can effectively reduce the image transmission time and delay. In order to ensure the continuity of the intraoperative image and add the breakpoint continuation function, the image can be continued from the breakpoint when the image is disconnected. With the development of the fifth generation mobile communication technology, 3D high-definition laparoscopic image transmission is expected to be further improved. The emergence of 5G network technology is particularly important for the development of 3D laparoscopic high-definition images in remote surgery.

4.2.4 Remote master-slave security processing mechanism

In the robot remote surgery, doctors and patients are in different physical environments. The security processing mechanism of the doctor's console and the patient's console of the remote surgery robot is mainly controlled by the communication transmission. In case of an unexpected communication situation, such as continuous packet loss on the network, the remote control boxes at both ends will immediately stop two-way signal transmission. The holding brake at all joints at both ends of the doctor's console and the patient's console of the surgical robot will be activated immediately to stop all movements of the robot. At the same time, an alarm signal will be sent, and the robot will enter the standby state, thus ensuring the safety of remote surgery. It is particularly important to ensure the safety and operability of remote surgery by ensuring the master-slave security processing mechanism between "doctors and patients."

5. Basic principle and configuration conditions of the master and slave end of the remote surgical robot

The remote surgical robot system integrates key technologies such as robot technology, communication technology, remote control technology, space mapping algorithm, and fault tolerance analysis. The intraoperative endoscope image is compressed by the image encoder and then transmitted to the decoder at the main hand end through the network for decoding. Then, the doctor can observe the transmitted surgical image through the display, so as to operate the main hand; the signals of each joint sensor in the master hand are collected and processed in real time and then output. The data packets are encapsulated by the master communication controller and sent to the slave hand *via* the dedicated Internet. The received data packets are verified and filtered by the slave controller at the hand end and sent to the robot motion controller. The motion controller performs motion calculation, and finally inputs the data information to the drivers of each motor, then controls the manipulator to complete the operation of the main end physician.

5.1 Master and slave control communication method for remote surgery

The Internet is the basis of communication. It has not only complex physical circuits, but also complex protocol families, verification mechanisms and network security mechanisms. The network delay mainly depends on the transmission distance and the physical link through which data transmission passes, including the number of routers and the processing time of routers. The transmission routes and routing routes of fixed transmission nodes are usually fixed. However, due to the sharing and competition of the network, the processing time and processing tasks of the router are changing, and the processing time of data packets on the router at different times is also changing. Therefore, data packet disorder, delay, and other problems will occur. Therefore, in order to meet the stringent requirements of surgical operation, it is necessary to use a dedicated network and solve the problem of data transmission fluctuations through delay compensation and filtering.

5.1.1 Network control model

The network control system is generally divided into two structures, direct control and indirect control. The main difference between them is the signal transmission mode. Both the direct control signal and the sensor signal are transmitted through the network, and there is no restriction on the transmission network. The network that transmits the two signal flows can be independent of each other. The remote end of the indirect control structure is an independent closed-loop control system. The actuator signal collected by the sensor is directly fed back to the control system at the remote end and no longer fed back to the main controller to reduce the impact of the network on signal transmission.

5.1.2 Construction and implementation of control system

There are many ways of data communication, including wireless or wired Internet, optical fiber, 5G communication, etc. Each communication method contains a variety of different communication protocols. The remote control system uses socket to complete the communication protocol. The transport layer is implemented based on TCP protocol. When packet loss occurs in network congestion, we directly receive the next group of data packets to ensure the reliability of remote control.

5.1.3 Quantitative analysis of control model

In order to meet the requirements of remote surgery, it is necessary to test and verify the proposed method. In order to quantitatively analyze the practicability of predictive filtering algorithm, we build a remote operation simulation platform and randomly introduce 10-30 ms delay into the master-slave tracking system. The master-slave tracking test is carried out in combination with the motion frequency of the human hand, and good prediction results are finally obtained [10].

5.2 Remote surgery stereo image transmission method

5.2.1 Video encoding method

Unlike local surgical robots, remote surgery requires the transmission of endoscopic high-definition images through the Internet. Under certain network bandwidth conditions, in order to ensure the real time of image transmission, image compression means are needed to reduce the amount of data transmitted, and image compression and decompression processing will introduce new delays. Common video coding modes include H.264/MPEG-AVC coding, H.265/MPEG-HEVC coding, etc [11].

Compared with H.264, in order to improve the compression and coding efficiency of high-definition video, H.265 adopts the ultra-large quadtree coding architecture, and uses three basic units, namely, coding unit (CU), prediction unit (PU), and transformation unit (TU), to implement the whole coding process, which improves the coding efficiency and effectively reduces the decoding time [12].

5.2.2 Stereo image transmission mode

Three-dimensional stereo images are composed of two cameras taking pictures of objects from different angles of view, and then interleaving the images with odd and even lines. The 3D stereo image synthesis process adopted by the remote surgery robot, At any time, the 3D stereo endoscope camera outputs two high-definition images (a) and (b) with a resolution of 1920 * 1080, scales the two images to an image (c) with a resolution of 1920 * 540, and then splices the two images to form a 1920 * 1080 Top-Bottom format high-definition image, which is then input to the image encoder for compression and remote network transmission. After receiving the image at the main hand end, through parameter adjustment, the two images spliced up and down are displayed alternately in odd and even rows to form a three-dimensional stereo image (d), and finally, the stereo image under the endoscope field of vision is displayed on the display at the main hand operation end.

5.2.3 Delay and optimization of remote surgery

Low transparency and large network delay of remote minimally invasive surgical robot will prolong the response time of surgeons. According to the experiment, when the delay of remote surgery exceeds 500 ms, the operation risk will be significantly increased [13]; According to the statistics of the transatlantic remote "Lindbergh operation," the delay doctors can tolerate is 330 ms. For the developer of robot equipment, a detailed quantitative description of the system delay will help to find deficiencies and continuously optimize, so the delay test of surgical robot is very meaningful.

The delay of the remote robot system is mainly composed of two parts: ① the sample-communication-execution delay between the master and slave hands; ② capture-transmission-display delay between the endoscope and the display. Therefore, it is necessary to measure the delay of these two parts separately. After continuous measurement and optimization of the test results, the final test results completely test the system delay of the remote surgical robot, and theoretically ensure that its reliability meets the use requirements.

5.2.4 Master and slave configuration of remote surgical robot

Based on the above test results, combined with the architecture of the minimally invasive surgical robot and the requirements for signal and video transmission, we designed a remote communication control system based on 5G/Internet dedicated line, which integrates the remote surgical robot.

The main terminal communication control box is the receiving and sending and control module of all kinds of information at the doctor's operating terminal under network conditions. It consists of a box, an image encoding and decoding unit, a power supply unit, a network communication unit, a motion control and signal processing unit, a status display unit, an interaction unit, an interface unit, etc. The functions of each unit are as follows:

Box: integrated with each component unit to facilitate overall transportation.

Image encoding and decoding unit: composed of image encoder, used for encoding and decoding stereo endoscope dual-channel images and transmitting them at both ends of remote surgery.

Power supply unit: It is a switch power supply conforming to medical specifications, which is used to supply power to all units inside the box.

Network communication unit: It is a special industrial computer used to transmit control signals at both ends of remote surgery and monitor the network status.

Motion control and signal processing unit: interacts with the network communication unit, can collect the motion information of the master hand, and can actively control the motion of the master hand.

Status display unit: used to display the working status of network communication unit and motion control and signal processing unit.

Interaction unit: human-computer interaction interface, which is used to set network connection, start/stop data transmission, etc., and can feedback the robot operation status to the operator through prompt tone, etc.

Interface unit: including power supply interface, network interface, video output interface, foot switch signal acquisition interface, robot main end operation data output interface, etc.

The main communication control workflow is to connect the interface of the main end of the robot itself and the main end medical monitor with the main end communication control box, and then connect the main end communication control box to the Internet through the RJ45 interface. At the same time, supply 220 V AC power through the interface unit, and start-up.

The slave communication control box is the receiving and sending and control module of all kinds of information at the slave end of the robot under network conditions. It is composed of box, image encoding and decoding unit, power supply unit, network communication unit, energy instrument control unit, status display unit, interaction unit, interface unit, etc. The functions of each unit are as follows.

Box, power supply unit, network communication unit and status display unit: the same as the main control box.

Image encoding and decoding unit: composed of image encoder, used for encoding and decoding stereo endoscope dual-channel images and transmitting them at both ends of remote surgery.

Energy instrument control unit: It is composed of PLC modules, which is used to simulate the control signal output by the main machine of the excitation energy tool.

Interaction unit: human-computer interaction interface, which is used to set network connection, start/stop data transmission, etc., and can feedback the robot operation status to the slave assistant through prompt tone.

Interface unit: including power supply interface, network interface, video input interface, robot slave operation data output interface, etc.

The work flow of the slave communication control box is as follows: connect the communication port of the slave robot to the slave communication box through the network cable, and then connect the slave communication control box to the Internet through the RJ45 interface. At the same time, supply 220 V AC power through the interface unit and start-up.

5.2.5 Use of remote surgical robot

After testing, in order to ensure the smoothness and security of remote operation, the average network delay should not exceed 30 ms, and two dedicated networks with a bandwidth of not less than 50 Mb should be provided to ensure network stability.

The remote surgical operation doctors should not only receive the operation training of local surgical robots, but also receive the operation training in the remote environment. The operating physician also needs to be familiar with the operation mode and operation specification of the robot, be able to know the meaning of various operation status prompts fed back by the robot in a timely and accurate manner, and intervene with the robot to ensure the safety of remote surgery.

The remote surgical operation assistant shall also receive sufficient local and remote surgical robot operation training of the system. The assistant also needs to be familiar with the operation mode and operation specification of the robot, be able to know the meaning of various operation status prompts fed back by the robot in time, and be able to accurately intervene the robot according to the surgical requirements to ensure the safety of remote surgery.

The assistant of the remote surgical robot should be familiar with the connection, setting, and testing processes of the robot, and the connection between the robot and each module should be accurate and reliable. A comprehensive test should be carried out 2 hours before the robot implements the remote operation to complete the initialization and operation test of the robot.

6. Network solution for remote surgery

The construction and networking scheme for remote surgery support is a critical technology that ensures the smooth development of remote surgery. Since the inception of the concept of remote surgery, the choice of network communication mode has been crucial to ensure stable, speedy, and efficient signal data transmission. Additionally, minimizing operational delays caused by remote communication and surgical failure due to remote signal interruption has been a top priority for designers and users of remote surgery systems. From the first proposal of remote surgery to the realization of the first remote surgery and the current boom in the field, the selection of an appropriate network communication mode remains a vital consideration for the advancement of remote surgery technology.

6.1 Traditional networking schemes

6.1.1 Dedicated fiber optic cable network solution

In 2001, Professor Jacques Marescaux in France completed the world's first remote surgery, Lindbergh surgery, through the Zeus robot system, using a dedicated submarine fiber optic cable transmission network. This network directly connects the master operator and the slave operator through a dedicated fiber optic cable. It has several advantages, including wide bandwidth, large capacity, good signal quality, and high reliability. However, the drawback of this network is the limitation of the point-to-point physical connection, which requires special erection and maintenance of the fiber optic cable dedicated line and is extremely expensive, making it not widely promoted.

6.1.2 Satellite communication network solution

The satellite communication network uses artificial earth satellites as relay stations to relay radio waves, allowing interconnection between two or more earth stations. This network has many advantages, including wide coverage, large communication capacity, good transmission quality, less geographical restrictions, convenient and rapid networking, and easy global seamless connection. However, the main disadvantages of satellite transmission are a delay of about 0.6 seconds for audio and video, high cost of satellite signal transceiver equipment and channel usage at the user end, and high professional requirements for maintenance personnel. Currently, the satellite communication networking method can provide more than a few megabytes of communication rate, mainly used for mobile medical emergency rescue equipment to participate in telemedicine.

6.1.3 ADSL Internet access networking program

This networking scheme refers to client network or equipment access to the Internet through asymmetric digital subscriber line (ADSL) and the use of the Internet to form an interconnected network. This type of networking can provide up to 3.5 Mbps uplink and up to 24 Mbps downlink, and the cost of access is usually between several hundred and several thousand dollars per year in various provinces and cities. Although the cost of this solution is lower than that of private network and fiber optic Internet access methods, the actual available bandwidth drops when public network resources are insufficient, and upstream and downstream bandwidths are inconsistent because the data streams pass through the public network and share the public network bandwidth with the other user data streams. Therefore, the bandwidth stability is poor with this networking method, which may adversely affect two-way audio and video interaction applications with high bandwidth stability requirements, such as non-smooth video. Nevertheless, the networking scheme still has the advantages of easy networking and low cost and is suitable for building a telemedicine system using software video among hospitals below the county level. Some of the hospitals' self-built teleconsultation systems using software video partially adopt this networking method, which is one of the most common Internet access methods for small institutions and individual users.

6.1.4 3G/4G communication networking scheme

This networking scheme means that both the user side and the data center use 3G/4G communication to connect to the Internet and achieve interconnection between them. When a business relationship is established between multiple users, the information flow is delivered to the destination device through the Internet. However, since the data stream must pass through both 3G/4G and public network bottlenecks while sharing the public network bandwidth, the actual available bandwidth is reduced when the 3G/4G signal is weak or public network resources are insufficient. The upstream and downstream bandwidth may also be asymmetric. Therefore, the bandwidth stability using this networking method is poor, which can negatively impact applications that require two-way audio/video interaction.

6.2 Emerging networking schemes for remote surgery: the optional 5G communication networking scheme

6.2.1 5G communication networking scheme

The latest generation of cellular mobile communication technology is 5G, which inherits the advantages of previous systems such as 4G (LTE-A, WiMax), 3G (UMTS, LTE), and 2G (GSM), and also adds new features. Compared to previous technologies, 5G technology offers high-speed data transmission, low-latency rates, high capacity, large-scale device connectivity, low cost, and low energy consumption. The development of 5G technology as a bearer network for new technologies has revolutionized the development of areas such as telesurgery.

The International Telecommunication Union (ITU) has identified three main application scenarios for 5G: enhanced mobile broadband, ultra-high reliability low-latency communication, and massive machine-like communication. The key performance indicators of 5G include high speed, low latency, and large connectivity. Enhanced mobile broadband (eMBB) provides a better application experience for mobile Internet users, while ultra-high reliability low-latency communication (uRLLC) is used for telemedicine, industrial control, autonomous driving, and other applications with high requirements for low latency. The most prominent features of 5G are high speed, low latency, and large connectivity, with user experience rates of up to 1Gbps, latency down to milliseconds, and user connectivity up to 1 million connections per square kilometer.

6.2.2 5G network architecture for remote surgery

The 5G remote surgery network communication system requires two-way network communication. One is for remotely controlling the robotic arm, and the other is for transmitting live surgical video feedback. To ensure the smooth progress of surgery, we adopt a dual 5G (or dual gigabit dedicated line) multi-guaranteed network, which ensures the stability, reliability, and low latency required for remote medical operations. To ensure the stability and reliability of the 5G access network, we use high-performance indoor distributed systems (Pico RRU) for 5G. We use dedicated 5G core network equipment to ensure low latency on both ends of the network, guaranteeing system independence and security. We use a new type of distributed Pico Site to provide indoor coverage and configure uninterruptible power supply (UPS) backup power to ensure reliable power supply. These measures ensure the stability and reliability of the 5G remote surgery network communication system, meeting the requirements for remote medical care.

The use of network slicing technology in the 5G network can greatly improve the speed and security of remote surgery. With the development of 5G technology, the slicing packet network (SPN) has emerged, supporting the next-generation transport network architecture, bandwidth, traffic patterns, slicing, latency, and time synchronization. The core advantage of the SPN network is its flexibility. By binding elastic ethernet or FlexE technology with SPN, a larger physical link can be divided into multiple smaller physical channels, ensuring quality of service and isolation between transport layers. The SPN technology is a fiber-optic network transmission technology architecture independently developed in China, which has been successfully applied in the transmission of China's 5G network, achieving the organic integration of TDM transmission technology and packet transmission technology, fully meeting the requirements of lossless and efficient 5G transport. The SPN transmission technology has the advantages of large bandwidth, ultra-low latency, ultra-high precision synchronization, flexible control, and network slicing, which are essential in 5G remote surgery communication. By adopting SPN technology, efficient, secure, and fast network transmission can be achieved, ensuring the stability and precision of remote surgery.

Communication plan during surgery: If possible, a video conferencing system or a 5G smart bedside car can be utilized to ensure voice and video communication between the surgical control and the controlled end. In the absence of this equipment, mobile phones can be used for voice communication between both parties. However, wireless or wired headphones should be provided for doctors to ensure convenience, real-time communication and to avoid external interference.

Quality of 5G remote surgery network communication and monitoring method for surgical equipment: During remote surgery, the network should be subjected to a PING test, and the network delay should be monitored in real time. Both test routes should be tested. To reduce the impact on the network, the size of the PING packet should be set to the smallest possible size. During the surgery, three safeguard plans should be implemented in the following order of priority: The first plan is to use 5G for both control and video transmission, the second plan is to use two dedicated 5G lines for transmission, and the third plan is to use two dedicated lines for transmission. The first plan should be adopted initially. If there are network quality problems resulting in increased delay or difficulty in controlling the robot, the second and third plans should be used.

Standards for diagnosing network and surgical equipment failures in 5G remote surgery: The ideal network delay for 5G during surgery should be within 30 milliseconds, and the delay for dedicated lines should be within 10 milliseconds. If the average delay of 5G or dedicated lines exceeds 50 milliseconds within 3 minutes, or if there is unstable jitter in the instantaneous delay, the fallback plan should be initiated. The switch between 5G and dedicated lines should be completed within 3 minutes to ensure the smooth completion of the surgery.

The fusion of aggregate network technology and quantum communication encryption technology ensures the security of surgical networks. By adopting heterogeneous multi-link aggregation transmission technology, data is split and transmitted across different networks at the transmission layer of the network, endowing the network with features such as multi-link parallel transmission, link weight adjustment, forward error correction encoding technology, network self-adaptation, and real-time determination of the total network bandwidth. This achieves lower latency, higher stability, and higher efficiency, fully exploiting the adaptability of the public network for data transmission. The implementation of this technology can greatly reduce the cost of remote surgery and promote the normalization process of remote surgery. In the process of applying quantum encryption communication technology, the project team combines quantum encryption communication technology with remote robotic surgery to achieve the theoretically "unconditionally secure" communication mode for remote laparoscopic surgery. By using quantum superposition states and entanglement effects, combined with quantum random number generators (QRNG), quantum key distribution devices (QKD), and other equipment, key resources are generated, distributed, and received for quantum key production, distribution, and reception, providing encrypted transmission for remote surgery.

6.2.3 Fiber optic private network configuration

A fiber optic private network configuration is a star-shaped network that connects user LANs or devices through a dedicated line at a single point. Multiple private networks can also form a tree-shaped network by cascading. Fiber optic private networks are usually constructed using synchronous digital hierarchy (SDH) technology and are physically isolated from public networks. Therefore, from an application perspective, they offer high security, stable bandwidth, and high standardization of terminal equipment interfaces. However, the disadvantage of this network configuration is its higher cost compared to Internet-based networking. This networking approach can provide fully optical transparent channels ranging from 2 Mbps to 10 Gbps and offers data, image, and audio transmission services for point-to-point and point-to-multipoint connections. It is suitable for networking remote medical systems between county-level hospitals or above in provinces and cities that require high-quality audio-video interaction, frequent usage, and large image data volume.

During the specific implementation process of remote surgery, a gigabit dedicated line with dual router access is used, relying on clear networking architecture of SDH, packet transport network (PTN), and optical transport network (OTN) equipment, which provides high-risk security operation guarantees. In terms of maintenance, it has a 7×24-hour full-time scheduling and maintenance capability, enabling quick fault repair and restoration. The above network guarantees should be deployed at least 1 day before the operation, and network debugging should be completed. After the network debugging is completed, it is necessary to perform joint debugging with the surgical robot to ensure that both 5G and the dedicated line can support the surgical tasks. The networking adopts a disaster recovery mechanism. The 5G equipment and the dedicated line are protected by main and standby transmission equipment, and the reliability of transmission is ensured using dual router and dual-loop methods. All equipment is protected by UPS for power supply, and in case the power supply cannot be guaranteed, dual power supply or oil machine protection should be considered.

6.2.4 Aggregation network technology

Aggregation network technology is composed of 5G fused communication terminals and cloud servers. The 2-channel 1920×1080P60 video signals of the endoscope are collected, and 3D signals are synthesized and encoded, and then transmitted through multiple 5G links *via* the aggregation transmission. The cloud server deploys the 5G fused communication system software, which provides the service-side function of heterogeneous multi-link aggregation transmission. In terms of aggregation network technology, the transmission of the surgical endoscope video signal and control signal uses heterogeneous multi-link network aggregation transmission technology to improve transmission efficiency and stability. The control command signal is issued by the main hand, connected to the 5G fused communication gateway next to the main hand through the aggregation link, and the gateway transmits the control signal through the network port to the 5G network for transmission. The cloud server deploys the 5G fused communication system software, which implements the service-side function of heterogeneous multi-link aggregation transmission in the kernel layer, supporting both uplink and downlink aggregations. Therefore, aggregation network technology has the advantages of signal stability, fast transmission speed, environmental independence, and strong universality, and has good application potential in future remote surgery.

6.2.5 Deterministic network

"Deterministic network" is a new technology that provides end-to-end network service quality assurance for different users and businesses, and can provide differentiated business services for remote surgery. Its determinism is reflected in three aspects: Firstly, security isolation determinism, achieved through logical or physical segmentation of the network using slicing technology, as well as measures such as user access authorization, data storage filtering, and transmission security checks to achieve security isolation. Secondly, latency and jitter determinism. In the 5G era, many network applications such as remote robotic surgery, autonomous driving, and VR games require end-to-end latency to be controlled within a few milliseconds, and jitter to be controlled within the range of seconds. Thirdly, bandwidth determinism. In the era of traffic, there are higher requirements for upstream and downstream bandwidth. Remote surgery has extremely strict requirements for network latency, jitter, packet loss, redundancy protection, and fast switching. Deterministic network is the key means to achieve these standards. It can cooperate with network slicing and edge computing to sink AI and other technologies to the grassroots level, promote the integration of data and 5G's "cloud-edge-end" functions, fully leverage the advantages and characteristics of 5G independent networking, adjust the network architecture, and meet the overall requirements of remote surgery. Therefore, deterministic network also has good application potential in future remote surgery.

7. Personnel and cost analysis of remote surgery

Generally, the cost of hospital medical services includes labor costs, fixed asset costs, material costs, administrative expenses, business expenses, and other expenses. Remote surgery involves special cost expenditures (such as remote networks) in addition to the general medical service costs.

7.1 Standard configuration for remote surgery resources

Remote Regional Medical Center

Equipment and software: remote surgical robot and its operating system, communication equipment, and data transmission system;

Personnel: one surgeon, one surgical assistant, one equipment maintenance personnel, and one communication transmission maintenance personnel.

Remote Primary Healthcare Institution

Equipment and software: remote surgical robot and its operating system, communication equipment, and data transmission system;

Personnel: two collaborating surgeons, one anesthesiologist, two nursing staff, one equipment maintenance personnel, and one communication transmission maintenance personnel.

7.2 Composition of remote surgery costs

Depreciation and maintenance costs of equipment (including regional medical center and primary healthcare institution equipment): equipment depreciation and maintenance costs of the remote surgical robot system;

Usage costs of specialized instruments and consumables: costs of instruments and disposable materials used multiple times during remote surgical procedures;

Personnel costs: costs of personnel such as the surgeon, surgical assistant, remote collaboration surgeon, nursing staff, anesthesiologist, equipment maintenance personnel, and communication transmission maintenance personnel;

Other costs: depreciation costs of the operating room and auxiliary equipment, and other related consumables.

7.3 Cost-benefit analysis of remote surgery for patients

The hospitalization costs of remote surgery patients include two types of costs: direct costs and indirect costs. Direct costs include medical and non-medical expenses. Medical expenses include various treatment-related expenses, the cost depreciation of the surgical robot system, and personnel costs of remote surgical physicians. Non-medical expenses include living, transportation, and accommodation expenses during hospitalization. Indirect costs include family members' lost income, patients' lost income, and other costs. For remote surgery patients, the structure of these costs is the same, but the amount of cost consumption will differ. Conducting remote surgery treatment will reduce the patient's indirect cost expenditure.

7.4 Economic analysis at the regional medical center level

Hospitals are the main body for introducing and using new medical technologies, and they are also the most commonly used perspective for economic analysis. For hospitals, the cost of remote surgery includes resource costs used during surgery (instrumentation and surgical supplies), drugs, food and lodging, and nursing, as well as indirect costs such as hospital management and operating expenses. Remote surgery is a medical activity that connects experts with patients and medical workers using computer communication technology and medical technology to achieve long-distance data, text, voice, and image data transmission. Considering the characteristics of remote medical services, the cost of remote medical services should include hardware costs, software costs, housing costs, labor costs, and operating costs.

1. Hardware costs refer to the relevant hardware equipment purchased for the remote medical service project at the regional medical center and the patient's primary healthcare institution.

2. Software costs refer to the development and purchase of software used for remote medical services at the regional medical center and the primary healthcare institution.

3. Housing costs refer to the cost of housing for the remote medical service project at the regional medical center and the primary healthcare institution.

4. Labor costs refer to the cost of human resources required for the remote medical service project at the regional medical center and the primary healthcare institution.

5. Operating costs refer to the costs incurred during the operation and maintenance of the remote medical service project at the regional medical center and the primary healthcare institution.

8. The future direction of telesurgery

The development and application of telesurgery robots has become a new trend worldwide, which helps solve the problem of telemedicine in special geographical areas and special situations, and has great prospects in the future [14].

8.1 The application in regions with scarce medical resources

As an important part of telemedicine, telesurgery can effectively improve the biased distribution of medical resources, coordinate medical resources, and increase the rate of patient treatment and medical resource utilization.

8.2 The application in the field of special environment

In military medicine, in 2009, the U.S. Army developed a complete surgical robot system based on the da Vinci system to cope with the wartime environment to achieve unmanned processing [15], including surgical robot system, management and display system, control and supervision system, monitoring system, equipment replacement system, equipment delivery system, and drug supply system. Although the system is not used in the clinic, the study of the system suggests that telemedicine will enter the era of fully remote surgery in an unmanned mode.

8.3 Driving the development of other areas of technology

Faced with complex cases requiring multidisciplinary surgery to resolve the disease, telesurgery can also be performed many-to-one, with two or even more control systems controlling the same patient. Combined multidisciplinary surgery solves surgical problems of neighboring organs with the same surgical orifice or combines different hospitals to perform remote surgery [16]. In addition, the development of telesurgery can simultaneously lead to the development of other telemedicine disciplines, such as telecare and telerehabilitation after telesurgery [17]. The Telecare Medical Information System (TMIS) utilizes wireless communication technology and smart devices, enabling patients to receive remote medical treatment from doctors via the internet without the need to visit the hospital, thus providing convenience for postoperative rehabilitation care following remote surgeries [18]. It combines healthcare and information technology to achieve electronic medical information management and remote collaboration. Doctors and nurses can record patients' medical information, and the system supports remote collaboration and consultations. Doctors can remotely access patients' imaging data, provide remote guidance and diagnostic opinions. TMIS also collects and analyzes medical data, generates reports for medical quality assessment and decision support, thereby improving the service quality and efficiency of healthcare institutions.

It can also promote the development of imaging medicine. Data conversion in telesurgery cannot be achieved without remote proximity systems in the field of imaging, which can present information about the surgical field of view and the surgical environment to the operator in an image-audio format to create a sense of presence [18]. A typical robotic telepresence system includes a light source, a digital image and audio acquisition and processing system, and an intelligent decision and control execution system. The remote presence system has evolved from a simple image-audio acquisition and processing system to an integrated system that incorporates surgical field of view, surgical environment, and other image-audio information with some learning and adaptive capabilities. The way forward now is to combine intraoperative images with patient-specific 3D models and to combine them with virtual/augmented reality imaging.

With limited medical resources in the deep sea and high altitudes, conventional medical resources may not be able to solve problems in a timely and effective manner in case of sudden surgical emergencies. The potential of telesurgery for applications in maritime aviation and space stations is enormous.

Telemedicine can help eliminate distance barriers and provide medical expertise to remote areas. Due to the relative shortage of surgeons and the need to explore new approaches to surgical education, surgical tele-mentoring may be a solution to enhance and improve surgical education models. Although remote robotic surgical teaching may not replace local surgical instructors, studies have demonstrated that it is a valuable tool for remote instruction in minimally invasive surgery.

Telesurgery can serve as a tele-education function. By remotely interrogating multiple surgical specialists and remotely training hands-on surgeons, the professionalism of new hand surgeons around the world can be more effectively enhanced. This can revolutionize surgical education by creating an interactive, scalable and accessible education system with support and guidance from experts around the world [19, 20].

9. Prospect

As an emerging breakthrough technology in the twenty-first century, remote robotic surgery technology has been classified as a major research project by many countries by virtue of its advanced real-time transmission technology and robotic surgery system. Artificial intelligence has great potential for development as a strategic development plan in China, and the development of autonomous surgical capabilities has received a great deal of attention from researchers as one of the development directions of surgical robots. Surgical robots have replaced surgeons into numerous dangerous environments to independently complete remote rescue and treatment work, and have played a significant role in national defense and military, major disasters, future battlefield, and aerospace fields. It is believed that with the increasing volume of remote surgery and further development of artificial intelligence, robotic systems capable of autonomously completing remote surgery will be further developed.

Acknowledgements

This work was supported by the National Natural Science Foundation of China (52122501), the Major Scientific and Technological Innovation Project of Shandong Province (2019JZZY021002), Qingdao People's Life Science and Technology Project (18-6-1-64-nsh), and the Taishan Scholar Program of Shandong Province (tsqn20161077). The sponsors played a role in the design and conduct of the study and collection of the data.

Author details

Haitao Niu
Department of Urology, The Affiliated Hospital of Qingdao University, Qingdao, China

*Address all correspondence to: niuht0532@126.com

References

[1] Becker RL, Specht CS, Jones R, et al. Use of remote video microscopy (telepathology) as an adjunct to neurosurgical frozen section consultation. Human Pathlogy. 1993;**24**(8):909-911

[2] Satava RM. Emerging medical applications of virtual reality: A surgeon's perspective. Artificial Intelligence in Medicine. 1994;**6**(4):281-288

[3] Marescaux J, Leroy J, Rubino F, et al. Transcontinental robot-assisted remote telesurgery: Feasibility and potential applications. Annals of Surgery. 2002;**235**(4):487-492

[4] Xu S, Perez M, Yang K, et al. Determination of the latency effects on surgical performance and the acceptable latency levels in telesurgery using the dV-trainer (®) simulator. Surgical Endoscopy. 2014;**28**(9):2569-2576

[5] Lacy AM, Bravo R, Otero-Piñeiro AM, et al. 5G-assisted telementored surgery. The British Journal of Surgery. 2019;**106**(12):1576-1579

[6] Zheng J, Wang Y, Zhang J, et al. 5G ultra-remote robot-assisted laparoscopic surgery in China. Surgical Endoscopy. 2020;**34**(11):5172-5180

[7] Rosser JCJR, Young SM, Kionsky J. Telementoring: An application whose time has come[J]. Surg Endosc. Surgical endoscopy. 2007;**21**(8):1458-1463

[8] Choi PJ, Oskouian RJ, Tubbs RS. Telesurgery: Past, Present, and Future[J]. Cureus. 2018;**10**(5):e2716

[9] Rutkowski TM. Robotic and virtual reality BCIs using spatial tactile and auditory oddball paradigms. Frontiers in Neurorobotics. 2016;**6**(10):20

[10] Xiong YG, Quek F. Hand motion gesture frequency properties and multimodal discourse analysis. 2006;**69**(3):353-371

[11] Video Developer Report 2019. Bitmovin. Retrieved 5 November 2019

[12] Ohm JR, Sullivan GJ, Schwarz H, et al. Comparison of the coding efficiency of video coding standards—Including high efficiency video coding (HEVC). IEEE Transactions on Circuits & Systems for Video Technology. 2012;**22**(12):1669-1684

[13] Perez M, Xu S, Chauhan S, et al. Impact of delay on telesurgical performance: Study on the robotic simulator dV-trainer. International Journal of Computer Assisted Radiology and Surgery. 2016;**11**(4):581-587

[14] Xia SB, Lu QS. Development status of telesurgery robotic system[J]. Chinese Journal of Traumatology. 2021

[15] Pablo GJ, et al. Trauma Pod: A semi-automated telerobotic surgical system[J]. The International Journal of Medical Robotics and Computer Assisted Surgery. 2009;**5**(2):136-146

[16] Doarn CR, et al. Determining the Threshold of Time-Delay for Teleoperation Accuracy and Efficiency in Relation to Telesurgery[J]. Telemedicine & E Health the Official Journal of the American Telemedicine Association; 2014

[17] Cazac C, Radu G. Telesurgery – an efficient interdisciplinary approach used to improve the health care system[J]. Journal of Medicine & Life. 2014;**7**(Spec Iss 3):137-141

[18] Zemitin N, Ortmaier T, Morel G. A new robot for force control in minimally

invasive surgery: IEEE/RSJ International Conference on Intelligent Robots & Systems, 2003[C]. 2004 IEEE/RSJ International Conference on Intelligent Robots and Systems (IROS)

[19] Bogen EM, Augestad KM, Patel HR, et al. Telementoring in education of laparoscopic surgeons: An emerging technology[J]. World J Gastrointest Endosc. 2014,**6**(5):148-155

[20] Mcintyre TP, Monahan TS, Villegas L, et al. Teleconferencing surgery enhances effective communication and enriches medical education[J]. Surgical Laparoscopy Endoscopy & Percutaneous Techniques. 2008;**18**(1):45-48

Chapter 9

Artificial Intelligence in Surgery, Surgical Subspecialties, and Related Disciplines

Ryan Yimeng Lee, Alyssa Imperatore Ziehm, Lauryn Ullrich and Stanislaw P. Stawicki

Abstract

Artificial intelligence (AI) and machine learning (ML) algorithms show promise in revolutionizing many aspects of surgical care. ML algorithms may be used to improve radiologic diagnosis of disease and predict peri-, intra-, and postoperative complications in patients based on their vital signs and other clinical characteristics. Computer vision may improve laparoscopic and minimally invasive surgical education by identifying and tracking the surgeon's movements and providing real-time performance feedback. Eventually, AI and ML may be used to perform operative interventions that were not previously possible (nanosurgery or endoluminal surgery) with the utilization of fully autonomous surgical robots. Overall, AI will impact every surgical subspecialty, and surgeons must be prepared to facilitate the use of this technology to optimize patient care. This chapter will review the applications of AI across different surgical disciplines, the risks and limitations associated with AI and ML, and the role surgeons will play in implementing this technology into their practice.

Keywords: artificial intelligence, machine learning, robotics, surgery, nanotechnology, nanosurgery, computer vision, autonomy

1. Introduction

Artificial intelligence (AI) and machine learning (ML) are rapidly transitioning from "experimental" into the "mainstream adoption" [1–3]. The current pace of progress appears to be accelerating, with an emerging number of potential applications of AI/ML in surgery and its various subspecialties [4]. These programs have shown promise in their capacity to process vast amounts of data, identify multivariate relationships within data, and reduce uncertainty of predictions to enable alternative options to certain tasks [5, 6]. Still, AI has not yet progressed to fully automating tasks due to certain limitations, such as the inability to understand common-sense scenarios, adjust to untrained circumstances, and make intuitive or ethical judgments—all necessary abilities required from a surgeon [7–10]. These complementary strengths suggest that the role of AI may be optimized by collaborating with human intelligence [11]. However, this has not stopped scholarly discussions from imagining what increasingly practical considerations of AI might look like in the future, including concepts such as "autonomous actions in surgery" [12].

In this chapter, we will explore current and potential future applications of AI/ML in the sphere of surgery, surgical subspecialties, and related disciplines of medicine. Each section of this chapter will outline specific aspects where we believe AI may play a role within the context of surgical care delivery.

2. Methods

For the purposes of this narrative review, we performed an exhaustive literature search, with primary source platforms being Google™ Scholar and PubMed. The primary search term was "surgery" with the following secondary terms—"artificial intelligence," "machine learning," "technology," and "subspecialty." Specific names of surgical specialties (e.g., orthopedics, neurosurgery, and vascular surgery) were also employed. The primary search term "surgery" in combination with each of the other keywords, in various iterations, resulted in more than 875,000 potential listings. Literature screening focused on sources with "full text" availability, limited to English language. In addition, various correspondences (e.g., Letters to Editor and Brief Communications) were excluded. This resulted in approximately 142,000 secondary literature results. The search was limited to original research and reviews within this group, with at least five citations (using Google™ Scholar). With these criteria, our final list of potentially suitable articles was fewer than 2000. A more intensive review of the tertiary phase of our article screening resulted in 96 articles with relevance to this review. After this, secondary sources (derived during in-depth review of our 96 most relevant articles and examining their respective reference lists) were added. Utilizing the above methodology, the resultant reference list includes 158 citations (**Figure 1**).

In the primary search, only studies with five or more citations were considered. Because newer studies tend to have fewer citations, this may introduce selection bias against newer studies that either address aspects of these concerns or bring up new ones. Given the rapidly evolving field of AI, future reviews could evaluate more novel studies for potential innovations.

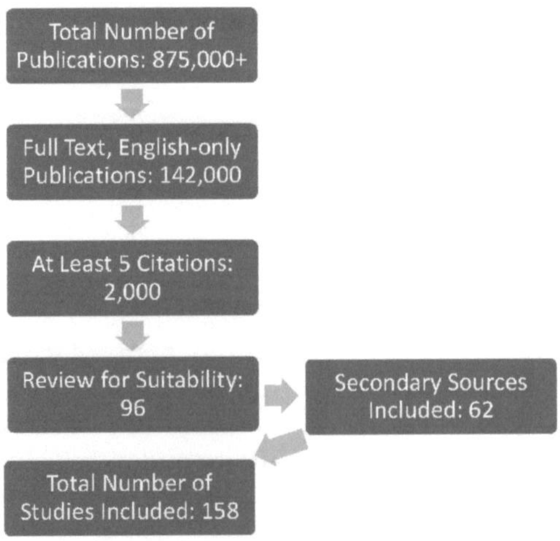

Figure 1.
Flowchart of the selection process for review articles.

2.1 Focused list of AI/ML applications across surgical specialties

A focused list of topics regarding the implication and application of AI and ML are presented below. AI is broadly defined as a system that can learn to think or act [13]. ML, which falls under the broad scope of AI, refers more specifically to an algorithm that adjusts itself based on detected patterns in data [13]. Deep learning is a subset of ML that uses neural networks to learn intricate relationships in data [14]. Each item will be presented briefly, with relevant literature sources provided accordingly. It is important to note that a complete review encompassing all applications of AI/ML and all specialties of surgery is beyond the scope of this chapter.

3. Perioperative risk assessment and surgical planning

Due to the ability to quickly and efficiently incorporate and compile large amounts of data, AI/ML paradigms are likely to be heavily involved in preoperative risk assessment in all fields of surgery. Through the collection of patient data and characteristics, such as weight, heart rate, blood pressure, comorbidities, and other factors, highly sophisticated models can be used in algorithms that predict the risk of the patient before undergoing a surgical procedure. With the ability to calculate risk, AI/ML may also bring the potential for appropriate mitigating strategies that could decrease patient morbidity and mortality [4, 15]. By utilizing large data sets organized by specific surgical procedures and procedure types, AI/ML-powered algorithms could be used to modify models that carry out statistical weight optimization for different variables associated with morbidity and/or mortality for each type of surgery, within a specific set of clinical circumstances (e.g., emergency versus nonemergency) or within a certain population (e.g., demographic). Assuming a representative sample, an effective AI/ML algorithm would allow surgeons and other perioperative medicine experts to input values for individual patients and return an objective preoperative risk assessment, leading to potential applications in precision medicine. For instance, there are multiple different bariatric surgeries available to patients, including sleeve gastrectomy, Roux-en-Y gastric bypass, adjustable gastric band, and biliopancreatic diversion [16]. Though sleeve gastrectomy is now the most common approach, each technique has trade-offs between cost, short-term morbidity, long-term morbidity, and long-term weight loss, and this can sometimes lead to complex decisions in choosing the optimal procedure [17]. Machine learning algorithms could help address this issue using preoperative data to provide individualized recommendations, potentially leading to more optimal bariatric surgery prescriptions [16]. Recent studies have investigated the use of similarly structured and implemented algorithms across many different types of surgeries and surgical challenges, from predicting preoperative risk of cardiac complications, identification of a difficult airway prior to intubation, and the general risk–benefit estimations of different procedural or surgical interventions [18–22]. When properly designed and implemented, such algorithms would allow for risk stratification and, thus, better preparation for adverse outcomes following surgery. Future improvements would increase the specificity and sensitivity of these algorithms, facilitating a more accurate prediction of perioperative risk. Additionally, AI algorithms may be able to provide quantitative predictions about outcomes with and without surgery, providing both surgeons and patients with the information for objective decision-making [23].

Additional preoperative risk assessment could take the form of dedicated ML analysis of the radiologic imaging [24]. Preoperative imaging is utilized before surgery to give surgeons more information about the patient's pathology and anatomy and is essential for preoperative planning. ML algorithms can be used in the preoperative setting to predict prognoses and augment surgical decision-making across various surgical specialties [25–27]. An example of the implementation of preoperative ML models is the utilization of computed tomography (CT) scans to diagnose lung cancer. Using ML to evaluate CT scans has shown comparable to even better sensitivities and specificities compared to radiologists [28]. Such models can be further augmented to provide data about each identified tumor and suggestions for surgical planning [29]. More widespread adoption of ML algorithms that read imaging could lead to advancements in surgical planning in interventions such as lumbar decompression in spinal stenosis to assessing characteristics of corneal endothelium in specular microscopy for treatment of corneal edema [20, 30]. The utilization of ML algorithms could transform how surgeons interpret CT scans preoperatively and could, in return, improve patient care and surgical outcomes.

Advances in the algorithmic interpretation of medical imaging have led to the emergence of radiomics, a field involving the analysis of medical imaging to provide information about the physiology or pathology of the disease [31]. Radiomics contributes an additional layer to how ML algorithms can interpret medical imaging and has shown unique promise in surgical oncology, where minute changes in image features can be associated with various prognoses. Typical features used in radiomic workflow may include the intensity of signals and the distribution of these signals [32]. Because benign and malignant tumors have different microenvironments and expression of specific markers, magnetic resonance imaging (MRI) radiomics shows promise in being able to differentiate malignant or benign tumors from normal tissue [32]. Radiomics could therefore improve patient outcomes through early identification of disease.

In terms of specific examples, radiomics can be used to determine axillary lymph node (ALN) metastases in patients with breast cancer. The most common site of breast cancer metastasis is to the axillary lymph nodes (ALN). Early detection of ALN metastases can inform the surgical management of breast cancer [33]. Based on the Z0011 clinical trial results, the current diagnostic procedure for ALN metastases for most patients is sentinel lymph node biopsy (SLNB) [34]. Although this procedure is less invasive than ALN dissection, SLNB still carries the risk of lymphedema, axillary paresthesia, and reduced range of motion in the involved upper extremity [35]. Furthermore, in some cases, SLNB has been shown to have false negative rates in the range of 5–10% [36]. Thus, finding more effective alternative ways to identify ALN metastases is increasingly important. Radiomics has shown the ability to identify malignant tissues and determine ALN metastases at a higher rate than radiologists [37]. In the future, radiologists equipped with radiomics capabilities may be able to more efficiently and more accurately identify ALN metastases, leading to more prompt medical and surgical therapeutic interventions. Evidence suggests that radiomics may be able to differentiate between different subtypes of cancer based on the unique molecular profile and the resulting appearance on imaging of each subtype [38]. The ability to specifically diagnose different subtypes of cancer from their respective radiologic imaging characteristics may allow surgeons to stratify patient prognoses and better determine medical and surgical management (e.g., precision medicine/surgery).

Preoperative uses of ML and AI could also improve patient outcomes for those who are awaiting organ transplants. More specifically, ML algorithms trained to analyze patient characteristics, such as age, sex, severity of disease, hemodynamic measurements, and other variables, could be used to predict waitlist mortality and posttransplant outcomes [39]. These programs could be used to improve patient outcomes more broadly through a more objective management of organ transplant waitlists and recipient match optimization. ML algorithms may also be used in the future in more direct applications to transplant surgery. For instance, in liver transplantation, graft-weight-to-recipient-body-weight (GW/RW) ratios <0.8% are associated with an increased risk of complications such as small-for-size syndrome [40]. Consequently, the estimation of graft weight in living donors is important for limiting adverse outcomes associated with graft size mismatch. Studies have been conducted on the potential use of ML models trained on donor age, sex, body mass index, CT scans, and other data to estimate the donor graft weight [40]. These models have the potential to greatly enhance the precision of graft weight estimation, improving outcomes of liver transplantation. Additionally, experiences learned from hepatic transplantation may be suitable for adoption across other areas of organ transplantation (e.g., kidney, pancreas, heart, and lung), similarly reducing various potentially

Source	**Year of publication**	**Country of origin**	**Surgical discipline**	**Studied AI/ML algorithms**	**Major findings relevant to this review**
Hashimoto et al.	2018	USA	All disciplines	ML surgical decision-making	AI in the form of ML, natural language processing, artificial neural networks, and computer vision has led to applications such as the detection of bleeding in tissue in video, analysis of Electronic Health Record (EHR) text, and predicting lung cancer staging based on diagnostic and therapeutic data
Loftus et al.	2020	USA	All disciplines	ML surgical decision-making	ML models may increase accuracy and reduce biases in surgical decision-making
Bihorac et al.	2019	USA	Major inpatient surgeries	ML preoperative risk of complications	ML algorithm using EHR data could predict the risk of certain complications and of mortality at 1-, 3-, 6-, 12-, and 24 months after surgery (Areas under the curve (AUCs) of 0.82 and 0.94)
Zhou et al.	2022	China	Thyroid surgery	ML preoperative risk of complications	ML algorithm using preoperative patient data and neck circumference could predict difficult airway intubation (AUCs of 0.812 and 0.848)
Wilson et al.	2021	USA	Orthopedic surgery, neurosurgery	ML preoperative determination of surgery candidacy	ML algorithm using lumbar MRI scans could predict spinal surgery candidacy (Area under the curve (AUC) of 0.88)

Source	Year of publication	Country of origin	Surgical discipline	Studied AI/ ML algorithms	Major findings relevant to this review
Bellini et al.	2021	Italy	Thoracic surgery	ML preoperative risk of complications	ML models can evaluate preoperative data to provide individualized preoperative risk of outcomes after lung cancer resection and identification of pulmonary nodules
Malani et al.	2023	India	Gynecologic surgery	ML preoperative detection of disease	ML models can evaluate imaging to determine the presence of disease for surgical intervention
Shoham et al.	2022	Israel	Dermatologic surgery	ML preoperative prediction of surgery complexity	ML model using preoperative patient and tumor data can predict the complexity of surgical resection of nonmelanoma skin cancer (AUC of 0.79)
Bian et al.	2023	China	Surgical oncology	ML analysis of imaging	ML radiomics model using CT scans can predict the presence of lymph node metastases in patients with pancreatic ductal adenocarcinoma with better accuracy than clinician alone ($p < 0.001$)
Etienne et al.	2020	France	Thoracic surgery	ML analysis of imaging, preoperative risk assessment	Multiple ML models can identify the presence of malignant nodules using patient CT scans
Fairchild et al.	2023	USA	Neurosurgery	ML analysis of imaging	ML model can identify the presence of difficult-to-detect brain metastases with 94% accuracy for prospectively diagnosed metastases and 80% accuracy for new metastases
Martin et al.	2022	USA	Orthopedic surgery	ML analysis of imaging, preoperative risk assessment	ML algorithms can detect the presence of fractures and automate the calculation of measurements such as coronal knee alignment and acetabular component inclination and version
Savage	2020	USA	Surgical oncology	ML analysis of imaging	ML algorithms can detect the presence of lung cancer at rates comparable to radiologists
Cui et al.	2021	China	Surgical oncology	ML analysis of imaging	ML model can identify the presence of lung cancer nodules (76.0% accuracy

Source	Year of publication	Country of origin	Surgical discipline	Studied AI/ML algorithms	Major findings relevant to this review
					with 0.004 false positives/scan when double-read) and provide information about number, coordinates, and suspicion of each nodule
Vigueras-Guillén et al.	2020	Netherlands	Ophthalmology	ML analysis of imaging	ML model can assess corneal endothelium density, coefficient of variation, and hexagonality using images from specular microscopy in 98.4% of specular images compared to 71.5% using previous software
Yu et al.	2021	China	Surgical oncology	ML analysis of imaging, radiomics	ML radiomics can predict the presence of axillary lymph node metastasis (AUCs of 0.88 and 0.87) and provide insight into tumor microenvironment (immune cells, methylation, and long noncoding RNAs (lncRNAs))
Chang et al.	2021	Taiwan	Neurosurgery	ML analysis of imaging, radiomics	ML radiomics can predict molecular subgroups of medulloblastoma based on differing MRI profiles of each subgroup (AUCs of 0.82, 0.72, and 0.78)
Hsich et al.	2019	USA	Transplant surgery	ML preoperative risk assessment	ML model evaluated which variables have high importance in predicting heart transplant waitlist mortality, including glomerular filtration rate (GFR), serum albumin, and extracorporeal membrane oxygenation (ECMO) usage
Giglio et al.	2023	Italy	Transplant surgery	ML preoperative surgical decision-making	ML models trained on donor characteristics and CT scans can accurately predict liver donor graft weight to optimize donor-recipient matching with less errors than other methods ($p < 0.001$)
Gujio-Rubio et al.	2020	Spain	Transplant surgery	ML preoperative risk assessment	ML algorithms for preoperative risk assessment show promise in liver, pancreas, kidney, heart, and lung transplantation

Table 1.
Summary of included studies on preoperative artificial intelligence/machine learning (AI/ML).

preventable complications, improving patient clinical outcomes, and maximizing effective utilization of organs (**Table 1**) [41].

4. Intraoperative surgical decision-making

Although AL/ML-based algorithms and approaches can greatly improve patient outcomes during preoperative use, perhaps the most promising and powerful use of these programs is their ability to improve intraoperative care. Algorithms trained on patient vital signs, various biometric and non-biometric characteristics, electrocardiography (EKG), and other data points could be utilized to help facilitate real-time reduction of various intraoperative risks, including those of hypertension, hypoxemia, massive hemorrhage, and other complications [42–44]. Loftus et al. write that this comprehensive analysis of patient parameters using AI is especially important for more complex disease states, such as frailty [45]. Though frailty is a multifactorial disease state affected by physical, cognitive, and social variables, frailty is currently diagnosed by a few physical, often subjective criteria. For instance, the Fried frailty phenotype assesses patients based on their recent physical activity, subjective feelings of exhaustion, walking speed, handgrip strength, and unintentional weight loss. Diagnosing frailty can therefore be inconsistent, even though frailty is known to increase morbidity, mortality, and risk of other comorbidities that also increase surgical risk. Through expert-led ML training on large sets, algorithms could be developed to better classify complex disease systems such as frailty or sepsis and improve intraoperative risk assessment [45]. These outputs could further allow for augmented decision-making, or the advanced application of highly sophisticated models that are trained on multiple iterations of the same surgical procedure type. This, in turn, could provide decision-making assistance for surgical teams performing same-type operation based on the patient's vital signs, procedural characteristics, the progression of the surgery, and various other potential characteristics [46]. For instance, if a machine learning model identifies that a certain constellation of parameters was associated with worse outcomes, it could potentially suggest that the surgical team addresses a specific aspect of patient care to improve the projected outcome, or perhaps to reduce various complication risks [4, 47–50]. Komorowski et al. showed the possibility of this type of AI through an algorithm that was able to suggest optimal treatment and dosing options for sepsis patients leading to lower patient mortality than human clinicians alone [51].

Surgery often places high demands on surgeons' cognition, creating an opportunity for ML/AI algorithms to reduce cognitive load and further identify ways to improve surgical outcomes [50, 52, 53].

4.1 Intraoperative pathology and histology determination

Clinical algorithms based on AI/ML have the potential to be highly helpful when healthcare professionals must quickly "make sense of" large amounts of aggregate/consolidated data, including text-based content [54–56]. One of the fields within the broader domain of "AI" that has gained particular interest in recent years is the so-called "computer vision" [57, 58]. Advancements in computer vision have been applied to object recognition, facial recognition, and action recognition, and potential applications of this technology in the area of surgery and related specialties are readily apparent [59]. This includes the use of AI to interpret radiologic imaging and a potentially important role in intraoperative histological analysis. The current procedure/workflow for intraoperative pathology in many oncologic surgeries involves the excision of a portion of the tumor, where the sample is then transported to the laboratory for preparation and interpretation by a pathologist. This process can take 20–30 min, prolonging the overall surgical procedure and also potentially delaying the diagnosis, where each additional step also contributes potential barriers to timely diagnosis [60]. Applications of "computer vision" could potentially address challenges associated with intraoperative interpretation of histology. Data are also emerging on the use of ML algorithms in analyzing images from Raman spectroscopy to identify malignant and benign tumors. The actual algorithm is functionally similar to the process used in radiologic analyses, but Raman spectroscopy imaging can be further processed to provide imaging more similar to hematoxylin and eosin (H&E) staining, which may better allow surgeons and pathologists to verify ML classifications of tissue samples [61]. Intraoperative pathology consultations are quite common in neurosurgical tumor procedures, breast cancer, hepatobiliary and pancreatic resections, lymph node dissections, and dermatopathology [62–66]. These procedures may also benefit from AI-aided streamlining of intraoperative histology and pathology in the future.

The use of computer vision algorithms in surgery can be further expanded to include the characterization of molecular tissue margins. When removing malignant tumors, patient outcomes are optimal with maximal resection of the tumor while sparing as much healthy tissue as possible. Positive margins, or cancerous cells that remain after incomplete resection, are associated with recurrence of cancer, leading to worse patient outcomes. Some estimates indicate that positive margins may be found in approximately 5% of liver and breast cancer resections, so identification of tumor margins is still a significant problem that must be addressed [67, 68]. As mentioned previously, Raman spectroscopy has already been used by pathologists to distinguish neoplastic and normal tissue based on differential Raman scattering, but future advancements could also lead to intraoperative Raman spectroscopy to determine tumor margins [69]. Like with other imaging modalities, computer vision algorithms in the future will be able to identify features such as positive margins. This could allow surgeons to identify tumor margins within the operating room without needing to

Source	Year of publication	Country of origin	Surgical discipline	Studied AI/ML algorithms	Major findings relevant to this review
Hatib et al.	2018	USA	All surgical disciplines	ML intraoperative risk assessment	ML model was able to predict intraoperative hypotension from the analysis of perioperative arterial pressure waveforms (area under the curve (AUC of 0.95 15 min before hypotensive event)
Lundberg et al.	2018	USA	All surgical disciplines	ML intraoperative risk assessment	ML model was able to predict intraoperative hypoxemia from preoperative patient characteristics, real-time ventilation settings, anesthetic agents, etc.(AUC of 0.76 compared to that of 0.60 with anesthesiologist's prediction)

Source	Year of publication	Country of origin	Surgical discipline	Studied AI/ ML algorithms	Major findings relevant to this review
Lee et al.	2022	Korea	All surgical disciplines	ML intraoperative risk assessment	ML model using pre- and intraoperative parameters (arterial pressure waveforms, oxygen saturation, and ST segment elevation) was able to accurately predict intraoperative massive transfusion (AUC of 0.972 compared to that of 0.824 using the benchmark model)
Loftus et al.	2019	USA	All surgical disciplines	ML intraoperative risk assessment	ML algorithms will be useful for modeling complex disease states (such as frailty and sepsis) for a more accurate intraoperative risk assessment
Yang et al.	2019	USA	All surgical disciplines	ML decision-making	ML decision support tools may be able to provide clinical decision-making in all aspects of medicine
Pappada et al.	2013	USA	Surgical critical care	ML decision-making	The ML model was able to predict glycemic trends in critically ill trauma and cardiothoracic surgery patients with 96.7% accuracy for normal glucose values and 53.6% accuracy for hyperglycemic episodes
Komorowski et al.	2018	UK	Surgical critical care	ML decision-making	The ML model was developed to recommend sepsis treatment strategy and dosage based on patient demographics, vital signs, laboratory values, medications received, etc., and patient mortality was the lowest when clinician treatments matched AI recommendations
Barth and Seamon	2015	USA	All surgical disciplines	ML decision-making	Situational awareness is vital for patient safety, and AI may help reduce cognitive load to increase situational awareness
De Melo et al.	2020	USA	All surgical disciplines	ML decision-making	Virtual assistants significantly decreased self-reported cognitive load in participants undergoing cognitively demanding tasks
Voulodimos et al.	2018	Greece	All surgical disciplines	Computer vision	Recent advancements in computer vision include object detection, face recognition, action recognition, and pose estimation
Hollon et al.	2020	USA	Neurosurgery	Computer vision	Computer vision models can analyze Raman spectroscopic

Source	Year of publication	Country of origin	Surgical discipline	Studied AI/ ML algorithms	Major findings relevant to this review
					images to aid real-time intraoperative brain tumor diagnosis (overall accuracy of 94.6% compared to that of 93.9% with pathologist interpretation)
Orringer et al.	2017	USA	Neurosurgery	Computer vision	Computer vision model can process Raman spectroscopy of brain tumor samples into simulated H&E staining and can be used to classify brain tumors (AUC of 0.984)
Daoust et al.	2021	Canada	Surgical oncology	Computer vision	Computer vision model validated on porcine tissue can identify tissue margins based on Raman spectroscopy with accuracy of 0.990 and 0.967

Table 2.
Summary of included studies on intraoperative artificial intelligence/machine learning (AI/ML).

wait for margins to be identified histologically, increasing efficiency and outcomes of tumor resection surgeries (**Table 2**).

5. Enhancement of laparoscopic and minimally invasive surgery

In addition to aiding in tumor resections, computer vision is likely to impact many other aspects of surgery, especially with the increased integration of minimally invasive and robotic surgery [70]. Computer vision ML algorithms in the future may be able to process real time the videos taken during minimally invasive surgery (MIS) and robotic surgery, providing the surgeon with a broad array of additional, structured, and potentially actionable information. For example, computer vision algorithms may be useful in enhancing laparoscopic images. Given the anatomy of the abdomen, one issue common to an entire range of laparoscopic video signals is the quality of images. Nonuniform lighting, light-absorbing surfaces and substances (e.g., blood), along with other reasons for low endoscopic visibility, may lead to increased surgical risk and decreased efficiency in the operating room (OR) [71]. Because of these potential setbacks, computer vision algorithms may be able to process laparoscopic images in real time, digitally increasing lighting, removing vapor haze, and potentially filling in aspects of the image that may be obscured due to low visibility [72]. These applications have the potential to greatly improve ease-of-use of laparoscopes during surgery, decreasing the risk of incorrect targeting and decreasing the amount of time spent operating.

Further integration of computer vision in surgery could even lead to better identification of important anatomical landmarks in minimally invasive and robotic surgery. As mentioned previously, computer vision has already been used to identify objects in images and faces in security videos, and a logical extension of these uses would be the capacity to identify important surgical landmarks. For instance, rates of bile duct injury in laparoscopic cholecystectomies (LCs) have been seen to hover around 0.45–0.8% [73, 74]. One of the most common causes of bile duct injury in LCs is misidentification of the common bile duct for the cystic duct [75]. An ML model trained on imaging data from laparoscopic surgeries was developed to identify critical anatomy in LCs in video with near-human accuracy, potentially leading to reduced risk of bile duct injury in LC in the future [76]. The largest challenge in building a model for this use would be the requirement for labeled video information. More specifically, any actionable model would need to be trained on many videos of laparoscopic surgeries in which the cystic duct is pre-identified in each of the thousands of frames within each training video. This formidable task is further complicated by the natural anatomical variations in human anatomy, necessitating the need for an even larger test data set of "normal variants" that can be encountered in the OR. Despite current limitations, it is likely only a matter of time before high fidelity models can be created, with significant resultant downstream benefits.

Of importance, AI/ML may also play a role as a component of augmented reality (AR) in surgery [77, 78]. One example with relatively mature application of AR is the area of spine surgeries, such as using the XVision Spine System (Augmedics, Arlington Heights, IL, USA) [79]. In this instance, AR-guided surgery works by using CT or MRI imaging to develop a three-dimensional (3D) model, then employing the AR program to overlay the model on the patient using AR glasses or other image projection modalities. Though this is a relatively new technology, initial studies investigating the use of AR systems in cadaveric pedicle screw placement indicate an absolute increase of accuracy from 88% (via fluoroscopy) to 94% (via AR guidance) [80]. In the immediate future, AR implementations will most likely be concentrated in orthopedic surgery and neurosurgery due to the relative immobility of bones and the spine compared to visceral organs. However, the potential increased use of peri- and intraoperative imaging in abdominal and thoracic surgeries may increase the viability of AR guidance in other operation theaters [81, 82].

5.1 Surgical education

Perhaps, the most significant benefit of AR in surgery is in medical education. Head-mounted devices used in AR have already proven useful in various aspects of medical education, including anatomy and surgery [83]. In the near future, AR may allow surgeons to practice various procedures anywhere in a low-stakes environment and decrease cognitive effort, allowing for a more sustained practice [84]. AR may eventually be used within the operating room as a teaching tool, allowing surgeons to manipulate personalized models of the patient's organs based on some of the techniques described previously. Thus, AR may become a valuable supplemental tool to train future surgeons and other specialists who want to practice procedures.

Machine Learning algorithms may play other essential roles in surgical education. Aspiring surgeons start their training with varying degrees of motor skill and learning abilities, with the use of ML algorithms in the future, students may be able to be classified based on generated learning curves. Gao et al. were able to analyze the proficiency of students performing various surgical tasks using an algorithm to predict the number of trials needed for each student to proficiently complete the task [85]. Similar algorithms in the future may be applied to planning surgical resources for students based on the need to optimize learning for all students within a surgical program. Other ML programs may be able to provide feedback to learners about specific skills. For instance, surgical skill is an important factor in patient outcomes, directly preventing complications and indirectly in mediating other elements such as the length of surgery [86]. Thus, measuring and improving surgical skills is important in improving patient care. However, there is a lack of practical objective assessments of surgical skill and dexterity. Currently, many assessments of surgical skills are subjective in nature [87]. AI algorithms may be able to address these concerns.

Video-based learning remains a promising learning method for surgical residents [88]. However, video-based review can be limited by having to parse through long videos, especially when reviewing multiple examples. Hashimoto et al. show that it is possible to develop a computer vision model capable of accurately identifying distinct phases of a surgery [89]. This technology allows surgeons to quickly find specific stages of an operation for more efficient review, and similar AI models have been validated in other types of surgeries as well [90]. While out of the scope of these studies, these models could be supplemented with AI that directly analyzes the surgeon's skills. For instance, an algorithm could be created to rate surgical motion economy within the operation theater, and by proxy surgical skill [91]. Using videos of surgeons performing the same procedure, the algorithm may be able to provide objective feedback on the motion economy and path length compared to other surgeons in a video database. AI programs that combine surgical phase recognition and surgical skill analysis could be used to indicate certain stages of the procedure where the surgeon could improve motion economy. Surgeons, especially those in training, may not be completely aware of unnecessary movements they are making during surgery, and these algorithms could provide an objective way to compare and teach motion economy. AI algorithms may be applied to similar measures, such as fluidity of motion, force application in laparoscopic surgery, or a combination of these factors. In the future, these algorithms may provide objective insight into surgical skills and dexterity, allowing for targeted practice of specific skills (**Table 3**).

Source	Year of publication	Country of origin	Surgical discipline	Studied AI/ML algorithms	Major findings relevant to this review
Kumar et al.	2015	USA	Minimally invasive surgery	Computer vision	Computer vision algorithms, especially with growing usage of surgical robots, may be used to decrease cognitive load through identification of intraoperative phases and segmentation of objects and people within the surgical theater
Xia et al.	2022	Canada	Minimally invasive surgery	Computer vision	Computer vision algorithm can enhance and refine laparoscopic images to optimize vision in occluded regions of the abdominal cavity
Ruiz-Fernandez et al.	2020	Spain	Minimally invasive surgery	Computer vision	Computer vision application was able to process imaging from laparoscopic surgeries to remove water vapor haze and improve visibility in dark areas
Owen et al.	2022	UK	Minimally invasive surgery	Computer vision	Computer vision algorithm developed to identify critical structures in laparoscopic surgeries 65–75% accuracy (compared to 70% baseline). Labels were verified by three expert surgeons afterward

Source	Year of publication	Country of origin	Surgical discipline	Studied AI/ ML algorithms	Major findings relevant to this review
Qian et al.	2019	USA	All surgical disciplines	Augmented reality	Augmented reality could innovate surgery in several ways, including surgical guidance during laparoscopic surgeries, overlay of tumor margins, feedback of distance between instrument and anatomical structures, and the planning of port placement
Gorpas et al.	2019	USA	Surgical oncology	Augmented reality	Augmented reality program can overlay fluorescence data within the da Vinci surgical robot for real-time identification of normal and malignant tissue
Peh et al.	2020	Germany	Spine surgery	Augmented reality	Augmented reality surgical navigation showed improved accuracy of thoracic and lumbar pedicle screw placement in cadavers compared to standard fluoroscopy-guided pedicle placement (94% vs. 88%)
Soler et al.	2004	France	Abdominal surgery	Augmented reality	Augmented reality shows promise in digestive surgery through 3D modeling of abdominal structures, overlay visualizations during operations, and planning of needle targeting
Rad et al.	2022		Thoracic surgery	Augmented reality	Augmented reality may be used in thoracic surgery to improve surgical training, enhance planning through visualization of structures, and provide visual assistance during surgery
Peden et al.	2016	UK	Surgical education	Augmented reality	Augmented reality in suturing skill development in suturing-naïve students has been shown to be more enjoyable than conventional learning with comparable skill development
Barteit et al.	2021	Germany	Surgical education	Augmented reality	Augmented and virtual reality surgical simulations of sleeve gastrectomy led to subjective decreased cognitive effort and decreased stress
Gao et al.	2020	USA	Surgical education	ML	ML model trained on initial completion times of suturing-naïve medical students was able to predict the number of trials needed for proficiency
Hashimoto et al.	2019	USA	Surgical education	Computer vision	Computer vision algorithm can identify the specific phase of laparoscopic sleeve gastrectomy with over 85% accuracy
Garrow et al.	2021	Germany	Surgical education	Computer vision	Computer vision algorithms have shown the ability to identify the specific phase of various surgeries including sleeve gastrectomy,

Source	Year of publication	Country of origin	Surgical discipline	Studied AI/ ML algorithms	Major findings relevant to this review
					laparoscopic cholecystectomy, and colorectal surgery
Azari et al.	2019	USA	Surgical education	Computer vision	Computer vision data for tracking surgeon hand movements during surgery were used to train an ML model for evaluating surgical skill, with measures of motion economy being most precise (R^2 = 0.64)

Table 3.
Summary of included studies on computer vision and augmented reality (AR).

6. Postoperative risk assessment

The use of ML and AI in postoperative risk assessment would work similar to peri- and intraoperative risk assessment using patient vital signs and characteristics. After performing a surgery, the surgeon must be able to triage patients by likelihood of postoperative complications. Improperly triaged high-risk patients may be sent to hospital floors where there is a high patient-to-clinician ratio, which can limit the frequency of patient assessments and lead to higher rates of morbidity and mortality [92]. Loftus et al. were able to develop an AI model capable of using pre- and perioperative labs and vital signs, intraoperative anesthesia variables (such as intraoperative high inspired oxygen fraction (FIo_2)), and postoperative evaluations (including scheduled postop location) to identify undertriaged patients at risk of postoperative complication [92]. In the future, similar technology could be integrated into the electronic health record and send mobile alerts to physicians, allowing for quicker alterations to patient care [93]. Because postoperative risk assessments may utilize more complete information, they have been shown to provide a more accurate prediction of postsurgical prognoses and complications [94, 95].

Machine learning models for postoperative care will also be better suited for predicting pain management needs of the surgical patient. Opiates are common medications prescribed for postoperative pain. However, the opioid epidemic affects over 3 million people in the USA, and it is estimated that 500,000 people in the USA are dependent on opiates [96]. Physicians are now much more aware of the risks of opioid addiction; therefore, opioid dependence and abuse are important considerations to make when prescribing opioids for postoperative pain. A few studies have investigated the use of ML to predict long-term opioid use. One study developed a model to predict long-term opioid use, defined as opioid prescriptions that were requested in addition to the original prescription, in patients who underwent elective hip arthroplasty. Internal validation indicated that the model had good predictive value for the testing cohorts in the study [97]. Other studies have looked at the use of similar algorithms in breast cancer surgery, anterior cruciate ligament (ACL) reconstruction, and joint arthroplasty [98–100]. While these studies did not utilize external validation, these proof-of-concept studies indicate that ML in the future may have utility in predicting long-term opioid use, allowing for more informed prescription of pain medications and potentially earlier identification of patients at risk for opioid dependence.

Machine learning algorithms may also be used for gait analysis in postoperative care. For most elective joint surgeries, postoperative assessment involves patient-reported outcome measures or performance-based metrics like the range of motion and mobility [101]. These assessment methods may introduce bias through subjective ratings of outcomes measures by the patient or through biased ratings of performance metrics by physicians [101]. Gait analysis using ML may be able to provide ancillary objective analysis of postsurgical outcomes. One study showed that an ML model incorporating walking speed, gait cycle, maximum force of a step, and other biomechanical variables was able to separate patients who had total knee arthroplasty with patients who underwent unicompartmental knee arthroplasty [102]. Other studies have shown similar potential in total knee arthroplasty and ACL reconstruction [103, 104]. Furthermore, computer vision can likely be leveraged to increase the power of these models. Currently, there exist programs that allow users to mark parts of the body in videos, such as the knees and elbows, and follow the motion of these structures throughout the video. However, manual input of data is time-consuming and prone to human error. To alleviate these concerns, multiple markerless models have been developed to map out patient gait, tracking the movement of anatomical structures such as the ankles, knees, hips, shoulders, head, and arms that do not require human input [105–107]. Based on gait estimation from video, future ML algorithms may be able to stratify patients based on how well they will regain function following surgery. Algorithms may also be able to identify which patients might experience recurring issues or may be at higher risk of falls based on their gait (**Table 4**) [108].

Source	Year of publication	Country of origin	Surgical discipline	Studied AI/ML algorithms	Major findings relevant to this review
Loftus et al.	2021	USA	Surgical critical care	ML postoperative risk assessment	ML algorithms trained on pre- and intraoperative patient data extracted from the hospital Electronic Health Record (EHR) were used to develop a model that could accurately identify critically ill patients who were undertriaged (Area under the receiver operating characteristic curve (AUROC) of 0.92)
Ren et al.	2022	USA	Surgical critical care	ML postoperative risk assessment	ML algorithm trained on real-time perioperative data extracted from hospital EHR could predict and alert physicians about categorized postoperative complications (AUC between 0.78 and 0.89 depending on complication predicted)
Shahian et al.	2012	USA	Cardiac surgery	ML postoperative risk assessment	ML models trained on data combining clinical and administrative data allowed for the analysis of perioperative and long-term postoperative data for accurate prediction of survival up to 2500 days post-CABG

Source	Year of publication	Country of origin	Surgical discipline	Studied AI/ ML algorithms	Major findings relevant to this review
Forte et al.	2022	Netherlands	Cardiac surgery	ML postoperative risk assessment	ML models implementing postoperative data were more accurately able to predict 30-day and 1-year mortality compared to models using just preoperative data (AUCs of 0.75 and 0.79 using pre- and postoperative data vs. areas under the curve (AUCs) of 0.70 and 0.69 using preoperative data only)
Kunze et al.	2021	USA	Orthopedic surgery	ML postoperative risk assessment	ML models trained preoperative data, including Harris hip score, age, body mass index (BMI), etc., were able to predict prolonged opioid use in patients after hip arthroscopy (AUC of 0.75)
Lötsch et al.	2018	Germany	Surgical oncology	ML postoperative risk assessment	ML models trained on clinical and psychological data (such as subjective answers to pain perception surveys) were able to accurately exclude the possibility of persistent pain (95% accuracy) following breast cancer surgery, although it was unable to predict patients who would experience persistent pain
Anderson et al.	2020	USA	Orthopedic surgery	ML postoperative risk assessment	ML model trained on preoperative demographic data, military employment data (such as rank and time deployed), and prescription data was able to predict patients at risk of long-term opioid use (AUC of 0.76) following ACL reconstruction surgery
Gabriel et al.	2022	USA	Orthopedic surgery	ML postoperative risk assessment	ML model trained on patient demographic data, comorbidities, and perioperative data (such as postoperative day 1 (POD1) morphine equivalents) was able to predict long-term opioid use (up to AUC of 0.94 with balanced bagging classifier)
Kokkotis et al.	2022	Greece	Orthopedic surgery	ML postoperative risk assessment	ML algorithms may be able to provide insight into gait and postoperative outcomes following total knee arthroplasty and ACL surgeries through the use of biomechanical measurements
Jones et al.	2016	UK	Orthopedic surgery	ML postoperative risk assessment	ML algorithm using biomechanical measurements was able to differentiate between patients who underwent total knee arthroplasty

Source	Year of publication	Country of origin	Surgical discipline	Studied AI/ML algorithms	Major findings relevant to this review
					and unicompartmental knee arthroplasty, and who had gaits much more similar to healthy patients
Martins et al.	2015	Portugal	Orthopedic surgery	ML postoperative risk assessment	ML model was used to determine gait differences based on three different assistive devices after total knee arthroscopy, allowing for the classification of the type of assistive device used
Kokkotis et al.	2022	Greece	Orthopedic surgery	ML postoperative risk assessment	ML model trained on ground reaction forces and biometric data allowed for the classification of ACL-deficient, ACL-reconstructed, and healthy patients with accuracy of up to 94.95%
Cao et al.	2017	USA	Orthopedic surgery	Computer vision	Convolutional neural network was implemented to create a program that could estimate human poses even with occlusion of feet or arms during motion
Chen et al.	2022	China	Orthopedic surgery	Computer vision	ML models could classify the type of gait based on computer vision-aided anatomical markers and calculations with up to 98% accuracy
Moro et al.	2022	Italy	Orthopedic surgery	Computer vision	Computer vision algorithm allows for automated gait analysis with biomechanical measurements comparable to manually marked video
Ng et al.	2020	Canada	Orthopedic surgery	Computer vision	Computer vision-aided models trained on human pose estimation and gait variables identified cadence, average margin of stability, and minimum margin of stability as factors significantly associated with falls during the study

Table 4.
Summary of included studies on postoperative artificial intelligence/machine learning (AI/ML).

7. Autonomous robots and artificial intelligence

While the aforementioned applications of AI/ML will greatly enhance surgical outcomes, the most impactful applications of AI will involve the development of autonomous robots that will be able to apply and expand on these algorithms. Robotic autonomy can be categorized based on the need for human involvement in robot function. Within this proposed scale: a 0 denotes a machine that has no inherent autonomy and is rather completely controlled by the operator, a 1 represents a robot that the operator controls but provides some degree of assistance, and 2–5 represent varying levels of autonomy; a 5 represents "true autonomy" of the machine without need for human intervention [109]. Currently, most surgical machines score at level 0 or 1, with machines such as the da Vinci surgical system and robotic endoscopic systems falling squarely in these categories [110]. Applications of level 2 automated robots, such as performing autonomous suturing, have been described [111]. At the current stage, automatons are limited to the autonomy of simple tasks, though there is a push to develop machines that may autonomously perform more complex tasks. Some experiments using phantom tissue have shown success using autonomous robots to ablate abnormal tissue or perform anastomosis of the small bowel, but these experiments were performed on phantom tissue in idealized experimental settings with low trial numbers [112]. Still, these proof-of-concept experiments show that higher-level autonomous robots might emerge sooner rather than later. These complex autonomous robots would integrate multiple sensory modalities, from computer vision to tactile sensation to proprioceptive or auditory information [113].

As AI gets more complicated, the process of training also becomes increasingly complex. Three main learning methods exist for visual-based learning for artificial intelligence: imitation learning, reinforcement learning, and transfer learning [114]. Imitation learning is a method of learning involving the observation of an expert performing the task. Based on the observed actions, the algorithm updates its knowledge (also known as policy) to be more like the demonstration [115]. In an ideal environment, imitation learning will lead to the most reproducible behavior [116]. The use of imitation learning in surgery is limited because of its inability to generalize behaviors. When environments are dissimilar to the demonstration environments, such as differing orientation of visceral organs or working with anatomical variations, the performance of imitation learning algorithms will be suboptimal [116]. This can be alleviated somewhat by dividing the imitation task into subtasks and training subtasks depending on starting circumstances. However, generalizability is still lower than in the other learning methods [115].

Reinforcement learning is another type of learning that is used in AI. This method of learning involves trial-and-error, where the agent performs its task and updates its actions based on the outcomes of its actions. An example of reinforcement learning is the training of the chess engine AlphaZero, in which the engine played many simulated games with itself and improved its playing ability based on the outcomes of each game [117]. Reinforcement learning is a powerful tool that is better able to generalize behaviors compared to imitation algorithms, but reinforcement requires many trials to optimize performance. Additionally, training a model in a real surgical environment is dangerous.

Fortunately, AI flaws can be circumvented via transfer learning, which essentially involves the agent learning through reinforcement learning in a simulated environment and transferring its knowledge to a real environment [114]. Using the simulation, the agent can quickly be trained on many trials before being transferred to real circumstances. Issues for transfer learning are readily apparent; when there is discordance between simulation and real environments, the performance of the model will be suboptimal. A few methods have been proposed to improve transfer learning outcomes. One method is simply improving the quality of the simulation. Computational simulations are much more efficient than physical manipulations of simulated environments, and improvements in computational power are enhancing virtual simulation environments to better model the real world. Other methods involve changing the policies of the agents to better adapt to circumstances that were not seen during simulation training. One proposed system involves the learning of multiple skill latents in simulation. Broadly defined, "skill latents" represent prelearned or predetermined "primitive skills" which can be subsequently combined within a "model-predictive control" environment to perform more complex tasks [118]. These skill latents can then be accessed and simulated in real time when situations arise that have not been seen before, and the skill latents that produce the optimal effect can be chosen for the agent's actions [118]. Instead of perfectly modeling the real world, this approach tries to make the AI's learning as flexible as possible and/or applicable. Because transfer learning models can be trained in simulation, and because these models can be adaptive, it is likely that autonomous surgical robots in the near future will use transfer learning models to navigate the surgical field (**Table 5**).

Source	**Year of publication**	**Country of origin**	**Surgical discipline**	**Studied AI/ML algorithms**	**Major findings relevant to this Review**
Shademan et al.	2016	USA	All surgical disciplines	Automation	An autonomous robot using computer vision and an automated suturing algorithm was able to perform suturing tasks on *ex vivo* and living porcine tissue
Hu et al.	2018	USA	Neurosurgery	Automation	Autonomous robot using computer vision algorithms was able to create a 3D reconstruction of the surgical cavity and successfully perform robotic ablation of a surgical phantom in seven out of ten trials
Tapia et al.	2020	Switzerland	All surgical disciplines	Automation	A proprioceptive liquid-metal stretch sensor was able to reconstruct deformation of soft actuators in real time
Hua et al.	2021	China	All surgical disciplines	Automation	Deep reinforcement learning, imitation learning, and transfer learning are the main methods to teach autonomous robots
Rivera et al.	2022	USA	All surgical disciplines	Automation	Machine learning through primitive imitation led to increased performance compared to other learning algorithms in two different primitive tasks
Kumar et al.	2022	USA	All surgical disciplines	Automation	Though imitation learning algorithms are very powerful in ideal settings, reinforcement learning is more optimal when there is sufficient noise in the data set for various different learning policies and tasks
Silver et al.	2018	USA	All surgical disciplines	Automation	Reinforcement learning algorithm was used to create a program capable of learning and optimizing performance in chess, shogi, and Go

Source	Year of publication	Country of origin	Surgical discipline	Studied AI/ML algorithms	Major findings relevant to this Review
He et al.	2018		All surgical disciples	Automation	Transfer learning algorithms involving prelearned skill latents could be successfully applied to complete new tasks (such as drawing and pushing an object)

Table 5.
Summary of included studies on autonomous robots.

8. Nanotechnology

One technological field that is gaining increased interest in recent years is nanotechnology. Nanotechnology refers to devices or machines on the scale of microns and encompasses a wide range of technologies, including nanosensors, nanoparticles, and nanobots [119]. Nanotechnology opens doors to new therapeutics for a variety of reasons. Most obviously, the size of these devices allows access to previously inaccessible spaces. Due to the nanoscale size of these machines, they have higher surface area-to-volume ratios, leading to increased reactivity, and quantum effects play a larger role in interactions compared to macroscale sizes [120]. While nanotechnology does not necessarily need to involve artificial intelligence, these two fields may work synergistically to help surgeons in the future provide interventions not previously possible.

Because "nano-machines" operate on a scale much smaller than conventional robots, nanotechnology can allow for better and more selective delivery of drugs, such as chemotherapy agents. For instance, nanoparticle capsules may protect agents from enzymatic degradation or unfavorable pH environments or allow drugs to cross the blood–brain barrier [121, 122]. Additionally, one of the most powerful aspects of nanotechnology is the increased specificity of drug delivery targeting. Attaching specific moieties to nanoparticles can allow for targeted binding and release of encapsulated contents [123]. This application has implications in cancer treatment. Although chemotherapeutic agents are useful in treating cancer, these drugs often cause a wide range of adverse effects due to systemic distribution of these drugs. Various nanoparticle vessels, including nanocrystals, liposomes, and carbon nanotubes, can be fitted with surface coatings allowing cell-specific delivery of cancer therapies, ultimately reducing side effects [121, 124, 125]. AI may further increase the specificity of nanoparticle drug delivery through analysis of patterns of biomarkers. Through the integration of AI in biomarker sensing, the presence of different groups and concentrations of certain biomarkers can allow for classification of disease type and stage, enabling targeted and modifiable release of drugs from nanocapsules [126]. The selectivity of nanoparticles can also be leveraged for targeted ablation therapy for certain cancers. For instance, synthetic high-density lipoprotein nanoparticles were used to facilitate the delivery of photothermal ablative agents to hepatocellular carcinoma cells in mouse models, reducing tumor burden and stimulating local immune response [127]. Similar technologies could be applied to other ablation techniques, including radiation, cryoablation, and electroporation, in a wide variety of cancers [128].

Besides use in surgical oncology, nanotechnology may allow surgeons to operate on a nanoscale. Atomic force microscopy (AFM) may be an integral part of nanosurgery in the future. At its core, AFM consists of a microscopic cantilever fitted with a tip along with a laser and photodetector. As the tip of the AFM traverses along a surface, such as tissue, changes in the surface will move the tip and cause deflections of the laser, which can be detected by the photodetector [129]. The use of AFM enables the detection of several angstroms of change [129]. Furthermore, the force applied by the tip to the surface can be used to touch, push, and cut the surface, providing the ability to manipulate membranes, proteins, and DNA [130–132]. Some experiments show the viability of using AFM to alter cell morphology and puncture cell membranes of individual cells [133]. Other uses of AFM in the future include signaling pathway identification, targeted drug delivery using specialized AFM tips, and disruption of cellular connections, such as dendrites, without interfering with cell bodies [130, 134]. Other potential "nano-machines" are limited only by human creativity and may include nanopropellors, nanowires, and "nanograbbers" (microscopic machines created by Leong et al. capable of performing *in vitro* biopsies) [134, 135].

Besides the direct manipulation of tissue, nanotechnology also makes possible a wide range of other surgeries. For instance, nanotechnology may increase the feasibility of islet transplantation in diabetes. While the results from the Edmonton protocol show that islet transplantation has promise in long-term glycemic control in type 1 diabetes, practicality of islet transplantation was limited by immune response against exogenous islet cells, causing gradual loss of islet function [136]. These concerns could be addressed by encapsulating islet cells with nanoparticles, with several approaches having been investigated to decrease immunogenicity of exogenous compounds [137–139]. Thus, alongside improving drug delivery, nanoparticle capsules may also be used to shield contents and suppress immune response.

Finally, nanoparticles may play roles in facilitating hemostasis and preventing infection after surgery. Many different hemostatic nanomaterials, such as mesoporous xerogels, polyphosphate-bound gold colloids, titanium dioxide (TiO_2) nanotubes, and many others, have peen proposed [140]. While additional properties of each nanomaterial differ, they are thought to function by providing scaffolding for coagulation factors [140]. Antimicrobial nanoparticles may also be used for infection control in surgery. Postoperative infection carries a high rate of morbidity. An estimated 11% of deaths in the intensive care unit (ICU) resulted from surgical site infections [141]. Because of this need, antimicrobial nanoparticles may be able to address postsurgical infection risk. Silver nanoparticles have shown promise in accumulating within bacteria and disrupting various cellular processes, such as DNA replication and protein translation [142]. Silver nanoparticles have the potential to improve infection control, especially in orthopedic surgery. Orthopedic implants are susceptible to colonization of biofilm-forming bacteria, which can lead to high risk of morbidities [143]. One concern is the dose-dependent toxicity on human tissue attributable to silver nanoparticle use [144]. However, studies have indicated that osteocytes may be more resilient to this specific type of toxicity. Though silver nanoparticles initially decrease Saos-2 (human osteosarcoma cell line) survivability, Saos-2 cells seem to adapt to silver nanoparticle exposure over the course of 35 days *in vitro* [143]. Given these findings, it is possible that silver nanoparticles may be used to coat orthopedic implants that reduce the effect of osteoblast function (**Table 6**).

Source	Year of publication	Country of origin	Surgical discipline	Studied AI/ML algorithms	Major findings relevant to this review
Roduner	2006	Germany	All surgical disciplines	Nanotechnology	Nanorobots have unique properties due to their microscopic size, including increased surface area-to-volume ratios and increased strength of quantum effects
Hofferberth et al.	2016	USA	Thoracic surgery	Nanotechnology	Nanotechnology may have numerous uses in thoracic surgery, such as nanoparticles mapping lymphatic drainage of malignant tumors, targeting tumor cells for drug delivery, and selective cell ablation
Krůpa et al.	2014	Czech Republic	Neurosurgery	Nanotechnology	Various nanotechnologies have shown promise in transporting drugs across the blood–brain barrier, allowing for targeted delivery into brain tumors
Zhang et al.	2013	China	Surgical oncology	Nanotechnology	Nanotechnology may be able to improve cancer care through encapsulated chemotherapy drugs, allowing for targeted distribution. Nanoparticles may also be able to increase intracellular accumulation of drugs within cancer cells
Xu et al.	2021	China	Surgical oncology, urology	Nanotechnology	Nanotechnology may be able to improve bladder cancer care through targeted intravesical delivery of various drugs
Khawaja	2011	Pakistan	Neurosurgery	Nanotechnology	Nanotechnology may improve glioblastoma multiforme outcomes through targeted chemotherapy delivery, thermo- and photo-therapy, and surgical nanorobots
Adir et al.	2020	Israel	Surgical oncology	Nanotechnology, ML	ML algorithms can be used to analyze complexes of biomarkers to classify various cellular disease states, allowing for targeted delivery of drugs via nanotechnology
Wang et al.	2021	China	Surgical oncology	Nanotechnology	Nanoplatforms may be able to improve the delivery of cancer drugs as seen in multiple studies
Binnig et al.	1986	USA	All surgical disciplines	Nanotechnology	Atomic force microscope that could measure vertical

Source	Year of publication	Country of origin	Surgical discipline	Studied AI/ML algorithms	Major findings relevant to this review
					displacement of the cantilever tip less than 1 Å was developed
Song et al.	2012	USA	All surgical disciplines	Nanotechnology	A modified atomic force microscope setup that would allow for mechanical manipulation of cellular samples, with possible applications to separating cellular junctions, was created
Li et al.	2005	USA	All surgical specialties	Nanotechnology	A modified atomic force microscope attached with specific antibodies was used to recognize cellular receptors and provide augmented reality feedback to the user, allowing for nanomanipulation of the sample
Wen and Goh	2004	Canada	All surgical specialties	Nanotechnology	Atomic force microscopy was able to incise a single collagen fibril
Yang et al.	2015	USA	All surgical specialties	Nanotechnology	Atomic force microscopy was used to penetrate fixed HaCaT cell membranes and disrupt intermediate filaments, leading to decreased intercellular connections
Brodie and Vasdev	2018	UK	All surgical specialties	Nanotechnology	Nanomachines, such as micropipettes to cleave dendritic connections or "micrograbbers" to biopsy-specific cells, may innovate nanosurgery in the future
Leong et al.	2009	USA	All surgical specialties	Nanotechnology	A tetherless, temperature-activated microgripper 190 μm when closed was able to take biopsy samples from *ex vivo* tissue samples
Im et al.	2012	South Korea	Surgical oncology	Nanotechnology	Coating rat allotransplanted islet cells with nanolayer shielding almost doubled survival against immune response (6.8 days vs. 3.6 days)
Park et al.	2018	South Korea	Surgical oncology	Nanotechnology	Nanolayer shielding of allotransplanted islet cells was validated in monkey models, with heparin nanoshielded islet grafts surviving average of 108 days vs. 68.5 days in the control

Source	Year of publication	Country of origin	Surgical discipline	Studied AI/ML algorithms	Major findings relevant to this review
Izadi et al.	2018	Iran	Surgical oncology	Nanotechnology	Nanolayer shielding of mouse islet cells with poly(ethylene glycol) was conjugated with Jagged-1 (JAG-1), which led to significant reduction in fasting blood glucose ($p < 0.01$)
Sun et al.	2018	China	Orthopedic surgery	Nanotechnology	Nanotechnology has enabled the development of many different kinds of synthetic hemostatic materials, including silica-based xerogels, self-assembled peptides, ethylene/propylene oxide gels, TiO_2 nanotubes, polyphosphate gold colloids, and others
Rai et al.	2012	India	All surgical disciplines	Nanotechnology	Silver nanoparticles have been shown in various studies to have broad-spectrum antimicrobial effects through disruption of various cellular processes
Castiglioni et al.	2017	Italy	Orthopedic surgery	Nanotechnology	High concentrations of silver nanoparticles initially reduced Saos-2 osteogenic cell numbers, but this reduction decreased over 35 days without impairing cellular differentiation

Table 6.
Summary of included studies on nanotechnology.

9. Limitations and concerns

Though AI shows great promise in changing many aspects of medical and surgical care, it is important to highlight the limitations of this technology. The construction of ML algorithms is reliant on large amounts of data to create generalizable algorithms that limit unnecessary data within the data set [145]. The classification of ML model algorithms can identify tumors from imaging. Both training and test data sets still require annotation, manpower, and time [12, 146]. These factors limit how quickly these algorithms can be generated. Additionally, ML algorithms identify patterns from input data without interpretation or critical analysis and may be prone to biases within the data set. There often exist biases in who participates in clinical trials, and this may lead to outputs that disproportionately segregate minorities and other groups which are not as well represented in the training data for the ML model [147, 148]. In some cases, minute changes or fluctuations in the input data can drastically affect the model field output [146]. In the same vein, poor data, such as poor video or image quality, can have deleterious effects on the quality of the model [149]. Because of this, standardization of imagining techniques and video characteristics is vital for model efficacy [146]. Verifying the integrity of these models is integral to maintaining patient autonomy. Faulty or biased recommendations made by AI models can affect a patient's ability to provide informed consent for their care [150]. Finally, there may be a risk for "adversarial attacks," defined as data inputted in the training set with the intention of biasing outputs [151]. Notably, potential methods for adversarial attacks have been identified for every type of machine learning model and may be as overt as modifying input data or as seemingly innocuous as rotating an image slightly [151, 152]. There may be many reasons for adversarial data input, from fraudulent reimbursement to altering research outcomes, so it is vital that methods are implemented to prevent intentional and unintentional biases in these models.

Ethical concerns surrounding the use of AI center around oversight and liability. It is important that AI is tested and verified before actual clinical use, but there are currently no governing body and no approval process for reviewing ML algorithms in clinical care, let alone for autonomous surgery [12]. This is especially important because of the "black-box" effect, which is especially prevalent in deep learning algorithms. Due to the existence of "hidden" layers in deep learning neural networks, it is often not entirely clear how the AI model arrives at its output, and this can limit how much trust physicians and patients put in the recommendations made by these algorithms [153]. Without entities to review these algorithms, AI will remain primarily experimental. There are many legal concerns regarding the use of AI in surgery. One of the most prominent concerns among physicians is liability [154, 155]. Currently, there is essentially no case law on the legality of AI in clinical settings [155]. Therefore, legal entities must establish how malpractice and liability are handled if complications occur because of the use of AI. Without answers to complex legal questions, the use of AI in surgery will be severely limited. According to Price et al., physicians are incentivized to minimize the use of AI under current law. Normally, a physician's actions are privileged under tort law if normal standard of care is followed [155]. However, if a physician follows AI recommendations that go against the current standard of care, even if the AI recommendation is correct, any resulting poor outcomes could lead to litigation [155]. Thus, under current law, the clinical use of AI will mostly be limited to confirming clinical decisions, greatly reducing the potential value of AI. Finally, in cases where data are stored on the cloud or in cases where data are crowd-sourced, there may be data privacy concerns [149]. Additionally, in shared data, there may be concerns about the ownership of uploaded data [149]. Thus, with each application of AI, terms must clearly delineate medicolegal terms, who owns uploaded data, and how models may be monetized.

10. Future implications for surgeons

Though important barriers must be addressed before AI/ML can be more broadly implemented in direct patient care, it is evident how powerful AI/ML can be in finding patterns and facilitating/directing clinical care in the future. While some surgeons may be concerned about AI replacing job opportunities in the future, AI should instead be seen as a dynamic tool for enhancing surgeons' abilities to provide optimal patient care. AI algorithms in the near future will potentially improve the diagnosis of conditions and enhance the prediction of complications. These algorithms can consolidate vast amounts of data—more than any surgeon could reasonably cognitively process—and thus may be ideal in helping surgeons identify patients at risk for certain complications, ultimately making surgeries safer for patients [156]. This is addition to many other benefits appreciated across immediately adjacent clinical and nonclinical fields, applications, and implementations. When properly leveraged, the use of AI will help decrease cognitive load and allow surgeons to focus more on other aspects of patient care.

Artificial intelligence may enhance many aspects of patient care in the future, but machines cannot replace the human aspect of medicine. Though AI will allow providers in the future to parse massive data sets and find patterns that would previously have been missed, AI does not diminish the need for human-human interaction and the surgeon-patient relationship [157]. The surgeon-patient relationship is still an essential aspect of care and is still vital in gaining the trust of the patient. Given the complex nature of ML algorithms, patients may not be willing to trust recommendations from AI, especially in the near future. Thus, surgeons will remain instrumental in the care of patients and can serve as advocates for the many uses of AI in the future. Though surgeons in the future may utilize AI to enhance diagnosis, medical management, and surgical procedures, it is critical that they do not solely rely on these algorithms. Reliance solely on AI may lead to the "deskilling" of providers and may lead to missing mistakes made by these algorithms [158].

Finally, while AI/ML may help enhance many other aspects and facets of patient care, it is critically important to remember that it is most likely surgeons will be ultimately responsible for interpreting patterns identified by AI and determining the role of AI in surgery. Therefore, it is vital for surgeons to work with data scientists, machine learning experts, and other healthcare team members to determine how AI can be utilized for optimal patient care. AI has the potential to be a powerful tool, but it will only be as helpful as the surgeons who wield it.

11. Conclusions

Artificial intelligence and machine learning have a myriad of uses in surgery in all surgical disciplines. AI may enhance disease diagnosis, help surgeons identify patients at risk of complications, and improve the ease of minimally invasive surgery. Furthermore, AI shows promise in improving surgical education and may eventually be used in fully autonomous surgery and nanosurgery. Despite its potential uses, AI is currently limited by large data requirements, concerns about the integrity of data input, and ethical and legal considerations. Surgeons should work to address these issues and take an active role in determining the best ways to implement AI to optimize patient care.

Author details

Ryan Yimeng Lee[1,2]*, Alyssa Imperatore Ziehm[3], Lauryn Ullrich[3] and Stanislaw P. Stawicki[4]

1 Lewis Katz School of Medicine at Temple University, Philadelphia, Pennsylvania, USA

2 St. Luke's University Health Network, Bethlehem, Pennsylvania, USA

3 Department of Surgery, Regional Level I Trauma Network, St. Luke's University Health Network, Bethlehem, Pennsylvania, USA

4 Department of Research and Innovation, St. Luke's University Health Network, Bethlehem, Pennsylvania, USA

*Address all correspondence to: ryan.lee0014@temple.edu

References

[1] Ibrahim A et al. Artificial intelligence in digital breast pathology: Techniques and applications. The Breast. 2020;**49**: 267-273

[2] Hua TK. A short review on machine learning. Authorea. 2022

[3] Lonsdale H, Jalali A, Gálvez JA, Ahumada LM, Simpao AF. Artificial intelligence in anesthesiology: Hype, hope, and hurdles. Anesthesia and Analgesia. 2020;**130**:1111-1113

[4] Hashimoto DA, Rosman G, Rus D, Meireles OR. Artificial intelligence in surgery: Promises and perils. Annals of Surgery. 2018;**268**(1):70-76

[5] Jarrahi MH. In the age of the smart artificial intelligence: AI's dual capacities for automating and informating work. Business Information Review. 2019; **36**(4):178-187

[6] Agrawal A, Gans JS, Goldfarb A. Artificial intelligence: The ambiguous labor market impact of automating prediction. Journal of Economic Perspectives. 2019;**33**(2): 31-50

[7] Guszcza J, Lewis H, Evans-Greenwood P. Cognitive collaboration: Why humans and computers think better together. Deloitte Review. 2017; **20**:8-29

[8] Brynjolfsson E, McAfee A. Winning the race with ever-smarter machines. MIT Sloan Management Review. 2012; **53**(2):53

[9] Jarrahi MH. Artificial intelligence and the future of work: Human-AI symbiosis in organizational decision making. Business Horizons. 2018;**61**(4): 577-586

[10] Goldfarb A, Lindsay J. Artificial Intelligence in War: Human Judgment as an Organizational Strength and a Strategic Liability. Brookings Institution; 2020

[11] De Luca G. The development of machine intelligence in a computational universe. Technology in Society. 2021; **65**:101553

[12] Gumbs AA et al. Artificial intelligence surgery: How do we get to autonomous actions in surgery? Sensors. 2021;**21**(16):5526

[13] Russel SJ, Norvig P. Artificial Intelligence a Modern Approach. Upper Saddle River, New Jersey, USA: Pearson Education Inc.; 2010

[14] LeCun Y, Bengio Y, Hinton G. Deep learning. Nature. 2015;**521**(7553): 436-444

[15] Loftus TJ et al. Artificial intelligence and surgical decision-making. JAMA Surgery. 2020;**155**(2):148-158

[16] Pereira SS, Guimarães M, Monteiro MP. Towards precision medicine in bariatric surgery prescription. Reviews in Endocrine and Metabolic Disorders. 2023:1-17

[17] Topart P. Obesity surgery: Which procedure should we choose and why? Journal of Visceral Surgery. 2023;**160**(2): S30-S37

[18] Bihorac A et al. MySurgeryRisk: Development and validation of a machine-learning risk algorithm for major complications and death after surgery. Annals of Surgery. 2019;**269**(4): 652

[19] Zhou C, Wang Y, Xue Q, Yang J, Zhu Y. Predicting difficult airway intubation in thyroid surgery using multiple machine learning and deep learning algorithms. Frontiers in Public Health. 2022;**10**:937471

[20] Wilson B et al. Predicting spinal surgery candidacy from imaging data using machine learning. Neurosurgery. 2021;**89**(1):116-121

[21] Bellini V, Valente M, Del Rio P, Bignami E. Artificial intelligence in thoracic surgery: A narrative review. Journal of Thoracic Disease. 2021;**13**(12): 6963

[22] Malani SN IV, Shrivastava D, Raka MS, Raka MS IV. A comprehensive review of the role of artificial intelligence in obstetrics and gynecology. Cureus. 2023;**15**(2):e34891

[23] Shoham G, Berl A, Shir-az O, Shabo S, Shalom A. Predicting Mohs surgery complexity by applying machine learning to patient demographics and tumor characteristics. Experimental Dermatology. 2022;**31**(7): 1029-1035

[24] Bian Y et al. Artificial intelligence to predict lymph node metastasis at CT in pancreatic ductal adenocarcinoma. Radiology. 2023; **306**(1):160-169

[25] Etienne H et al. Artificial intelligence in thoracic surgery: Past, present, perspective and limits. European Respiratory Review. 2020;**29**(157): 200010

[26] Fairchild AT et al. A deep learning-based computer aided detection (CAD) system for difficult-to-detect brain metastases. International Journal of Radiation Oncology* Biology* Physics. 2023;**115**(3):779-793

[27] Martin RK, Ley C, Pareek A, Groll A, Tischer T, Seil R. Artificial intelligence and machine learning: An introduction for orthopaedic surgeons. Knee Surgery, Sports Traumatology, Arthroscopy. 2022;**30**:1-4

[28] Savage N. How AI is improving cancer diagnostics. Nature. 2020; **579**(7800):S14-S14

[29] Cui X et al. Performance of a deep learning-based lung nodule detection system as an alternative reader in a Chinese lung cancer screening program. European Journal of Radiology. 2022; **146**:110068

[30] Vigueras-Guillén JP, van Rooij J, Engel A, Lemij HG, van Vliet LJ, Vermeer KA. Deep learning for assessing the corneal endothelium from specular microscopy images up to 1 year after ultrathin-DSAEK surgery. Translational Vision Science & Technology. 2020; **9**(2):49-49

[31] Koçak B, Durmaz EŞ, Ateş E, Kılıçkesmez Ö. Radiomics with artificial intelligence: A practical guide for beginners. Diagnostic and Interventional Radiology. 2019;**25**(6):485

[32] Shur JD et al. Radiomics in oncology: A practical guide. Radiographics. 2021; **41**(6):1717-1732

[33] Zhang Y et al. Risk factors for axillary lymph node metastases in clinical stage T1-2N0M0 breast cancer patients. Medicine. 2019;**98**(40):e17481

[34] Giuliano AE et al. Effect of axillary dissection vs no axillary dissection on 10-year overall survival among women with invasive breast cancer and sentinel node metastasis: The ACOSOG Z0011 (Alliance) randomized clinical trial. JAMA. 2017;**318**(10):918-926

[35] Wilke LG et al. Surgical complications associated with sentinel lymph node biopsy: Results from a prospective international cooperative group trial. Annals of Surgical Oncology. 2006;**13**:491-500

[36] Wang Y et al. Improved false negative rate of axillary status using sentinel lymph node biopsy and ultrasound-suspicious lymph node sampling in patients with early breast cancer. BMC Cancer. 2015;**15**(1):1-7

[37] Yu Y et al. Magnetic resonance imaging radiomics predicts preoperative axillary lymph node metastasis to support surgical decisions and is associated with tumor microenvironment in invasive breast cancer: A machine learning, multicenter study. eBioMedicine. 2021;**69**:103460

[38] Chang F-C et al. Magnetic resonance radiomics features and prognosticators in different molecular subtypes of pediatric Medulloblastoma. PLoS One. 2021;**16**(7):e0255500

[39] Hsich EM et al. Variables of importance in the scientific registry of transplant recipients database predictive of heart transplant waitlist mortality. American Journal of Transplantation. 2019;**19**(7):2067-2076

[40] Giglio MC et al. Machine learning improves the accuracy of graft weight prediction in living donor liver transplantation. Liver Transplantation. 2022;**29**(2):172-183

[41] Guijo-Rubio D, Gutiérrez PA, Hervás-Martínez C. Machine learning methods in organ transplantation. Current Opinion in Organ Transplantation. 2020;**25**(4):399-405

[42] Hatib F et al. Machine-learning algorithm to predict hypotension based on high-fidelity arterial pressure waveform analysis. Anesthesiology. 2018;**129**(4):663-674

[43] Lundberg SM et al. Explainable machine-learning predictions for the prevention of hypoxaemia during surgery. Nature Biomedical Engineering. 2018;**2**(10):749-760

[44] Lee SM et al. Development and validation of a prediction model for need for massive transfusion during surgery using intraoperative hemodynamic monitoring data. JAMA Network Open. 2022;**5**(12):e2246637-e2246637

[45] Loftus TJ, Upchurch GR, Bihorac A. Use of artificial intelligence to represent emergent systems and augment surgical decision-making. JAMA Surgery. 2019; **154**(9):791-792

[46] Yang Q, Steinfeld A, Zimmerman J. Unremarkable AI: Fitting intelligent decision support into critical, clinical decision-making processes. In: Proceedings of the 2019 CHI Conference on Human Factors in Computing Systems. Scotland, UK: Association for Computing Machinery Special Interest Group on Computer-Human Interaction in Glasgow; 2019. pp. 1-11

[47] Stawicki S. Fundamentals of Patient Safety in Medicine and Surgery. New Delhi, India: Wolters Kluwer (India) Pvt. Ltd; 2015

[48] Laessig MA et al. Potential implementations of blockchain technology in patient safety: A high-level overview. In: Blockchain in Healthcare: From Disruption to Integration. Cham, Switzerland: Springer; 2023. pp. 117-140

[49] Pappada SM et al. Evaluation of a model for glycemic prediction in

critically ill surgical patients. PLoS One. 2013;**8**(7):e69475

[50] Barth N, Seamon MJ. Situation awareness in patient safety. Fundamentals of Patient Safety in Medicine and Surgery. 2015;**15**:105

[51] Komorowski M, Celi LA, Badawi O, Gordon AC, Faisal AA. The artificial intelligence clinician learns optimal treatment strategies for sepsis in intensive care. Nature Medicine. 2018; **24**(11):1716-1720

[52] Ehrmann DE et al. Evaluating and reducing cognitive load should be a priority for machine learning in healthcare. Nature Medicine. 2022;**28**(7): 1331-1333

[53] De Melo CM, Kim K, Norouzi N, Bruder G, Welch G. Reducing cognitive load and improving warfighter problem solving with intelligent virtual assistants. Frontiers in Psychology. 2020; **11**:554706

[54] Lee LW, Dabirian A, McCarthy IP, Kietzmann J. Making sense of text: Artificial intelligence-enabled content analysis. European Journal of Marketing. 2020;**54**:615-644

[55] Ofli F et al. Combining human computing and machine learning to make sense of big (aerial) data for disaster response. Big Data. 2016;**4**(1): 47-59

[56] Özdemir V, Hekim N. Birth of industry 5.0: Making sense of big data with artificial intelligence, "the internet of things" and next-generation technology policy. Omics: A Journal of Integrative Biology. 2018;**22**(1): 65-76

[57] Vyborny CJ, Giger ML. Computer vision and artificial intelligence in mammography. AJR. American Journal of Roentgenology. 1994;**162**(3):699-708

[58] Li X, Shi Y. Computer vision imaging based on artificial intelligence. In: 2018 International Conference on Virtual Reality and Intelligent Systems (ICVRIS). Hunan, China: IEEE; 2018. pp. 22-25

[59] Voulodimos A, Doulamis N, Doulamis A, Protopapadakis E. Deep learning for computer vision: A brief review. Computational Intelligence and Neuroscience. 2018;**2018**:7068349

[60] Hollon TC et al. Near real-time intraoperative brain tumor diagnosis using stimulated Raman histology and deep neural networks. Nature Medicine. 2020;**26**(1):52-58

[61] Orringer DA et al. Rapid intraoperative histology of unprocessed surgical specimens via fibre-laser-based stimulated Raman scattering microscopy. Nature Biomedical Engineering. 2017;**1**(2):0027

[62] Mahe E et al. Intraoperative pathology consultation: Error, cause and impact. Canadian Journal of Surgery. 2013;**56**(3):E13

[63] Chen SB, Novoa RA. Artificial intelligence for dermatopathology: Current trends and the road ahead. Seminars in Diagnostic Pathology. Elsevier. 2022;**39**(4):298-304

[64] Bari H, Wadhwani S, Dasari BV. Role of artificial intelligence in hepatobiliary and pancreatic surgery. World Journal of Gastrointestinal Surgery. 2021;**13**(1):7

[65] Robertson S, Azizpour H, Smith K, Hartman J. Digital image analysis in breast pathology—From image

processing techniques to artificial intelligence. Translational Research. 2018;**194**:19-35

[66] Golden JA. Deep learning algorithms for detection of lymph node metastases from breast cancer: Helping artificial intelligence be seen. JAMA. 2017; **318**(22):2184-2186

[67] Hotsinpiller W, Everett A, Richman J, Parker C, Boggs D. Rates of margin positive resection with breast conservation for invasive breast cancer using the NCDB. The Breast. 2021;**60**: 86-89

[68] Choti MA et al. Trends in long-term survival following liver resection for hepatic colorectal metastases. Annals of Surgery. 2002;**235**(6):759

[69] Daoust F et al. Handheld macroscopic Raman spectroscopy imaging instrument for machine-learning-based molecular tissue margins characterization. Journal of Biomedical Optics. 2021;**26**(2):022911

[70] Kumar S, Singhal P, Krovi VN. Computer-vision-based decision support in surgical robotics. IEEE Design & Test. 2015;**32**(5):89-97

[71] Xia W, Chen E, Pautler S, Peters T. Laparoscopic image enhancement based on distributed retinex optimization with refined information fusion. Neurocomputing. 2022;**483**:460-473

[72] Ruiz-Fernández D, Galiana-Merino JJ, de Ramón-Fernández A, Vives-Boix V, Enríquez-Buendía P. A dcp-based method for improving laparoscopic images. Journal of Medical Systems. 2020;**44**:1-9

[73] Pesce A, Portale TR, Minutolo V, Scilletta R, Destri GL, Puleo S. Bile duct injury during laparoscopic cholecystectomy without intraoperative cholangiography: A retrospective study on 1,100 selected patients. Digestive Surgery. 2012;**29**(4):310-314

[74] Karvonen J, Gullichsen R, Laine S, Salminen P, Grönroos JM. Bile duct injuries during laparoscopic cholecystectomy: Primary and long-term results from a single institution. Surgical Endoscopy. 2007;**21**:1069-1073

[75] Moghul F, Kashyap S. Bile Duct Injury. Treasure Island (FL): StatPearls Publishing; 2022

[76] Owen D, Grammatikopoulou M, Luengo I, Stoyanov D. Automated identification of critical structures in laparoscopic cholecystectomy. International Journal of Computer Assisted Radiology and Surgery. 2022; **17**(12):2173-2181

[77] Qian L, Wu JY, DiMaio SP, Navab N, Kazanzides P. A review of augmented reality in robotic-assisted surgery. IEEE Transactions on Medical Robotics and Bionics. 2019;**2**(1):1-16

[78] Gorpas D et al. Autofluorescence lifetime augmented reality as a means for real-time robotic surgery guidance in human patients. Scientific Reports. 2019; **9**(1):1187

[79] Dibble CF, Molina CA. Device profile of the XVision-spine (XVS) augmented-reality surgical navigation system: Overview of its safety and efficacy. Expert Review of Medical Devices. 2021;**18**(1):1-8

[80] Peh S et al. Accuracy of augmented reality surgical navigation for minimally invasive pedicle screw insertion in the thoracic and lumbar spine with a new tracking device. The Spine Journal. 2020; **20**(4):629-637

[81] Soler L et al. Virtual reality and augmented reality in digestive surgery. In: Third IEEE and ACM International Symposium on Mixed and Augmented Reality. Arlington, VA, USA: IEEE; 2004. pp. 278-279

[82] Arjomandi Rad A et al. Extended, virtual and augmented reality in thoracic surgery: A systematic review. Interactive Cardio Vascular and Thoracic Surgery. 2022;**34**(2):201-211

[83] Peden RG, Mercer R, Tatham AJ. The use of head-mounted display eyeglasses for teaching surgical skills: A prospective randomised study. International Journal of Surgery. 2016; **34**:169-173

[84] Barteit S, Lanfermann L, Bärnighausen T, Neuhann F, Beiersmann C. Augmented, mixed, and virtual reality-based head-mounted devices for medical education: Systematic review. JMIR Serious Games. 2021;**9**(3):e29080

[85] Gao Y, Kruger U, Intes X, Schwaitzberg S, De S. A machine learning approach to predict surgical learning curves. Surgery. 2020;**167**(2): 321-327

[86] Cheng H et al. Prolonged operative duration is associated with complications: A systematic review and meta-analysis. Journal of Surgical Research. 2018;**229**: 134-144

[87] Darzi A, Smith S, Taffinder N. Assessing operative skill: Needs to become more objective. BMJ. 1999;**318**: 887-888

[88] Hu Y-Y et al. Complementing operating room teaching with video-based coaching. JAMA Surgery. 2017; **152**(4):318-325

[89] Hashimoto DA et al. Computer vision analysis of intraoperative video: Automated recognition of operative steps in laparoscopic sleeve gastrectomy. Annals of Surgery. 2019; **270**(3):414

[90] Garrow CR et al. Machine learning for surgical phase recognition: A systematic review. Annals of Surgery. 2021;**273**(4):684-693

[91] Azari DP et al. Modeling surgical technical skill using expert assessment for automated computer rating. Annals of Surgery. 2019;**269**(3):574

[92] Loftus TJ et al. Association of postoperative undertriage to hospital wards with mortality and morbidity. JAMA Network Open. 2021;**4**(11): e2131669-e2131669

[93] Ren Y et al. Performance of a machine learning algorithm using electronic health record data to predict postoperative complications and report on a mobile platform. JAMA Network Open. 2022;**5**(5):e2211973-e2211973

[94] Shahian DM et al. Predictors of long-term survival after coronary artery bypass grafting surgery: Results from the Society of Thoracic Surgeons adult cardiac surgery database (the ASCERT study). Circulation. 2012;**125**(12): 1491-1500

[95] Forte JC et al. Comparison of machine learning models including preoperative, intraoperative, and postoperative data and mortality after cardiac surgery. JAMA Network Open. 2022;**5**(10):e2237970-e2237970

[96] Azadfard M, Huecker MR, Leaming JM. Opioid Addiction. Treasure Island (FL): StatPearls Publishing; 2022

[97] Kunze KN, Polce EM, Alter TD, Nho SJ. Machine learning algorithms predict prolonged opioid use in opioid-naïve primary hip arthroscopy patients. JAAOS Global Research & Reviews. 2021;**5**(5):e21

[98] Lötsch J et al. Machine-learning-derived classifier predicts absence of persistent pain after breast cancer surgery with high accuracy. Breast Cancer Research and Treatment. 2018; **171**:399-411

[99] Anderson AB, Grazal CF, Balazs GC, Potter BK, Dickens JF, Forsberg JA. Can predictive modeling tools identify patients at high risk of prolonged opioid use after ACL reconstruction? Clinical Orthopaedics and Related Research. 2020;**478**(7):1603

[100] Gabriel RA et al. Machine learning approach to predicting persistent opioid use following lower extremity joint arthroplasty. Regional Anesthesia & Pain Medicine. 2022;**47**(5):313-319

[101] Kokkotis C et al. Identifying gait-related functional outcomes in post-knee surgery patients using machine learning: A systematic review. International Journal of Environmental Research and Public Health. 2022;**20**(1):448

[102] Jones G et al. Gait comparison of unicompartmental and total knee arthroplasties with healthy controls. The Bone & Joint Journal. 2016;**98**(10_Supple_B):16-21

[103] Martins M, Santos C, Costa L, Frizera A. Feature reduction with PCA/KPCA for gait classification with different assistive devices. International Journal of Intelligent Computing and Cybernetics. 2015;**8**(4):363-382

[104] Kokkotis C et al. Leveraging explainable machine learning to identify gait biomechanical parameters associated with anterior cruciate ligament injury. Scientific Reports. 2022; **12**(1):6647

[105] Cao Z, Simon T, Wei S-E, Sheikh Y. Realtime multi-person 2d pose estimation using part affinity fields. In: Proceedings of the IEEE Conference on Computer Vision and Pattern Recognition. Honolulu, HI, USA: IEEE; 2017. pp. 7291-7299

[106] Chen B et al. Computer vision and machine learning-based gait pattern recognition for flat fall prediction. Sensors. 2022;**22**(20):7960

[107] Kwon J, Lee Y, Lee J. Comparative study of markerless vision-based gait analyses for person Re-identification. Sensors. 2021;**21**(24):8208

[108] Ng K-D, Mehdizadeh S, Iaboni A, Mansfield A, Flint A, Taati B. Measuring gait variables using computer vision to assess mobility and fall risk in older adults with dementia. IEEE Journal of Translational Engineering in Health and Medicine. 2020;**8**:1-9

[109] Yang G-Z et al. Medical robotics—Regulatory, ethical, and legal considerations for increasing levels of autonomy. Science Robotics. 2017;**2**: eaam8638

[110] Saeidi H et al. Autonomous robotic laparoscopic surgery for intestinal anastomosis. Science Robotics. 2022; **7**(62):eabj2908

[111] Shademan A, Decker RS, Opfermann JD, Leonard S, Krieger A, Kim PC. Supervised autonomous robotic soft tissue surgery. Science Translational Medicine. 2016;**8**(337):337ra64

[112] Hu D, Gong Y, Seibel EJ, Sekhar LN, Hannaford B. Semi-autonomous

image-guided brain tumour resection using an integrated robotic system: A bench-top study. The International Journal of Medical Robotics and Computer Assisted Surgery. 2018;**14**(1):e1872

[113] Tapia J, Knoop E, Mutný M, Otaduy MA, Bächer M. Makesense: Automated sensor design for proprioceptive soft robots. Soft Robotics. 2020;7(3):332-345

[114] Hua J, Zeng L, Li G, Ju Z. Learning for a robot: Deep reinforcement learning, imitation learning, transfer learning. Sensors. 2021;**21**(4):1278

[115] Rivera C, Popek KM, Ashcraft C, Staley EW, Katyal KD, Paulhamus BL. Learning generalizable behaviors from demonstration. Frontiers in Neurorobotics. 2022;**16**:932652

[116] Kumar A, Hong J, Singh A, Levine S. When should we prefer offline reinforcement learning over behavioral cloning? arXiv. Vol. abs/2204.05618. 2022

[117] Silver D et al. A general reinforcement learning algorithm that masters chess, shogi, and go through self-play. Science. 2018;**362**(6419): 1140-1144

[118] He Z et al. Zero-shot skill composition and simulation-to-real transfer by learning task representations. arXiv. Vol. abs/1810.02422. 2018

[119] Tan A et al. Nanotechnology and regenerative therapeutics in plastic surgery: The next frontier. Journal of Plastic, Reconstructive & Aesthetic Surgery. 2016;**69**(1):1-13

[120] Roduner E. Size matters: Why nanomaterials are different. Chemical Society Reviews. 2006;**35**(7):583-592

[121] Hofferberth SC, Grinstaff MW, Colson YL. Nanotechnology applications in thoracic surgery. European Journal of Cardio-Thoracic Surgery. 2016;**50**(1):6-16

[122] Krůpa P, Řehák S, Diaz-Garcia D, Filip S. Nanotechnology–new trends in the treatment of brain tumours. Acta Medica. 2015;**57**(4):142-150

[123] Zhang G, Zeng X, Li P. Nanomaterials in cancer-therapy drug delivery system. Journal of Biomedical Nanotechnology. 2013;**9**(5):741-750

[124] Xu Y et al. Application of nanotechnology in the diagnosis and treatment of bladder cancer. Journal of Nanobiotechnology. 2021;**19**:1-18

[125] Khawaja AM. The legacy of nanotechnology: Revolution and prospects in neurosurgery. International Journal of Surgery. 2011;**9**(8):608-614

[126] Adir O et al. Integrating artificial intelligence and nanotechnology for precision cancer medicine. Advanced Materials. 2020;**32**(13):1901989

[127] Wang J et al. Hepatocellular carcinoma growth retardation and PD-1 blockade therapy potentiation with synthetic high-density lipoprotein. Nano Letters. 2019;**19**(8):5266-5276

[128] Wang K et al. Combination of ablation and immunotherapy for hepatocellular carcinoma: Where we are and where to go. Frontiers in Immunology. 2021;**12**:792781

[129] Binnig G, Quate CF, Gerber C. Atomic force microscope. Physical Review Letters. 1986;**56**(9):930

[130] Song B, Yang R, Xi N, Patterson KC, Qu C, Lai KWC. Cellular-level surgery using nano robots. Journal of Laboratory Automation. 2012;**17**(6):425-434

[131] Li G, Xi N, Wang DH. In situ sensing and manipulation of molecules in biological samples using a nanorobotic system. Nanomedicine: Nanotechnology, Biology and Medicine. 2005;**1**(1):31-40

[132] Wen CK, Goh MC. AFM nanodissection reveals internal structural details of single collagen fibrils. Nano Letters. 2004;**4**(1):129-132

[133] Yang R et al. Cellular level robotic surgery: Nanodissection of intermediate filaments in live keratinocytes. Nanomedicine: Nanotechnology, Biology and Medicine. 2015;**11**(1):137-145

[134] Brodie A, Vasdev N. The future of robotic surgery. The Annals of The Royal College of Surgeons of England. 2018; **100**(Supplement 7):4-13

[135] Leong TG, Randall CL, Benson BR, Bassik N, Stern GM, Gracias DH. Tetherless thermobiochemically actuated microgrippers. Proceedings of the National Academy of Sciences. 2009; **106**(3):703-708

[136] Shapiro AJ et al. International trial of the Edmonton protocol for islet transplantation. New England Journal of Medicine. 2006;**355**(13):1318-1330

[137] Im B-H et al. The effects of 8-arm PEG-catechol/heparin shielding system and immunosuppressive drug, FK506 on the survival of intraportally allotransplanted islets. Biomaterials. 2013;**34**(8):2098-2106

[138] Park H et al. Polymeric nano-shielded islets with heparin-polyethylene glycol in a non-human primate model. Biomaterials. 2018;**171**:164-177

[139] Izadi Z et al. Tolerance induction by surface immobilization of Jagged-1 for immunoprotection of pancreatic islets. Biomaterials. 2018;**182**:191-201

[140] Sun H et al. Nanotechnology-enabled materials for hemostatic and anti-infection treatments in orthopedic surgery. International Journal of Nanomedicine. 2018;**13**:8325

[141] Zabaglo M, Sharman T. Postoperative Wound Infection. Treasure Island (FL): StatPearls Publishing; 2021

[142] Rai MK, Deshmukh S, Ingle A, Gade A. Silver nanoparticles: The powerful nanoweapon against multidrug-resistant bacteria. Journal of Applied Microbiology. 2012;**112**(5): 841-852

[143] Castiglioni S, Cazzaniga A, Locatelli L, Maier JA. Silver nanoparticles in orthopedic applications: New insights on their effects on osteogenic cells. Nanomaterials. 2017; 7(6):124

[144] Herzog F et al. Mimicking exposures to acute and lifetime concentrations of inhaled silver nanoparticles by two different in vitro approaches. Beilstein Journal of Nanotechnology. 2014;**5**(1):1357-1370

[145] Khalsa RK, Khashkhusha A, Zaidi S, Harky A, Bashir M. Artificial intelligence and cardiac surgery during COVID-19 era. Journal of Cardiac Surgery. 2021; **36**(5):1729-1733

[146] Rampat R et al. Artificial intelligence in cornea, refractive surgery, and cataract: Basic principles, clinical applications, and future directions. Asia-Pacific journal of ophthalmology (Philadelphia, Pa.). 2021; **10**(3):268

[147] Murthy VH, Krumholz HM, Gross CP. Participation in cancer clinical trials: Race-, sex-, and age-based

disparities. JAMA. 2004;**291**(22): 2720-2726

[148] Crawford K, Calo R. There is a blind spot in AI research. Nature. 2016; **538**(7625):311-313

[149] Wang DD et al. 3D printing, computational modeling, and artificial intelligence for structural heart disease. Cardiovascular Imaging. 2021;**14**(1): 41-60

[150] Murphy D, Saleh D. Artificial intelligence in plastic surgery: What is it? Where are we now? What is on the horizon? The Annals of The Royal College of Surgeons of England. 2020; **102**(8):577-580

[151] Finlayson SG, Bowers JD, Ito J, Zittrain JL, Beam AL, Kohane IS. Adversarial attacks on medical machine learning. Science. 2019;**363**(6433): 1287-1289

[152] Biggio B, Roli F. Wild patterns: Ten years after the rise of adversarial machine learning. In: Proceedings of the 2018 ACM SIGSAC Conference on Computer and Communications Security. New York, NY, USA: Association for Computing Machinery; 2018. pp. 2154-2156

[153] Cutillo CM et al. Machine intelligence in healthcare—Perspectives on trustworthiness, explainability, usability, and transparency. NPJ Digital Medicine. 2020;**3**(1):47

[154] Pecqueux M et al. The use and future perspective of artificial intelligence—A survey among German surgeons. Frontiers in Public Health. 2022;**10**:982335

[155] Price WN, Gerke S, Cohen IG. Potential liability for physicians using artificial intelligence. JAMA. 2019; **322**(18):1765-1766

[156] Bahl M, Barzilay R, Yedidia AB, Locascio NJ, Yu L, Lehman CD. High-risk breast lesions: A machine learning model to predict pathologic upgrade and reduce unnecessary surgical excision. Radiology. 2018;**286**(3):810-818

[157] Hashimoto DA, Witkowski E, Gao L, Meireles O, Rosman G. Artificial intelligence in anesthesiology: Current techniques, clinical applications, and limitations. Anesthesiology. 2020;**132**(2): 379-394

[158] Myers TG, Ramkumar PN, Ricciardi BF, Urish KL, Kipper J, Ketonis C. Artificial intelligence and orthopaedics: An introduction for clinicians. The Journal of bone and joint surgery American. 2020;**102**(9):830

Chapter 10

Artificial Intelligence: Development and Applications in Neurosurgery

Raivat Shah, Vanessa Reese, Martin Oselkin and Stanislaw P. Stawicki

Abstract

The last decade has witnessed a significant increase in the relevance of artificial intelligence (AI) in neuroscience. Gaining notoriety from its potential to revolutionize medical decision making, data analytics, and clinical workflows, AI is poised to be increasingly implemented into neurosurgical practice. However, certain considerations pose significant challenges to its immediate and widespread implementation. Hence, this chapter will explore current developments in AI as it pertains to the field of clinical neuroscience, with a primary focus on neurosurgery. Additionally included is a brief discussion of important economic and ethical considerations related to the feasibility and implementation of AI-based technologies in neurosciences, including future horizons such as the operational integrations of human and non-human capabilities.

Keywords: artificial intelligence, neurosurgery, machine learning, deep learning, neural networks, telemedicine, robotic neurosurgery

1. Introduction

Beginning with Harvey Cushing's work in the early 1900s, modern neurosurgical advancements are often entwined with parallel developments in both medical and non-medical technologies [1]. Just as the application of microscopy, endoscopy, computed tomography (CT), magnetic resonance imaging (MRI), and ultrasound in neurosurgery have revolutionized and transformed the field, artificial intelligence (AI) is poised to do the same [2]. The past decade has witnessed exponential growth in research seeking to reconcile AI and neurosurgery, with primary goals of improving patient outcomes and enhancing quality of care. Academic interest toward the intersection of the two fields is very evident, with literature search permutations of the phrase "neurosurgery and AI" revealing over 20,000 absolute publications in the last 10 years on the PubMed database [3]. As AI grows in sophistication, ease of applicability, and prominence, it may grow and develop to be intrinsically tied with neurosurgical care in the future. This chapter will provide an overview of the current thoughts and applications of AI in neurosurgery within pre-, intra-, and postoperative contexts, evaluate the nuances of AI functionality in both developmental and use stages, consider implementation costs, feasibility, and limitations. We will also discuss any misconceptions related to the integration of AI within neurosurgery, with a focus on dispelling both exuberantly optimistic and overly negative views.

2. Methods

A literature search was performed using Google Scholar ™ search keywords of "artificial intelligence in medicine," "robotic neurosurgery," "artificial intelligence and neurosurgery," and "cost of artificial intelligence in medicine." This keyword search was mirrored in PubMed. The PubMed database and Google Scholar ™ were also searched for information on the basic information and explanation of artificial intelligence technologies, using the keywords "machine learning and neurosurgery," "neural networks in neurosurgery," and "deep learning in neurosurgery." There were no de facto inclusion criteria and no specific time limitation or time frame to the articles being utilized; rather, the articles were included based on relevance or relation to artificial intelligence use in medicine and the neuroscience field.

3. Artificial intelligence development and use: woos and woes

Artificial intelligence is an emerging field broadly defined as a set of technologies capable of incorporating human behavior and intelligence into machines and systems [4]. Due to its potential scope in diagnostic efficacy and treatment recommendations, AI is poised to be increasingly implemented into healthcare and clinical practice. However, a better understanding of what AI entails is warranted.

3.1 Machine learning

A discussion of AI in neurosurgery would be incomplete without a basic understanding of machine learning (ML), a subfield of AI [5]. The accelerated increase in computerization of patient data in healthcare has resulted in vast quantities of information beyond what can be reasonably digested by traditional methods of statistical analysis, commonly referred to as "big data" [6]. However, the emergence of ML has unlocked new possibilities for the extraction and identification of potentially valuable patterns from not only past data, but also created a framework for predicting future data trends [7–9]. The predictive potential of ML can only be harnessed when the model can be presented with large quantities of annotated data [10]. For instance, in radiographic imaging, ML is able to treat each computerized picture element, or pixel, as its own unique variable. Thus, when fed large quantities of data, the ML algorithm can *learn* at a degree of complexity (e.g., trace contours of fracture lines, parenchymal opacities, etc.) and a scale that is beyond natural human capabilities [10].

Machine learning subdomains have traditionally been grouped into two large categories: supervised and unsupervised learning. The former uses annotated datasets to train an algorithm to predict outcomes on unseen data; unsupervised learning, however, uses ML to cluster datasets without using labels, enabling the extraction of unknown features that may be useful for categorizing and predicting relevant clinical outputs without human intervention [11]. Nevertheless, many ML models in healthcare have been shown to demonstrate performance no better than conventional statistical methods [12, 13]. It should be repeatedly emphasized that the field of ML, in addition to being new, still possesses many fundamental weaknesses that limit its immediate widespread applicability.

Using diagnostic testing to determine the presence or absence of disease is an essential process in clinical medicine. In these scenarios, test results are oftentimes obtained as continuous values, which require conversion and interpretation into dichotomous groups to determine the presence or absence of a disease [14]. A key stage in this process involves defining a cut-off value, or reference value, to differentiate normal from abnormal conditions. The receiver operating characteristic (ROC) curve, the primary tool used for this determination, classifies a patient's disease state as positive or negative based on test outcomes, simultaneously identifying the optimal cut-off value with the best diagnostic performance [14]. The area under the curve (AUC) serves as a singular, scalar value summarizing the overall performance of a binary classifier [15]. This measure provides an aggregate evaluation of performance across all potential classification thresholds. In essence, the AUC measures the two-dimensional area beneath the ROC curve from points (0,0) to [1,1]. An AUC of 1.0 signifies perfect, error-free classification, whereas an AUC of 0.5, comparable to a random classification method like a coin toss, holds no diagnostic value. Typically, an AUC exceeding 0.8 is deemed acceptable in non-medical contexts, and an AUC surpassing 0.9 is considered excellent [16].

Nonetheless, it is crucial to underscore that strong performance as indicated by AUC values greater than 0.80 does not necessarily guarantee a robust model. If machine learning algorithms have not been cross-validated with novel datasets, they risk being overfit to past data, compromising their generalizability [14]. Thus, when attempting to leverage the model to predict performance on unseen data, the ML model may, at best, only offer slight gains compared to traditional statistical analysis [12, 13, 17–19]. Additionally, the robustness of any given ML model is directly dependent on the quality and quantity of data fed. If biases from differences in data collection methodologies are present in a dataset, both generalizability and performance of the model are negatively impacted [10]. Furthermore, the AUC is often presented with a 95% confidence interval because the data obtained from the sample are not fixed values but rather influenced by statistical errors. Finally, the use of real-world data inherently introduces corruptions in the dataset, also known as "noise." Random noise in input datasets can confound ML tasks of classification, clustering, and association analysis in addition to increasing model complexity and time of learning, all of which can degrade the performance of the learning algorithm as noise cannot be easily distinguished from desired inputs unless appropriately pre-processed before introduction to the model [20, 21]. In other words, despite impressive AUC values, such models may lack reliability when applied to new, unseen data, underscoring the critical importance of rigorous validation processes in the development of diagnostic tools.

3.2 Neural networks

The basic functional unit of the nervous system is the neuron [22]. Neurons function by receiving an input, processing the signal, and generating an output signal [23, 24]. Anatomically speaking, neurons are capable of consolidating up to thousands of neurotransmitter-driven synaptic inputs simultaneously via dendritic extensions, processing a highly transformed version of the original inputs in the soma, and producing a singular output through its axon in the form of an action potential [25]. Importantly, neuronal outputs are not generated at a fixed rate but rather are a function of whether or not the signal summation (excitatory - inhibitory inputs) exceeds a predefined threshold value in order to successfully depolarize the neuron and induce an action potential [26–28]. After traveling through the axon, the action potential signal is transmitted to a multiplicity of neurons synapsed at the axon terminal.

Broadly speaking, artificial neural networks (ANNs) model the biological principles of neuronal signaling in order to stratify and solve complex, nonlinear problems [29]. Considered a subfield of ML, ANNs refer to a digital machine learning algorithm based upon the concept of a biological neuron. Comparatively, where neurons rely on neurotransmitter signaling inputs ANNs leverage binary, categorical, or numeric data sets [5]. Transformation of input signals at the soma into an action potential is akin to an ANN arithmetic-based calculation of inputs into an output [30].

Although the theory underlying ANNs was first developed in the 1980s, premier advances in computational power and training data acquisition at scale have enabled its extensive application in recent years. In neurosurgery, ANNs have grown to be increasingly utilized in diagnostics, prognostics, and management [31]. Deep learning (DL) is yet another class of algorithms increasingly studied in the literature. Although similar to neural networks in principle, the term "deep" refers to the increasing depth of layers present in the neural network – typically accepted to imply at least three layers [32].

The ability to analyze non-linear data by ANNs is ideal for assisting neurosurgeons in clinical decision-making [33]. In particular, ANNs have been widely demonstrated to be superior to traditional analytical methods, especially as it pertains to clinical imaging tasks [34]. Even so, significant challenges still exist which limit the widespread use of ANNs and DL in neurosurgery and medicine at large, including insufficient data, obscured interpretability, reliability of data, high threshold of processing power, and data privacy [3].

3.3 Natural language processing

Natural language processing (NLP) is another subfield that falls under the scope of ML. As its name implies, the goal of NLP is to better enable human-computer communication by leveraging natural human language to better perform data abstraction processes [35]. In other words, the computer functions to *understand* human-generated text inputs by breaking down sentences into their constituent parts and applying algorithms to derive meaningful outputs. There are two primary divisions within the field of NLP: rules-based models and machine-based models. A rules-based model boasts minimal set-up costs, however is burdensome to scale for large datasets and inflexible as language usage evolves over time; conversely, machine-based models are preferable for large datasets as it can circumvent the rigidity of rules-based model while adapting to evolutions in human lexicon over time [36]. Three methodological approaches that dominate the application of NLP to neurosurgery are classification, annotation, and prediction [37]. Classification involves providing further diagnostic information, and informing the surgeon's decision making in the preoperative phase. Annotation entails automatizing the annotation of a large amount of data (e.g., radiological images) by identifying specific phenotypes related to a disease condition, enabling the NLP algorithm to train on much larger amounts of data and better extrapolate clinical outcomes. Prediction exploits previous data (e.g., free text notes) to predict patient surgical outcomes and enable the neurosurgeon to arrange the resources necessary for their care accordingly. Machine-based NLP as applied to neurosurgery and medicine at scale remains in its infantile stages, though its possibilities rise with the emergence of Large Language Models.

3.4 Large language models

Large Language Models (LLMs) like ChatGPT, developed by OpenAI, are a new wave of AI technology that have profound implications for diverse fields, including healthcare. Educated on a colossal quantity of textual data, these models grasp the delicate intricacies and nuances of human language, thereby equipping them to form pertinent and contextually relevant responses to a broad spectrum of prompts [38].

In March 2023, the performance of ChatGPT and GPT-4 was assessed on a 500-question mock neurosurgical written boards examination. Using Self-Assessment Exam 1 from the American Board of Neurological Surgery (ABNS), Ali et al. fed questions in single best answer, multiple-choice format. ChatGPT and GPT-4 achieved scores of 73.4 and 83.4%, respectively, relative to the question bank user average of 73.7% [39]. Both the question bank users and the LLMs exceeded the previous year's passing threshold of 69%, demonstrating the models' potential technical utility [39].

In a clinical context, including neurosurgery, LLMs could serve multiple purposes. Firstly, they could play a significant role in patient education, simplifying complex neurosurgical procedures, and providing insights into the recovery process in an accessible language [40]. Secondly, these models could help facilitate medical research, from identifying new hypotheses to aiding in clinical decision-making by providing summaries of recent research, medical literature, or guideline updates relevant to specific cases [41].

Another promising application lies in the realm of medical documentation. LLMs could help transcribe doctor-patient conversations, draft surgical reports, or summarize patient histories, thereby streamlining administrative tasks and allowing physicians to focus more on patient care [42]. Continuing Medical Education could also benefit from LLMs. By simulating complex clinical scenarios or generating case studies, these models could serve as an effective teaching tool for medical trainees [43].

4. Preoperative applications

The goal of the preoperative phase of care is to prepare both the neurosurgeon and the patient for a potential operation through means of diagnosis, surgical candidacy stratification, selection of treatment, and informed consent. AI is increasingly entering these realms as a potential adjunct to clinical practice.

4.1 Patient selection

A quantitative means of evaluating an individual patient outcome preoperatively is highly desirable in improving surgical decision-making. At the present moment, clinical outcome judgment is heavily reliant on the individual neurosurgeon. Prognostic indices in use today, though easily applicable, lack adequate predictive performance primarily due to the streamlining of numerical data to categorical data [44, 45]. Conversely, ML, by its very nature, could circumvent such a simplification.

Until now, previous literature has compared neurosurgical patient outcome predictive performance between ML algorithms, classical logistic regressions, prognostic indices, and neurosurgeons with differential results. Against classical logistic regressions, ML models have demonstrated superior performance in predictions of successful endoscopic third ventriculostomy, postoperative ventricular peritoneal shunt infection, mortality after embolization of AVMs, patient satisfaction after laminectomy for lumbar spinal stenosis, in-hospital mortality in patients with traumatic brain injury, cerebral vasospasm after aneurysmal subarachnoid hemorrhage, and outcomes after a burr-hole procedure for a chronic subdural hematoma [45–52]. Against current logistic regression prognostic indices for prediction of successful endoscopic third ventriculostomy (ETV) 6 months postoperatively, ANNs have demonstrated superior performance [45]. Masoudi et al. found that for ETV prediction 6 months postoperative, their multi-layer perceptron ANN demonstrated an AUC of 0.913 compared to a logistic regression AUC of 0.819 [53]. Some ML models have shown better performance compared to prognostic indices predicting outcome after stereotactic radiosurgery for cerebral arteriovenous malformation (AVM) with AUCs of 0.70–0.71 vs. 0.57–0.69 [44, 52]. A random forest classifier (RFC), a class of ML model achieved an AUC of 0.80, with 0.34 sensitivity, 0.95 specificity, 0.73 positive predictive value, 0.80 negative predictive value, and 0.79 accuracy for the prediction of traumatic brain injury in children following a cranial CT of the brain, demonstrating a substantial alternative to the currently used nomogram for the prediction of intracranial injury following CT in children with TBI [54].

Some recent studies have investigated the differences in ML and clinician performance in predicting neurosurgical outcomes in patients. Emblem et al. found that against fuzzy C-means, a class of ML model, neuroradiologists performed similarly in survival predictions for newly diagnosed glioma patients [55]. Emblem et al. also discovered that a support vector machine (SVM) model combined with perfusion-weighted magnetic resonance (MR) imaging better predicted survival in glioblastoma patients compared to neuroradiologists [56]. Currently, although especially experienced neurosurgeons have been demonstrated to exhibit strong patient survival prediction skills in patients with high-grade glioma undergoing surgery on group-wide metrics, they often missed on the individual level [57]. Hence, future AI tools could help bridge this gap by supporting neurosurgeons' insights in the prediction of patient survival.

4.2 Diagnostics

Both LLMs and ML have utilization within diagnostics. LLMs can serve as an adjunct to the patient evaluation process by suggesting rarer diagnoses and interventions that the physician may not have typically considered. These can be incorporated with the overall clinical picture as appropriate. The potential scope of which ML can be applied to diagnostics is largely divided between three categories: classification, detection, and segmentation. Classification involves algorithmic stratification of data inputs into categories (e.g., normal, abnormal). Detection entails visual localization of an area of interest (e.g., lesion). Segmentation implies outlining a target area using a precise, pixel-wise boundary [58]. The following categories will elucidate the various areas through which general ML and deep learning (DL) models have been applied to neurodiagnostics.

4.3 Intracranial hemorrhage

Earlier efforts were able to determine important correlations between imaging characteristics, the presence of intracranial hemorrhage (ICH), and patient outcomes [59–61]. Today, approved commercial software for ICH detection exists on the market with clinical uses including triage and early warning systems, double reading, and hemorrhage type classification. Boasting a validated sensitivity of 88.7 to 96.2% and a specificity of 92.3 to 99.0%, Aidoc for ICH, an FDA-approved DL tool, is one of the industry's leading support systems for evaluation and warning notification of unenhanced head CT images of ICHs [62–66]. Aidoc for ICH and other DL learning models have been demonstrated to produce inconsistencies in performance when applied to non-native trained clinical sites [64, 67]. Thus, further studies have sought to investigate alternatives including competing commercial software in addition to independently developed models. For instance, McLouth et al. and Rava et al. have validated the diagnostic capabilities of other DL ICH tools such as CINA v1.0 and Canon's ^{AUTO}Stroke Solution ICH across hospital sites in the United States, finding high accuracy and specificity with medium sensitivity thresholds [68, 69]. Wang et al., winners of the 2019-RSNA Brain CT Hemorrhage Challenge, developed a convolutional neural network (CNN) using a diverse array of datasets sourced from three institutions that achieved accuracy levels similar to that of senior radiologists [67]. Despite the outstanding results of the algorithm, it is important to note that the CNN model's applicability in clinical settings is currently limited by (1) the lack of patient clinical information in the RSNA-challenge provided datasets, thereby obscuring the confounding effects of scanner type, cause of bleeding, and patient demographics, (2) its inapplicability to MRI imaging which is oftentimes crucial for ICH screening and diagnosis, and (3) external validation data are lacking [67].

4.4 Stroke

In the past decade, deep learning applications in stroke imaging have dramatically risen, likely as a byproduct of higher stroke imaging volume with the arrival of endovascular thrombectomy in addition to the increasing acknowledgement of the emergent nature of the disease process [58]. DL applications to stroke imaging can be divided into three areas. (1) Alberta Stroke Program Early CT Score (ASPECTS) measurement, (2) large vessel occlusion (LVO) detection, and (3) infarct prognostication.

ASPECTS is a 10-point topographical quantitative grading scale widely used to guide acute stroke treatment by measuring 10 regions within the middle cerebral artery (MCA) territory for early signs of ischemia [70, 71]. Many commercial DL tools designed to perform automated ASPECTS evaluation have been tested in clinical settings, demonstrating variable results. One study found that three neuroradiologists showed a higher correlation with infarct core than e-ASPECTS (Brainomix) (r = 0.71, 0.76, 0.80, compared to 0.59) while another study found that RAPID ASPECTS (iSchemaView) displayed higher correlation than two neuroradiologists from between symptom onset and imaging until 4 hours post-symptom [72, 73]. These results suggest that automated ASPECTS evaluation may continue to be implemented as an adjunct to current neuroradiological diagnostics. The efficacy of ASPECTS analysis depends on the software utilized and established ground truth.

Early identification of large vessel occlusion (LVO) in the early stages of admission can mitigate the probability of the patient suffering from the long-term implications of stroke and rescue life. A 2019 study developed a U-Net architecture DL tool designed to detect the hyperdense MCA sign in noncontrast head CT scans from a local Hong Kong population and achieved a high sensitivity (.930), though relatively lower specificity accuracy and AUC [74]. Automated LVO detection on CT angiograms (CTA) has become integral to many stroke centers. Viz-AI, a commercial CNN-based solution, has demonstrated 82% sensitivity and 94% specificity for LVO detection [71].

The ability to accurately and reliably predict posttreatment stroke outcomes can aid the neurosurgeon in selecting patients for thrombectomy or other neuroendovascular procedures and developing a plan of care precisely tailored to the individual patient. Recent stroke thrombectomy trials utilizing automated perfusion CT and MR imaging have revolutionized the modern care of stroke patients. The now commercially available Rapid.AI perfusion product, which employs a threshold-based segmentation method, resulted in a 3-fold reduction in severe disability and death when used to select patients for thrombectomy [75]. However, CT perfusion (CTP) maps have historically been unreliable and threshold-based approaches may fail to fully capture the complexity of infarct evolution. Processing this data under a DL system, one can take into account other biomarkers and patient-specific factors for better prognostication. One study validated a CNN designed to identify and predict post-treatment MRI final lesion volume, achieving a modified ROC-AUC of 0.88 [76]. Nishi et al. used a U-Net DL tool to assess clinical post-treatment outcomes of LVO patients using pretreatment diffusion-weighted image data of patients who underwent mechanical thrombectomy, finding an ROC-AUC of 0.81 [77].

4.5 Intracranial aneurysms

Intracranial aneurysms (IAs) are commonplace in the population, with a global estimated prevalence between 2 and 5% [78]. Although most of these aneurysms are asymptomatic, they carry the risk of rupture which if realized leads to a subarachnoid hemorrhage – a prognosis producing a dramatic case fatality of 50% [79]. Thus, there is great interest in the rapid and accurate identification of unruptured intracranial aneurysms on brain imaging.

At the present moment, intra-arterial digital subtraction angiography (IADSA) is the gold-standard for the diagnosis of intracranial aneurysms, with computed tomography angiography (CTA), magnetic resonance angiography (MRA), and transcranial Doppler sonography also shown to be effective diagnostic tests [80]. Time-of-flight MR angiography (TOF-MRA) is a non-invasive, non-contrast enhanced technique that enables discrimination between vessels and stationary tissues by inducing blood inflow effects [81]. Due to the absence of ionizing radiation or intravenous contrast agents, time-of-flight MR angiography (TOF-MRA) is typically the first modality of choice for aneurysm screening. Hence, many inroads for DL applications have been explored in this area.

Nakao et al. developed a computer-assisted detection (CAD) deep CNN architecture combined with a maximum intensity projection (MIP) algorithm trained on 450 patients worth of TOF-MRA scans. The team achieved a high sensitivity of 94.2% (98/104) and only 2.9 false positives per case [82]. Faron et al. similarly developed a CNN model finding an overall sensitivity of 90% with a false positive rate of 6.1%. More consequently, the Faron team further found that there was no significant difference in aneurysm detection performance between the CNN model and two blinded diagnostic neuroradiologists, with an overall increase in human detection sensitivity when combining their detection hits with the CNN model's hits (reader 1: 98% vs. 95%, $P = 0.280$; reader 2: 97% vs. 94%, $P = 0.333$) [83].

Ueda et al. developed a ResNet architecture algorithm fed with 683 TOF-MRA patient scans and achieved a sensitivity of 91% (592 of 649) and 93% (74 of 80) for their internal and external data sets, respectively [84]. More interestingly, the model improved aneurysm detection in their retrospectively collected TOF-MRA scans by 4.8% (31 of 649) and 13% (10 of 80), respectively, compared to the initial radiologist-interpreted assessments.

Until recently, machine-learning algorithms largely focused on MRA imaging. However, more recent efforts were expanded to include CT-based imaging approaches. In 2020, Shi et al. developed a 3D CNN trained on 1177 digital subtraction angiography verified bone-removal CTA cases, which when tested on a cohort of suspected acute ischemic stroke (AIS) patients found that the model could exclude IA-negative cases with 99.0% confidence [85]. Limitations in their study include a relatively small sample of positive cases in the validation cohorts as well as the experimentally reasonable exclusion of CTA data with head trauma and arteriovenous malformation/fistula (AVM/AVF). In 2021, Yang et al. proposed a 3D CNN algorithm for detecting cerebral aneurysms using head CTA images, achieving a very high sensitivity of 97.5% (633 of 649) while revealing 8 intracranial aneurysms overlooked in initial reports [86]. When the model was paired with expert radiologists, their overall weighted alternative free-response receiver operating characteristic (wAFROC) curve improved by 0.01 ($P < .05$), demonstrating the viability for physician-machine adjunct usage.

4.6 Neuro-oncology

For over a century, neurosurgeons have played an essential role in the management of cancers afflicting the central nervous system (CNS). As the tenth leading cause of death for both men and women, accurate clinical evaluation of disease progression, and early detection of brain tumors using effective brain imaging techniques is paramount to improving patient outcomes. Historically, the preoperative phase involved manual segmentation of brain tumors and small related brain structures by the neurosurgeon – a laborious task [87]. Hence, many automated solutions have been explored, with the broadest categories for automated brain tumor segmentation of MR images including (i) intensity-based, (ii) ML-based, and (iii) hybrid-based approaches.

The intensity-based approaches are among the most conventional methods used in brain tumor segmentation, relying on a basic analysis of pixel values within the spatial domain. The thresholding technique, for instance, functions by binarizing the MR image by pixel intensity relative to an intensity threshold [87]. This technique, however, suffers from many limitations including sensitivity to noise and intensity non-homogeneity. Also classified as an intensity-based approach, the region-based method involves using pre-defined pixel/voxel conditions to extract intensity information by locating a region following seed point selection and connecting pixels with similar intensity values; many studies have recently improved upon this technique but suffer from limitations such as inability to remove noise, subjective manual setting of parameters, and annotation bias [88–92]. Most existing methods rely on such fully supervised methods [93].

Largely due to the aforementioned constraints and inflexibility, ML-based approaches to brain tumor segmentation have increasingly been explored, both in traditional ML as well as DL forms. Many recent studies leveraging traditional ML models have shown equal or superior performance relative to the conventional intensity-based models, though observing limitations in some studies such as subjective user-directed pixel label refinement of segmentation results, sensitivity to noise and distortions, non-uniform intensity distribution, and extraction of redundant features [94–96].

In the past decade, interest toward deep learning as applied to brain tumor segmentation has soared in popularity due to its anticipated superior performance compared to more conventional models of data abstraction. Many studies have relied on extracting 2D patches from 3D MR images to use as inputs for the 2D CNN [97–109]. Though CNNs have generally demonstrated improved performance compared to its intensity-approach counterparts, model training is often time-consuming as a large amount of training data, parameters, and processing power are required. Furthermore, 3D contextual information is often bypassed in 2D CNNs, thus spurring the development of 3D CNNs in recent years [110–115]. Although 3D CNNs enable better exploitation of 3D features from MR image information data, high computational resources (i.e. high network intensiveness and memory consumption) limit its widespread applicability. Thus, 2.5D deep neural networks (DNNs) approaches have been explored; Wang et al. validated a cascaded 2.5D model which improved segmentation accuracy by striking a balance between memory consumption and model complexity, demonstrating superior inference compared to already established models such as DeepMedic and ScaleNet [116–118].

Recently, Pham et al. introduced a hybrid metaheuristic-ML model to circumvent sensitivity to noise, intensity non-uniformity, and trapping into local minima and dependency on initial clustering centroids [119]. However, this model suffered from decreases in performance, though its introduction spurred the development of many hybrid models to find an optimal balance between each efficiency metric [96, 119–122]. Other hybrid approaches such as DL-traditional ML and ML-contour based models, though better than conventional methods, have not observed overall efficiency greater than the metaheuristic-ML hybrid [87]. At the present moment, the literature indicates that deep learning based and hybrid-based metaheuristic models are the most efficient and reliable methods available, though its widespread application requires further validation. Despite improvements in deep learning models as applied to brain tumor segmentation, it is imperative to note that limitations in tumor morphological uncertainty, low contrast resolution, annotation biases during data labeling, and imbalanced voxel distribution persist. Thus, advances in AI can aid the neurosurgeon in various brain tumor segmentation contexts though neurosurgeons should remain cautious when using DL models to inform his or her clinical judgment.

4.7 Spine

From the genesis of AI applications in surgery spine has been a site of significant innovation in ML and DL models, generating opportunities for applications in scoliosis quantification, vertebral fracture detection, and vertebral body segmentation.

The Cobb measuring method is the gold standard for quantification of the scoliotic curve [123]. With the digitalization of computerized radiography, most surgeons opt to use built-in computer software such as the Picture Archiving and Communications System (PACS); despite the proven efficiency of the software relative to the traditional "manual" method of Cobb angle measurement, systems like PACS use software (e.g., Surgimap) which requires users to manually select the upper and lower ends of vertebral bodies inherently introduces human error [123–127]. Hence, Cobb angle measurement has been an area of significant AI exploration.

Caesarendra et al. utilized a deep CNN to measure the Cobb angle of patients diagnosed with adolescent idiopathic scoliosis, producing accuracies up to 93.6% which demonstrates a high reliability compared to neurosurgeons' measurement (intraclass correlation coefficient > 0.95) [123]. Sun et al. assessed DL models based upon CNNs designed to segment each vertebra and locate the vertebral corners, finding a very high intraclass correlation coefficient (ICC) of 0.994, with a Pearson correlation coefficient and mean absolute error between the model and orthopedic annotation of 0.990 and 2.2° ± 2.0° [128]. These results are especially promising in cases where the Cobb angle does not exceed 90°.

AI applications in vertebral fracture detection have generated tremendous interest due to the relative ease in algorithmic-driven image discrimination relative to other neurosurgical contexts. Many studies have evaluated both ML and DL models in the context of fracture detection. Tomita et al. utilized a deep neural network to detect osteoporotic vertebral fractures trained upon 1432 CT scans, finding an ROC-AUC between 0.909 and 0.918 with an F-score of 90.8% and accuracy of 89.2%, measures approximately equivalent to radiologists [129]. Small et al. tested C-spine, an FDA-approved CNN developed by Aidoc to detect cervical spine fractures, finding an accuracy, sensitivity, and specificity for the CNN and radiologists of 92 vs. 95%, 76 vs. 93%, and 97 vs. 96%, respectively [130]. Derkatch et al. trained a CNN binary classifier fed with dual-energy x-ray absorptiometry data to vertebral compression fractures, which yielded an ROC-AUC of 0.94 with a sensitivity of 87.4% and a specificity of 88.4% [131]. Thus, these data suggest that ML and DL models can serve as an accessory to the radiologist and the neurosurgeon in vertebral fracture detection.

Currently, only a few semi-automatic methods for disc and vertebral labeling exist and are widely utilized. However, these methods are inundated with subjectivity due to the presence of user-directed input. Hence, many studies have sought to develop alternative methods to enhance accuracy and efficiency in radiological evaluation. Lehnen et al. demonstrated the feasibility of using a single CNN to identify various degenerative changes of the lumbar spine from MR images, finding high diagnostic accuracy for intervertebral disc detection/labeling (100%), spinal canal stenosis (98%), and nerve root compressions (91%) as well as moderately high diagnostic accuracy for disc herniations (87%), extrusions (86%), bulgings (76%), and spondylolisthesis (87.61%) [132]. However, the generalizability of their study is limited by a small sample size and exclusion of patients over 70 years old. Furthermore, the use of CNNs for spine segmentation is not particularly novel; in 2018, Whitehead et al. trained a cascade of CNNs and achieved Dice scores of 0.832 and 0.865 for vertebrae and discs, respectively [133]. Huang et al. developed a DL tool appropriately named Spine Explorer which quickly and automatically segments and measures lumbar MR images, achieving a near perfect mean Intersection-over-Union (IoU) of 94.7 and 92.6% for the vertebra and disc, respectively [134]. A year later, Shen et al. expanded the scope of Spine Explorer to include the paraspinal muscles and the spinal canal, finding IoU values of 83.3 to 88.4% and 82.1%, respectively [135]. However, both studies using Spine Explorer suffered from a low patient sample size. Recently, Cheng et al. developed a two-stage MultiResUNet DL model for the automatic segmentation of specific intervertebral discs, which yielded a segmentation accuracy of 94%, potentially indicating its eminence over other DL models, such as the U-Net, CNN-based, Attention U-Net, and standard MultiResUNet models [136].

Spine imaging findings are often insufficient in the determination of the underlying cause of lower back pain (LBP) and are often not of clinical significance due to the high frequency of asymptomatic presenting patients. NLP algorithms, however, can bridge the gap in data abstraction in the relationship between spine imaging findings and LBP. Tan et al. developed an NLP to identify lumbar spine imaging findings related to LBP on x-ray and MR radiology reports, demonstrating a significantly greater sensitivity (0.94, compared to 0.83 for rules-based), a higher overall AUC (0.98, compared to 0.90 for rules-based), and comparable specificity (0.97 vs. 0.95 for rules-based) when compared to the rules-based model [36]. Miotto et al. developed a convolutional neural network which, after training on manual free-text clinical notes on LBP patients, was able to discriminate between acute and chronic LBP (AUC of 0.98 and F score of 0.70), demonstrating the potential for systematization of patient symptomatology [137].

5. Intraoperative applications

The intraoperative phase of patient care revolves around optimizing the neurosurgeon's functionality and performance in the operating room (OR). AI's role intraoperatively includes augmented reality (AR), ML for pathology and neurooncologic applications, using algorithms to automate identification of intraoperative injuries based on the operative note.

Augmented reality has a myriad of intraoperative uses in both cranial and spinal procedures. From the cerebrovascular standpoint, AR has been used to decrease the craniotomy size and delineate aneurysm architecture for safer aneurysm clipping [138]. AR has also been used to superimpose white matter tracts onto the surgical field as well as identify eloquent brain regions during tumor resections [139]. The implementation of AR was shown to result in significantly greater rates of total resection with better preservation of critical functions such as vision, speech, and motor [139]. Head-up AR microscope displays with navigation were found to be more accurate than traditional microscopy with navigation based on fiducial or automatic intraoperative CT registration in the setting of transsphenoidal surgeries [140]. Rychen et al. described the successful use of AR to fuse CTA, DSA, and TOF MRI imaging with neuronavigation for superficial temporal artery to middle cerebral artery (STA-MCA) bypass operations [141]. Perhaps one of the most impressive features of these applications is that augmented reality is formulated to work with current microscopes and neuronavigation systems that are commonly used for neurosurgical procedures, rather than requiring an entirely new device.

Resection margins are of the utmost importance in the resection of malignant tumors as remnants of malignant tissue led to the recurrence of disease and decreased survival. Real time analysis of resection margins typically requires an experienced neuropathologist, as well as a processor well versed in chemistry [142]. ML was employed to process samples through the High Resolution Magic Angle Spinning Nuclear Magnetic Resonance (HRMAS NMR) methodology, with high accuracy (median AUC of 85.6% and AUPR of 93.4%) [142]. Jabarkheel et al. established the use of Raman spectroscopy to accurately differentiate benign and malignant tissue intraoperatively in pediatric tumor resections [143].

Spinal procedures also utilize AR to aid in the precise placement of pedicle screws, superimposing trajectories into the surgical field [144]. Computer-assisted navigation (CAN) has a wide range of uses from tumor resection to deformity correction. When utilized for screw placement, CAN reduces the need for fluoroscopic guidance thus decreasing radiation exposure. CAN also increases operative efficiency, which diminishes the operative time and patient exposure to anesthesia [145].

Another promising AI application in spinal surgery is robotics. The SpineAssist (MAZOR Robotics Inc., Caesarea, Israel), ROSA (Medtech, SA, Montpellier, France), the Excelsius GPS Robot (Globus Medical, Inc., Audubon, PA), and the Da Vinci Surgical System (Intuitive Surgical, Sunnyvale, CA) are the four most studied robotic systems available [145]. Each has its strengths and weaknesses, and it is worth mentioning that all of these systems are still ultimately controlled by the surgeon. Prospective trials on the SpineAssist system demonstrate up to 99% accuracy with pedicle screw placement, as opposed to the 92% accuracy rate achieved with navigation alone [145]. The robot mounts directly onto the spinous process or other bony landmark and easily interfaces with a CAN system. Retrospective trials and case reports for the ROSA and Excelsius machines show increased accuracy of pedicle screw placement, however the difference was not statistically significant for the ROSA system [145]. Both systems are freestanding which removes the issue of incorrect landmark fixation that can occur with the SpineAssist system, and the Excelsius decreases total radiation exposure. The ROSA, initially created for intracranial neurosurgery, uses a camera and a percutaneous pin system placed over bony landmarks that the robot arm follows. In terms of efficiency, the ROSA is less efficient than current methodologies, adding over 70 minutes to the operative time [145]. Lastly, the Da Vinci system is the most widely used surgical robot though not typically used for and not approved for neurosurgical applications such as spinal instrumentation. Current thinking on potential neurosurgical applications of this device are anterior lumbar fusions [145]. Further randomized trials are needed and likely some adjustments to the systems in order to truly harness the advantages they offer.

6. Postoperative applications

The goals of the postoperative phase of care include predicting prognosis, identifying potential postoperative complications, and optimizing variables for enhanced aftercare and recovery. A study by Arvind et al. demonstrated that ANN and LR are superior to the American Society of Anesthesiologist (ASA) class in predicting the incidence of the cardiac, wound, VTE, and mortality in patients undergoing anterior cervical discectomy and fusion (ACDF) [146]. Similarly, Kim et al. found ANN and LR to be more accurate than ASA classification for predicting the same complications in posterior lumbar fusion [147]. AI has also allowed for greater distinction between disease progression versus tumor necrosis from radiation therapy in gliomas [144, 148].

Follow up in the postoperative phase can be simplified using telemedicine with smart phone apps, video conferencing or simple phone communication. A prospective trial by Reider Demer et al. found that telemedicine postoperative follow up for patients who underwent elective intracranial neurosurgery was a safe and effective alternative to in-office visits [149]. What's more, the patients preferred the convenience of telemedicine visits.

It has been estimated that doctors spend up to 50% of their time on documentation, and nurses 20% [150]. Moreover, the initiation of the twenty first Century Cures Act has created a great need for methods to quickly produce summaries and communications that are easily understood [151]. Once further refined, LLMs could be invaluable tools to help fill this gap by generating rudimentary plain language medical information that can be modified by clinicians. They can also be used to generate authorization letters and various other types of documentation based on keywords. This would drastically reduce the amount of time spent on documentation and allow physicians as well as other medical providers to devote more of their time to patient care.

7. Cost, feasibility, and limitations

7.1 Cost and feasibility

Successful integration of any new process or technology is dependent upon the ease of implementation, as well as the overall cost of the technology versus the revenue and benefit it generates. The United States leads in health care spending but has the worst outcomes when compared to nations such as Canada, Germany, the United Kingdom, Australia, Japan, Denmark, France, the Netherlands, Switzerland, and Sweden [152]. Health care spending is estimated to comprise nearly 20% of the US gross domestic product in 2025, which equates to $5.3 trillion [145]. Neurosurgery is among the most expensive medical specialties, with the average procedure and hospitalization costing $21,825 to $22,924 depending on the volume of the medical center [153]. The cost of a spinal fusion is 12 times greater than it was 30 years ago [145]. This in combination with the emergence of value-based care and changing reimbursement patterns has led to increased research into cost saving methodologies. AI applications associated with this research include risk adjusted reimbursement models, predictive models of hospital length of stay, and predictors of patients more suitable for outpatient procedures. Within the neurosurgical realm, these studies have focused on spinal surgeries and there is a paucity of data on the intracranial surgical aspects of neurosurgery [154]. A meta-analysis of AI economic studies performed by Khanna et al. revealed that most of the research is focused on either diagnosis or treatment aspects throughout all medicine and the studies lack consideration of purchase and maintenance costs associated with AI, as well as few if any comparisons to alternative technologies [152].

Though investigation into the financial aspects of AI use in neurosurgery is on the rise, no study to date has produced a thorough net present value assessment within a large-scale experimental design [154]. Externally validated studies conducted on a larger scale with robust cost and net gain/loss calculations are necessary to accurately determine the feasibility and true value of the integration of AI into neurosurgery from a financial standpoint. This is particularly important being that the mean cost of an AI system ranges from $20,000 to $1 million, depending upon the system. The more complex the system, the greater the cost, albeit there are minimal viable products available in the $8000 to $15,000 price range [155].

Maintenance and continued operation represent a significant investment as well. AI systems require a staff of project managers, software engineers, data scientists, and software developers. A project manager will cost between $1200 to $4600 per month. Software engineers and data scientists contribute $600 to $1500 per day and $500 to $1100 per day in cost respectively. The annual salary of an in-house data scientist averages $94,000 while a software developer has an annual salary of $80,000 [156]. Additionally, health networks incur an average cost of $15,000 to recruit candidates to fill these positions, as well as the cost to train the staff [156]. Outsourcing the maintenance and operation of the system offers a more frugal alternative to in-house staffing, however, there can be a lack of continuity and immediate availability with the remote staff.

Reimbursement for AI is still in its relative infancy as payers only began to approve coverage of AI use in late 2020 [157]. Currently, eight image-based assistive or autonomous AI devices are approved by Center for Medicare and Medicaid (CMS) for repayment, with two of the technologies holding surgical utility (**Table 1**). The criteria for repayment is very specific and quite complex, with payments ultimately only covering a maximum of 65% of the actual expense [158]. Compensation is based on Current Procedural Terminology (CPT) codes or New Technology Add-on Payments (NTAPs), which have a reimbursement limit of 3 years [157, 158]. In Europe, AI is not routinely covered and not recognized as a separately reimbursable expense. Several suggested payment models including gainsharing models, outcome incentivization, and advance market commitments have been proposed as the potential for abuse/fraud or underutilization in underserved areas with per use payments has been recognized as a legitimate concern [157].

Ultimately, the future integration of AI into the field of neurosurgery will depend heavily upon whether the increase in efficiency and performance result in a tangible improvement in patient outcomes while providing a net cost savings to health networks. If AI is proven to be a substantial solution, reassessment of reimbursements and insurance coverage are likely to follow.

Manufacturer	System	Description/Use	Payment mechanism
Digital diagnostics	IDX-DR	Deep learning algorithm to diagnose diabetic retinopathy from fundoscopic images in the outpatient setting	CPT
viz.ai	Viz LVO	Radiological computer-assisted triage and notification software that analyzes CT images of the brain and notifies hospital staff when a suspected large-vessel occlusion (LVO) is identified	NTAP
Rapid AI	Rapid LVO	AI-guided medical imaging acquisition system intended to assist medical professionals in the acquisition of cardiac ultrasound images.	NTAP
Caption health	Caption guidance		NTAP
viz.ai	Viz SDH	Radiological computer-assisted triage and notification software that analyzes CT images of the brain and notifies hospital staff when a suspected subdural hematoma is identified	NTAP
Rapid AI	Rapid aspects	Computer-aided diagnostic device characterizing brain tissue abnormalities on brain CT images	NTAP
AIDoc	Briefcase for PE	Radiological computer-assisted triage and notification software that analyzes CT images of the chest and notifies hospital staff when a suspected pulmonary embolism is identified	NTAP
PROCEPT BioRobotics Corporation	The AQUABEAM system	Autonomous tissue removal robot for the treatment of lower urinary tract symptoms due to benign prostatic hyperplasia (BPH).	NTAP

Table 1.
Modified from paying for artificial intelligence in medicine. Parikh and Helmchen [157].

7.2 Limitations

The remarkable growth and promise of AI in neurosurgery are not without limitations and concerns that must be taken into account. Firstly, it is imperative to consider that potentially substantial ML-driven improvements in performance are distinct from clinically significant improvements. Although ML models may offer drastic improvements in big data prediction problems, many medical prediction scenarios tend to be intrinsically linear and binary; in such cases, it is unlikely ML models will offer substantial improvements in discrimination and be of clinical value to the neurosurgeon [12, 23]. In short, the efficacy of ML algorithms boils down to the ability to predict future outcomes based on past data.

A primary concern with LLMs is their current inability to fully comprehend context or exercise judgment, which causes significant misinterpretations along with the potential to disseminate incorrect and potentially harmful information [159]. LLMs lack a mechanism for discriminating against biased or false information and cannot inform the end user that the information provided is incorrect. This concern is further compounded by the lack of transparency in the decision-making processes of LLMs like GPT-4. These models can offer explanations as to how and why they make certain decisions upon request, but these justifications are formed post-hoc [160]. This makes it impossible to verify if the explanations accurately represent the model's actual decision-making process. Even more problematic is that when probed for an explanation, GPT-4 may provide contradictory information to its previous statements [159, 160]. The lack of reliability and reproducibility necessitates constant human oversight to ensure accuracy. Specific to medicine, clinicians would be required to fact check these tools, which could easily negate any time savings LLMs may offer. Intellectual property matters are another issue with LLMs. These tools not only pull data and property from creators without consent, but some have also created and cited false references [150].

Furthermore, there is a tendency for bias, violations of privacy, and inherent logistical difficulties with the global utilization of AI. Datasets used to train algorithms are predominantly composed of information representing the majority and common conditions. This model bias can negatively impact racial and ethnic minority groups, genders, and socioeconomically disadvantaged peoples, in addition to diminishing the ability to recognize difficult anatomy [161, 162]. A study by Kamulageya et al. found that the AI dermatologic algorithm Skin Image Search was woefully inaccurate when presented images of pathology in Ugandan patients with dark (Fitzpatrick 6) skin types [163]. The company website boasts an accuracy of 80% and but was found to only be 17% accurate when presented with darker skin tones [163]. Facial recognition algorithms have also been found to have diminished capabilities with both gender and race, performing the worst with females of darker skin tones [164]. These very groups already suffer from diminished access to care and undertreatment of disease in comparison to non-disadvantaged people. Model variance, which stems from insufficient data from minority groups also furthers the bias of AI algorithms. Differences in practices, equipment, and coding also decrease the generalization of AI algorithms. Designing algorithms with the global population in mind, analyzing performance on a subgroup basis, as well as externally validating the algorithms are ways to combat this [162].

Obtaining large quantities of patient data to train AI systems is difficult due to the necessary privacy protections added to patient data [161]. Inappropriate access to data sets and algorithms poses significant ethical, security, and privacy concerns. Algorithms can be manipulated by the addition of noise or altered data to produce harmful or deleterious effects on the system. Ensuring data privacy and security while allowing users and developers to learn and improve upon the technology is key to moving AI forward.

On a global scale, challenges to telesurgery include lags in connection speeds and the potential for delays and disconnections. The introduction of 5G technology has been touted as a possible remedy, however this remains to be seen [165]. Another consideration to this includes the cost of these systems and the maintenance [165, 166]. Will lower to middle income countries, which are in the greatest need of assistance, share in the cost or will the burden fall on the higher income nations? While this will reduce medical tourism to a point, this will still remain unless the infrastructure for preoperative and postoperative care is created within the countries in need. A likely solution for remote regions would involve smartphone apps for pre- and post-operative care and medical tourism over a shorter distance for operative and immediate aftercare until the patient is sufficiently recovered. With any AI solution to be implemented in a low to middle income country, the obstacles of infrastructure (electricity, wifi, phone lines, etc.), and governance for AI will need to be overcome on a broad scale.

Frequently stated worries are overreliance on technology, the loss of jobs, and physician disapproval. Most technologies being created are intended to assist and prevent fatigue, and skills must be maintained in order to properly utilize the technology. While there are solutions that involve autonomous actions to be handled solely by AI technology, patients themselves are not in favor of operations or procedures in which a surgeon is not involved. A cross-sectional study conducted by Palmisciano et al. found that while the majority of patient respondents thought AI use was appropriate for image interpretation/preoperative planning or indicating potential complications (76.7 and 82.2% respectively), only 17.7% of these patients approved of AI performing an entire operation [167]. Physicians themselves are also quite welcoming of AI integration into neurosurgery. A survey of neurosurgeons, anesthetists, nurses, and operating room practitioners conducted by Horsfall et al. revealed that the majority of respondents viewed the use of AI in various aspects of neurosurgery favorably [167].

The responses were 62% in favor of use for imaging interpretation, 82% approved of use for operative planning, 70% use for coordinating the surgical team, 85% in favor of AI generated real time alerts to complications or hazards, and 66% approved of autonomous surgery by AI. Members of the Congress of Neurological Surgeons and European Association of the Neurosurgical Societies were polled by Staartjes and colleagues regarding the use of ML in neurosurgery. The results demonstrated that 28.8% of respondents used ML in clinical practice and 31.1% used ML for research [168].

8. The future of AI in neurosurgery

Future directions of AI integration into the field of neurosurgery involve both simple and complex solutions, some with global implications. The rise of telemedicine during the COVID-19 pandemic resulted in expanded applications which can be further built upon to partially address the global shortage of neurosurgeons [165]. Approximately 39 countries do not have access to neurosurgical care [3]. Smartphone apps can be used for postoperative follow up, obviating the need to travel prolonged distances to receive continued evaluation. Telesurgery has garnered significant interest, as the potential to decrease transportation costs, improve logistics, and reduce the carbon footprint associated with medical tourism is great. Conceptualized iterations involve an operative suite with robotic equipment that will be controlled by surgeons in a control room. Given the paucity of neurosurgeons relative to the population in need globally, it has been proposed that a general surgeon be at the control room adjacent to the patient, while a neurosurgeon is at the helm in a remote control room [165]. This also has implications for military use as surgeons would be able to care for patients in war zones remotely rather than risking their lives in the field [165].

Within the operating room, the push toward improved logistics and ergonomics as well as minimal to no contact procedures continues. Technologies to merge the microscope view, navigation imaging, and virtual or augmented reality screen into a single device such as surgical glasses are being developed [165]. There are a few augmented reality glasses (HoloLens, xvision Spine System) designed for surgical planning that are already commercially available [169]. The glasses project 3-D models of the patient's anatomy (based on preoperative CT scans) directly into the surgical field, and can be controlled in a contactless manner with hand gestures and voice commands [169]. Magnetic navigation systems are being piloted for contactless endovascular operations [3].

9. Conclusion

This chapter broadly elucidated the scope of artificial intelligence in the field of neurosurgery. At the current moment, AI has successfully been introduced in some clinical settings, especially in the realm of diagnostics. With the increasing capacity of ML and ANNs to abstract patient information and produce clinically relevant results, it appears likely that AI will continue to be increasingly integrated within neurosurgery. In particular, a trend prioritizing the transition from fully supervised and rules-based methods toward self, partially, and semi-supervised algorithms is observed in deep learning, although the latter possesses its own set of limitations.

Furthermore, the literature has demonstrated ad nauseam that when ML and ANN algorithms are tested prospectively on novel patient datasets, they perform, at best, equivalent to expert neurosurgeons in diagnostic examples. Thus, notions suggesting a diminishing scope of the neurosurgeon due to the emergence of AI should be dispelled. Rather, AI can serve to function as an adjunct to the neurosurgeon by playing a supportive role in the pre-, intra-, and postoperative phases of care. An ideal world for the neurosurgical patient of the future is one in which they are treated by a neurosurgeon clinically informed by artificial intelligence.

Yet, there are certain issues to be addressed prior to the overwhelming adoption of AI. In order to make this a truly feasible and applicable solution on a wide scale, uniform (or at least interchangeable) and globally generalizable, externally validated products are needed. Robust studies to fully elucidate the entire cost versus the cost savings from increased efficiency and improved clinical results must be conducted. This will help to inform both healthcare networks and payers on the true value of AI, thus facilitating the creation of a framework for reimbursement and funding methods. In short, greater communication and consensus among developers, healthcare systems, physicians, and payers will allow for the true potential of AI to be realized as a health solution.

Author details

Raivat Shah[1], Vanessa Reese[2]*, Martin Oselkin[3] and Stanislaw P. Stawicki[4]

1 Muhlenberg College, Allentown, PA, United States

2 Department of Research and Innovation, St. Luke's University Health Network, Bethlehem, PA, United States

3 Department of Neurosciences, St. Luke's University Health Network, Bethlehem, PA, United States

4 Department of General Surgery, St. Luke's University Health Network, Bethlehem, PA, United States

*Address all correspondence to: vanessa.reese@sluhn.org

References

[1] Bliss M. Harvey Cushing: A Life in Surgery. Oxford, United Kingdom: Oxford University Press; 2007

[2] Panesar SS, Kliot M, Parrish R, Fernandez-Miranda J, Cagle Y, Britz GW. Promises and perils of artificial intelligence in neurosurgery. Neurosurgery. 2020;**87**(1):33-44. DOI: 10.1093/neuros/nyz471

[3] Mofatteh M. Neurosurgery and artificial intelligence. AIMS Neuroscience. 2021;**8**(4):477-495. DOI: 10.3934/Neuroscience.2021025

[4] Sarker IH. AI-based modeling: Techniques, applications and research issues towards automation, intelligent and smart systems. SN Computer Science. 2022;**3**(2):158. DOI: 10.1007/s42979-022-01043-x

[5] Choi RY, Coyner AS, Kalpathy-Cramer J, Chiang MF, Campbell JP. Introduction to machine learning, neural networks, and deep learning. Translational Vision Science & Technology. 2020;**9**(2):14. DOI: 10.1167/tvst.9.2.14

[6] Niño M, Illarramendi A. Understanding big data: Antecedents, origin and later development. DYNA New Technologies. 2015;**2**:1-8. DOI: 10.6036/NT7835

[7] Janiesch C, Zschech P, Heinrich K. Machine learning and deep learning. Electronic Markets. 2021;**31**(3):685-695. DOI: 10.1007/s12525-021-00475-2

[8] Na KS. Prediction of future cognitive impairment among the community elderly: A machine-learning based approach. Scientific Reports. 2019;**9**(1):3335. DOI: 10.1038/s41598-019-39478-7

[9] Stawicki S. Application of financial analysis techniques to vital sign data: A novel method of trend interpretation in the intensive care unit. OPUS 12 Scientist. 2007;**1**(1):14-16

[10] Obermeyer Z, Emanuel EJ. Predicting the future — Big data, machine learning, and clinical medicine. The New England Journal of Medicine. 2016;**375**(13):1216-1219. DOI: 10.1056/NEJMp1606181

[11] Lee J, Warner E, Shaikhouni S, et al. Unsupervised machine learning for identifying important visual features through bag-of-words using histopathology data from chronic kidney disease. Scientific Reports. 2022;**12**(1):4832. DOI: 10.1038/s41598-022-08974-8

[12] Gravesteijn BY, Nieboer D, Ercole A, et al. Machine learning algorithms performed no better than regression models for prognostication in traumatic brain injury. Journal of Clinical Epidemiology. 2020;**122**:95-107. DOI: 10.1016/j.jclinepi.2020.03.005

[13] Christodoulou E, Ma J, Collins GS, Steyerberg EW, Verbakel JY, Van Calster B. A systematic review shows no performance benefit of machine learning over logistic regression for clinical prediction models. Journal of Clinical Epidemiology. 2019;**110**:12-22. DOI: 10.1016/j.jclinepi.2019.02.004

[14] Nahm FS. Receiver operating characteristic curve: Overview and practical use for clinicians. Korean Journal of Anesthesiology. 2022;**75**(1):25-36. DOI: 10.4097/kja.21209

[15] Fawcett T. An introduction to ROC analysis. Pattern Recognition Letters. 2006;**27**(8):861-874. DOI: 10.1016/j.patrec.2005.10.010

[16] Muller MP, Tomlinson G, Marrie TJ, et al. Can routine laboratory tests discriminate between severe acute respiratory syndrome and other causes of community-acquired pneumonia? Clinical Infectious Diseases. 2005;**40**(8):1079-1086. DOI: 10.1086/428577

[17] Victor Volovici, Ewout W Steyerberg, Maryse C Cnossen, Iain K Haitsma, Clemens M F Dirven, Andrew I R Maas, Hester F Lingsma; Evolution of evidence and guideline recommendations for the medical management of severe traumatic brain injury, Journal of Neurotrauma. 2019; 36(22):3183-3189. Available from: https://www.liebertpub.com/doi/10.1089/neu.2019.6474 [Accessed: December 14, 2022]

[18] Uddin S, Khan A, Hossain ME, Moni MA. Comparing different supervised machine learning algorithms for disease prediction. BMC Medical Informatics and Decision Making. 2019;**19**(1):281. DOI: 10.1186/s12911-019-1004-8

[19] Abràmoff MD, Lavin PT, Birch M, Shah N, Folk JC. Pivotal trial of an autonomous AI-based diagnostic system for detection of diabetic retinopathy in primary care offices. npj Digital Medicine. 2018;**1**(1):1-8. DOI: 10.1038/s41746-018-0040-6

[20] Zhu X, Wu X. Class noise vs. attribute noise: A quantitative study. Artificial Intelligence Review. 2004;**22**(3):177-210. DOI: 10.1007/s10462-004-0751-8

[21] Gupta S, Gupta A. Dealing with noise problem in machine learning data-sets: A systematic review. Procedia Computer Science. 2019;**161**:466-474. DOI: 10.1016/j.procs.2019.11.146

[22] What are the parts of the nervous system? Published October 1, 2018. Available from: https://www.nichd.nih.gov/health/topics/neuro/conditioninfo/parts [Accessed: April 6, 2023]

[23] Shepherd GM. The Synaptic Organization of the Brain. 5th ed. Vol. xiv. Oxford, United Kingdom: Oxford University Press; 2004. p. 719. DOI: 10.1093/acprof:oso/9780195159561.001.1

[24] Ebersole JS, Pedley TA. Current Practice of Clinical Electroencephalography. Philadelphia, Pennsylvania: Lippincott Williams & Wilkins; 2003

[25] Reyes A. Influence of dendritic conductances on the input-output properties of neurons. Annual Review of Neuroscience. 2001;**24**:653-675. DOI: 10.1146/annurev.neuro.24.1.653

[26] Purves D, Augustine GJ, Fitzpatrick D, et al. Excitatory and inhibitory postsynaptic potentials. Neuroscience, 2nd Ed. Sunderland (MA): Sinauer Associates; 2001. Available from: https://www.ncbi.nlm.nih.gov/books/NBK11117/ [Accessed: January 28, 2023]

[27] McCulloch WS, Pitts W. A logical calculus of the ideas immanent in nervous activity. Bulletin of Mathematical Biology. 1990;**52**(1):99-115. DOI: 10.1007/BF02459570

[28] Han SH, Kim KW, Kim S, Youn YC. Artificial neural network: Understanding the basic concepts without mathematics. Dementia Neurocognitive Disorder. 2018;**17**(3):83-89. DOI: 10.12779/dnd.2018.17.3.83

[29] Indolia S, Goswami AK, Mishra SP, Asopa P. Conceptual understanding of convolutional neural network- a deep learning approach. Procedia Computer Science. 2018;**132**:679-688. DOI: 10.1016/j.procs.2018.05.069

[30] Sarker IH. Deep learning: A comprehensive overview on techniques, taxonomy, applications and research directions. SN Computer Science. 2021;**2**(6):420. DOI: 10.1007/s42979-021-00815-1

[31] Harbaugh RE. Editorial. Artificial neural networks for neurosurgical diagnosis, prognosis, and management. Neurosurgical Focus. 2018;**45**(5):E3. DOI: 10.3171/2018.8.FOCUS18438

[32] AI vs. Machine Learning vs. Deep Learning vs. Neural Networks: What's the Difference? Published January 19, 2022. Available from: https://www.ibm.com/cloud/blog/ai-vs-machine-learning-vs-deep-learning-vs-neural-networks [Accessed: February 26, 2023]

[33] Azimi P, Mohammadi HR, Benzel EC, Shahzadi S, Azhari S, Montazeri A. Artificial neural networks in neurosurgery. Journal of Neurology, Neurosurgery, and Psychiatry. 2015;**86**(3):251-256. DOI: 10.1136/jnnp-2014-307807

[34] Yang S, Zhu F, Ling X, Liu Q and Zhao P; Intelligent health care: Applications of deep learning in computational medicine. Frontiers in Genetics. 2021; 12:607471; [Accessed: February 8, 2023]. Available from: https://www.frontiersin.org/articles/10.3389/fgene.2021.607471/full

[35] Khurana D, Koli A, Khatter K, Singh S. Natural language processing: State of the art, current trends and challenges. Multimedia Tools and Applications. 2023;**82**(3):3713-3744. DOI: 10.1007/s11042-022-13428-4

[36] Tan WK, Hassanpour S, Heagerty PJ, et al. Comparison of natural language processing rules-based and machine-learning systems to identify lumbar spine imaging findings related to low back pain. Academic Radiology. 2018;**25**(11):1422-1432. DOI: 10.1016/j.acra.2018.03.008

[37] Bacco L, Russo F, Ambrosio L, et al. Natural language processing in low back pain and spine diseases: A systematic review. Frontiers in Surgery 2022; 9, 957085. Available from: https://www.frontiersin.org/articles/10.3389/fsurg.2022.957085 [Accessed: February 23, 2023]

[38] Dave T, Athaluri SA, Singh S. ChatGPT in medicine: An overview of its applications, advantages, limitations, future prospects, and ethical considerations. Frontiers in Artificial Intelligence. 2023;**6**:1169595. DOI: 10.3389/frai.2023.1169595

[39] Ali R, Tang OY, Connolly ID, et al. Performance of ChatGPT and GPT-4 on neurosurgery written board examinations. Neurosurgery. 2023;**00**: 1-13. DOI: 10.1101/2023.03.25.23287743

[40] Blease C, Kharko A, Annoni M, Gaab J, Locher C. Machine learning in clinical psychology and psychotherapy education: A mixed methods pilot survey of postgraduate students at a Swiss university, Frontiers in Public Health 2021;9, 623088. Available from: https://www.frontiersin.org/articles/10.3389/fpubh.2021.623088 [Accessed: July 31, 2023]

[41] Shickel B, Tighe P, Bihorac A, Rashidi P. Deep EHR: A survey of recent advances in deep learning techniques for electronic health record (EHR) analysis. IEEE Journal of Biomedical and Health Informatics. 2018;**22**(5):1589-1604. DOI: 10.1109/JBHI.2017.2767063

[42] Kumah-Crystal YA, Pirtle CJ, Whyte HM, Goode ES, Anders SH, Lehmann CU. Electronic health record interactions through voice: A review. Applied Clinical Informatics. 2018;**9**(3):541-552. DOI: 10.1055/s-0038-1666844

[43] Wartman SA, Combs CD. Medical education must move from the information age to the age of artificial intelligence. Academic Medicine: Journal of the Association of American Medical Colleges. 2018;**93**(8):1107-1109. DOI: 10.1097/ACM.0000000000002044

[44] Oermann EK, Rubinsteyn A, Ding D, et al. Using a machine learning approach to predict outcomes after radiosurgery for cerebral arteriovenous malformations. Scientific Reports. 2016;**6**(1):21161. DOI: 10.1038/srep21161

[45] Azimi P, Mohammadi HR. Predicting endoscopic third ventriculostomy success in childhood hydrocephalus: An artificial neural network analysis: Clinical article. Journal of Neurosurgery. Pediatrics. 2014;**13**(4):426-432. DOI: 10.3171/2013.12.PEDS13423

[46] Habibi Z, Ertiaei A, Nikdad MS, et al. Predicting ventriculoperitoneal shunt infection in children with hydrocephalus using artificial neural network. Child's Nervous System. 2016;**32**(11):2143-2151. DOI: 10.1007/s00381-016-3248-2

[47] Hamed Asadi, Hong Kuan Kok, Seamus Looby, Paul Brennan, Alan O'Hare, John Thornton; Outcomes and complications after endovascular treatment of brain arteriovenous malformations: A prognostication attempt using artificial intelligence. 2016, World Neurosurgery; 96, 562-569.e1; Available from: https://www.sciencedirect.com/science/article/pii/S1878875016309160 [Accessed: December 14, 2022]

[48] Parisa Azimi, Edward C Benzel, Sohrab Shahzadi, Shirzad Azhari, Hasan Reza Mohammadi; Use of artificial neural networks to predict surgical satisfaction in patients with lumbar spinal canal stenosis: Journal of Neurosurgery: Spine, 20, 3 (2014), 300-305. https://thejns.org/spine/view/journals/j-neurosurg-spine/20/3/article-p300.xml [Accessed: December 14, 2022]

[49] Shi HY, Hwang SL, Lee KT, Lin CL. In-hospital mortality after traumatic brain injury surgery: A nationwide population-based comparison of mortality predictors used in artificial neural network and logistic regression models: Clinical article. Journal of Neurosurgery. 2013;**118**(4):746-752. DOI: 10.3171/2013.1.JNS121130

[50] Travis M Dumont, Anand I Rughani, Bruce I Tranmer; Prediction of symptomatic cerebral vasospasm after aneurysmal subarachnoid hemorrhage with an artificial neural network: Feasibility and comparison with logistic regression models. World Neurosurgery. 2011;**75**(1):57-63. Available from: https://www.sciencedirect.com/science/article/pii/S187887501000358X [Accessed: December 14, 2022]

[51] Abouzari M, Rashidi A, Zandi-Toghani M, Behzadi M, Asadollahi M. Chronic subdural hematoma outcome prediction using logistic regression and an artificial neural network. Neurosurgical Review. 2009;**32**(4):479-484. DOI: 10.1007/s10143-009-0215-3

[52] Senders JT, Staples PC, Karhade AV, et al. Machine learning and neurosurgical outcome prediction: A systematic review. World Neurosurgery. 2018;**109**:476-486.e1. DOI: 10.1016/j.wneu.2017.09.149

[53] Masoudi MS, Rezaei E, Tahmouresi A, et al. Prediction of 6 months endoscopic third ventriculostomy success rate in patients with hydrocephalus using a multi-layer perceptron network. Clinical Neurology and Neurosurgery. 2022;**219**:107295. DOI: 10.1016/j.clineuro.2022.107295

[54] Tunthanathip T, Duangsuwan J, Wattanakitrungroj N, Tongman S, Phuenpathom N. Comparison of intracranial injury predictability between machine learning algorithms and the nomogram in pediatric traumatic brain injury. Neurosurgical Focus. 2021;**51**(5):E7. DOI: 10.3171/2021.8.FOCUS2155

[55] Emblem KE, Nedregaard B, Hald JK, Nome T, Due-Tonnessen P, Bjornerud A. Automatic glioma characterization from dynamic susceptibility contrast imaging: Brain tumor segmentation using knowledge-based fuzzy clustering. Journal of Magnetic Resonance Imaging. 2009;**30**(1):1-10. DOI: 10.1002/jmri.21815

[56] Emblem KE, Pinho MC, Zöllner FG, et al. A generic support vector machine model for preoperative glioma survival associations. Radiology. 2015;**275**(1):228-234. DOI: 10.1148/radiol.14140770

[57] Sagberg LM, Jakola AS, Reinertsen I, Solheim O. How well do neurosurgeons predict survival in patients with high-grade glioma? Neurosurgical Review. 2022;**45**(1):865-872. DOI: 10.1007/s10143-021-01613-2

[58] Kaka H, Zhang E, Khan N. Artificial intelligence and deep learning in neuroradiology: Exploring the new frontier. Canadian Association of Radiologists Journal. 2021;**72**(1):35-44. DOI: 10.1177/0846537120954293

[59] Matsoukas S, Scaggiante J, Schuldt BR, et al. Accuracy of artificial intelligence for the detection of intracranial hemorrhage and chronic cerebral microbleeds: A systematic review and pooled analysis. Radiology Medicine (Torino). 2022;**127**(10):1106-1123. DOI: 10.1007/s11547-022-01530-4

[60] Stawicki SP, Wojda TR, Nuschke JD, et al. Prognostication of traumatic brain injury outcomes in older trauma patients: A novel risk assessment tool based on initial cranial CT findings. International Journal of Critical Illness and Injury Science. 2017;**7**(1):23. DOI: 10.4103/IJCIIS.IJCIIS_2_17

[61] Ye H, Gao F, Yin Y, et al. Precise diagnosis of intracranial hemorrhage and subtypes using a three-dimensional joint convolutional and recurrent neural network. European Radiology. 2019;**29**(11):6191-6201. DOI: 10.1007/s00330-019-06163-2

[62] Intracranial Hemorrhage (ICH), Aidoc. Available from: www.AIforRadiology.com/ [Accessed: February 6, 2023]

[63] Ginat DT. Analysis of head CT scans flagged by deep learning software for acute intracranial hemorrhage. Neuroradiology. 2020;**62**(3):335-340. DOI: 10.1007/s00234-019-02330-w

[64] Voter AF, Meram E, Garrett JW, Yu JPJ. Diagnostic accuracy and failure mode analysis of a deep learning algorithm for the detection of intracranial hemorrhage. Journal of the American College of Radiology. 2021;**18**(8):1143-1152. DOI: 10.1016/j.jacr.2021.03.005

[65] Smith J. Radiological Computer Aided Triage and Notification Software (510(k) Number K180647), U. FDA, Editor. Philadelphia, PA; 2018

[66] Ojeda P, Zawaideh M, Mossa-Basha M, Haynor D. The utility of deep learning: Evaluation of a convolutional neural network for detection of intracranial bleeds on non-contrast head computed tomography studies. In: Medical Imaging 2019: Image Processing. Vol. 10949. San Diego, California, USA: SPIE; 2019. pp. 899-906. DOI: 10.1117/12.2513167

[67] Wang X, Liang G, Zhang Y, Blanton H, Bessinger Z, Jacobs N. I nconsistent performance of deep learning models on mammogram classification. Journal of the American College of Radiology. 2020;**17**(6):796-803. DOI: 10.1016/j.jacr.2020.01.006

[68] McLouth J, Elstrott S, Chaibi Y, et al. Validation of a deep learning tool in the detection of intracranial hemorrhage and large vessel occlusion. Frontiers in Neurology 2021;12, 656112. Available from: https://www.frontiersin.org/articles/10.3389/fneur.2021.656112 [Accessed: February 6, 2023]

[69] Rava RA, Seymour SE, LaQue ME, et al. Assessment of an artificial intelligence algorithm for detection of intracranial hemorrhage. World Neurosurgery. 2021;**150**:e209-e217. DOI: 10.1016/j.wneu.2021.02.134

[70] Pop NO, Tit DM, Diaconu CC, et al. The Alberta stroke program early CT score (ASPECTS): A predictor of mortality in acute ischemic stroke. Experimental and Therapeutic Medicine. 2021;**22**(6):1371. DOI: 10.3892/etm.2021.10805

[71] Soun JE, Chow DS, Nagamine M, et al. Artificial intelligence and acute stroke imaging. AJNR. American Journal of Neuroradiology. 2021;**42**(1):2-11. DOI: 10.3174/ajnr.A6883

[72] Guberina N, Dietrich U, Radbruch A, et al. Detection of early infarction signs with machine learning-based diagnosis by means of the Alberta stroke program early CT score (ASPECTS) in the clinical routine. Neuroradiology. 2018;**60**(9):889-901. DOI: 10.1007/s00234-018-2066-5

[73] Maegerlein C, Fischer J, Mönch S, et al. Automated calculation of the Alberta stroke program early CT score: Feasibility and reliability. Radiology. 2019;**291**(1):141-148. DOI: 10.1148/radiol.2019181228

[74] You J, Yu PLH, Tsang ACO, Tsui ELH, Woo PPS, Leung GKK. Automated computer evaluation of acute ischemic stroke and large vessel occlusion. arXiv. 2019;**4**:1-8. DOI: 10.48550/arXiv.1906.08059

[75] Albers GW, Marks MP, Kemp S, et al. Thrombectomy for stroke at 6 to 16 hours with selection by perfusion imaging. The New England Journal of Medicine. 2018;**378**(8):708-718. DOI: 10.1056/NEJMoa1713973

[76] Nielsen A, Hansen MB, Tietze A, Mouridsen K. Prediction of tissue outcome and assessment of treatment effect in acute ischemic stroke using deep learning. Stroke. 2018;**49**(6):1394-1401. DOI: 10.1161/STROKEAHA.117.019740

[77] Nishi H, Oishi N, Ishii A, et al. Deep learning-derived high-level neuroimaging features predict clinical outcomes for large vessel occlusion. Stroke. 2020;**51**(5):1484-1492. DOI: 10.1161/STROKEAHA.119.028101

[78] Liu J, Zou X, Zhao Y, et al. Prevalence and risk factors for unruptured intracranial aneurysms in the population at high risk for aneurysm in the rural areas of Tianjin. Frontiers in Neurology 2022; 13, 853054. Available from: https://www.frontiersin.org/articles/10.3389/fneur.2022.853054 [Accessed: April 6, 2023]

[79] van Gijn J, Kerr RS, Rinkel GJE. Subarachnoid haemorrhage. The Lancet. 2007;**369**(9558):306-318. DOI: 10.1016/S0140-6736(07)60153-6

[80] Keedy A. An overview of intracranial aneurysms. McGill Journal of Medicine. 2006;**9**(2):141-146

[81] Tang H, Hu N, Yuan Y, et al. Accelerated time-of-flight magnetic resonance angiography with sparse

undersampling and iterative reconstruction for the evaluation of intracranial arteries. Korean Journal of Radiology. 2019;**20**(2):265-274. DOI: 10.3348/kjr.2017.0634

[82] Nakao T, Hanaoka S, Nomura Y, et al. Deep neural network-based computer-assisted detection of cerebral aneurysms in MR angiography. Journal of Magnetic Resonance Imaging (JMRI). 2018;**47**(4):948-953. DOI: 10.1002/jmri.25842

[83] Faron A, Sichtermann T, Teichert N, et al. Performance of a deep-learning neural network to detect intracranial aneurysms from 3D TOF-MRA compared to human readers. Clinical Neuroradiology. 2020;**30**(3):591-598. DOI: 10.1007/s00062-019-00809-w

[84] Ueda D, Yamamoto A, Nishimori M, et al. Deep learning for MR angiography: Automated detection of cerebral aneurysms. Radiology. 2019;**290**(1):187-194. DOI: 10.1148/radiol.2018180901

[85] Shi Z, Miao C, Schoepf UJ, et al. A clinically applicable deep-learning model for detecting intracranial aneurysm in computed tomography angiography images. Nature Communications. 2020;**11**(1):6090. DOI: 10.1038/s41467-020-19527-w

[86] Yang J, Xie M, Hu C, et al. Deep learning for detecting cerebral aneurysms with CT angiography. Radiology. 2021;**298**(1):155-163. DOI: 10.1148/radiol.2020192154

[87] Fawzi A, Achuthan A, Belaton B. Brain image segmentation in recent years: A narrative review. Brain Sciences. 2021;**11**(8):1055. DOI: 10.3390/brainsci11081055

[88] Virupakshappa AB. Cognition-based MRI brain tumor segmentation technique using modified level set method. Cognition, Technology & Work. 2019;**21**(3):357-369. DOI: 10.1007/s10111-018-0472-4

[89] Ilunga-Mbuyamba E, Avina-Cervantes JG, Garcia-Perez A, et al. Localized active contour model with background intensity compensation applied on automatic MR brain tumor segmentation. Neurocomputing. 2017;**220**:84-97. DOI: 10.1016/j.neucom.2016.07.057

[90] Kermi A, Andjouh K, Zidane F. Fully automated brain tumour segmentation system in 3D-MRI using symmetry analysis of brain and level sets. IET Image Processing. 2018;**12**(11):1964-1971. DOI: 10.1049/iet-ipr.2017.1124

[91] Achuthan A, Rajeswari M. Segmentation of hippocampus guided by assembled and weighted coherent point drift registration. Journal of King Saud University - Computer and Information Sciences. 2021;**33**(8):1008-1017. DOI: 10.1016/j.jksuci.2019.06.011

[92] Safavian N, Batouli SAH, Oghabian MA. An automatic level set method for hippocampus segmentation in MR images. Computer Methods in Biomechanics and Biomedical Engineering: Imaging & Visualization. 2020;**8**(4):400-410. DOI: 10.1080/21681163.2019.1706054

[93] Liu Z, Tong L, Chen L, et al. Deep learning based brain tumor segmentation: A survey. Complex & Intelligent Systems. 2023;**9**(1):1001-1026. DOI: 10.1007/s40747-022-00815-5

[94] Chen G, Li Q, Shi F, Rekik I, Pan Z. RFDCR: Automated brain lesion segmentation using cascaded random forests with dense conditional random fields. NeuroImage. 2020;**211**:116620. DOI: 10.1016/j.neuroimage.2020.116620

[95] Nitta GR, Sravani T, Nitta S, Muthu B. Dominant gray level based K-means algorithm for MRI images. Health Technology. 2020;**10**(1):281-287. DOI: 10.1007/s12553-018-00293-1

[96] Mohammadreza Soltaninejad, Guang Yang, Tryphon Lambrou, Nigel Allinson, Timothy L Jones, Thomas R Barrick, Franklyn A Howe, Xujiong Ye; Supervised learning based multimodal MRI brain tumour segmentation using texture features from supervoxels. Computer Methods and Programs in Biomedicine. 2018;157:69-84; Available from: https://www.sciencedirect.com/science/article/pii/S016926071731355X?via%3Dihub [Accessed: February 25, 2023]

[97] Gunasekara SR, Kaldera HNTK, Dissanayake MB. A systematic approach for MRI brain tumor localization and segmentation using deep learning and active contouring. Journal of Healthcare Engineering. 2021;**2021**:e6695108. DOI: 10.1155/2021/6695108

[98] Ribalta Lorenzo P, Nalepa J, Bobek-Billewicz B, et al. Segmenting brain tumors from FLAIR MRI using fully convolutional neural networks. Computer Methods and Programs in Biomedicine. 2019;**176**:135-148. DOI: 10.1016/j.cmpb.2019.05.006

[99] Wu D, Ding Y, Zhang M, Yang Q, Qin Z. Multi-features refinement and aggregation for medical brain segmentation. IEEE Access. 2020;**8**:57483-57496. DOI: 10.1109/ACCESS.2020.2981380

[100] Silva CA, Pinto A, Pereira S, Lopes A. Multi-stage deep layer aggregation for brain tumor segmentation. In: Crimi A, Bakas S, editors. Brainlesion: Glioma, Multiple Sclerosis, Stroke and Traumatic Brain Injuries. Lecture Notes in Computer Science. New York City, New York: Springer International Publishing; 2021. pp. 179-188. DOI: 10.1007/978-3-030-72087-2_16

[101] Cui S, Mao L, Jiang J, Liu C, Xiong S. Automatic semantic segmentation of brain gliomas from MRI images using a deep cascaded neural network. Journal of Healthcare Engineering. 2018;**2018**:e4940593. DOI: 10.1155/2018/4940593

[102] Chen H, Qin Z, Ding Y, Tian L, Qin Z. Brain tumor segmentation with deep convolutional symmetric neural network. Neurocomputing. 2020;**392**:305-313. DOI: 10.1016/j.neucom.2019.01.111

[103] Guo Z, Li X, Huang H, Guo N, Li Q. Deep learning-based image segmentation on multimodal medical imaging. IEEE Transactions on Radiation and Plasma Medical Sciences. 2019;**3**(2):162-169. DOI: 10.1109/TRPMS.2018.2890359

[104] Sajid S, Hussain S, Sarwar A. Brain tumor detection and segmentation in MR images using deep learning. Arabian Journal for Science and Engineering. 2019;**44**(11):9249-9261. DOI: 10.1007/s13369-019-03967-8

[105] Li H, Li A, Wang M. A novel end-to-end brain tumor segmentation method using improved fully convolutional networks. Computers in Biology and Medicine. 2019;**108**:150-160. DOI: 10.1016/j.compbiomed.2019.03.014

[106] Iqbal S, Ghani MU, Saba T, Rehman A. Brain tumor segmentation in multi-spectral MRI using convolutional neural networks (CNN). Microscopy Research and Technique. 2018;**81**(4):419-427. DOI: 10.1002/jemt.22994

[107] Chen L, Bentley P, Mori K, Misawa K, Fujiwara M, Rueckert D.

DRINet for medical image segmentation. IEEE Transactions on Medical Imaging. 2018;**37**(11):2453-2462. DOI: 10.1109/TMI.2018.2835303

[108] Moeskops P, de Bresser J, Kuijf HJ, et al. Evaluation of a deep learning approach for the segmentation of brain tissues and white matter hyperintensities of presumed vascular origin in MRI. NeuroImage: Clinical. 2018;**17**:251-262. DOI: 10.1016/j.nicl.2017.10.007

[109] Mohammad Havaei, Axel Davy, David Warde-Farley, Antoine Biard, Aaron Courville, Yoshua Bengio, Chris Pal, Pierre-Marc Jodoin, Hugo Larochelle; Brain tumor segmentation with deep neural networks. Medical Image Analysis; 2017; 35; 18-31; Available from: https://www.sciencedirect.com/science/article/pii/S1361841516300330?via%3Dihub [Accessed: February 26, 2023]

[110] Myronenko A. 3D MRI brain tumor segmentation using autoencoder regularization. In: Crimi A, Bakas S, Kuijf H, Keyvan F, Reyes M, van Walsum T, editors. Brainlesion: Glioma, Multiple Sclerosis, Stroke and Traumatic Brain Injuries. Lecture Notes in Computer Science. New York City, New York: Springer International Publishing; 2019. pp. 311-320. DOI: 10.1007/978-3-030-11726-9_28

[111] Shubhangi Nema, Akshay Dudhane, Subrahmanyam Murala, Srivatsava Naidu; RescueNet: An unpaired GAN for brain tumor segmentation, Biomedical Signal Processing and Control. 2020; 55, 101641; Available from: https://www.sciencedirect.com/science/article/pii/S1746809419302228?via%3Dihub [Accessed: February 26, 2023]

[112] Baid U, Talbar S, Rane S, et al. A novel approach for fully automatic intra-tumor segmentation with 3D U-net architecture for gliomas. Frontiers in Computational Neuroscience 2020; 14, 10. Available from: https://www.frontiersin.org/articles/10.3389/fncom.2020.00010 [Accessed: February 26, 2023]

[113] Zhou Z, He Z, Shi M, Du J, Chen D. 3D dense connectivity network with atrous convolutional feature pyramid for brain tumor segmentation in magnetic resonance imaging of human heads. Computers in Biology and Medicine. 2020;**121**:103766. DOI: 10.1016/j.compbiomed.2020.103766

[114] Sun J, Peng Y, Guo Y, Li D. Segmentation of the multimodal brain tumor image used the multi-pathway architecture method based on 3D FCN. Neurocomputing. 2021;**423**:34-45. DOI: 10.1016/j.neucom.2020.10.031

[115] Ramzan F, Khan MUG, Iqbal S, Saba T, Rehman A. Volumetric segmentation of brain regions from MRI scans using 3D convolutional neural networks. IEEE Access. 2020;**8**:103697-103709. DOI: 10.1109/ACCESS.2020.2998901

[116] Wang G, Li W, Ourselin S, Vercauteren T. Automatic brain tumor segmentation based on cascaded convolutional neural networks with uncertainty estimation. Frontiers in Computational Neuroscience 2019;13, 56. Available from: https://www.frontiersin.org/articles/10.3389/fncom.2019.00056 [Accessed: February 26, 2023]

[117] Kamnitsas K, Ledig C, Newcombe VFJ, et al. Efficient multi-scale 3D CNN with fully connected CRF for accurate brain lesion segmentation. Medical Image Analysis. 2017;**36**:61-78. DOI: 10.1016/j.media.2016.10.004

[118] Fidon L, Li W, Garcia-Peraza-Herrera LC, et al. Scalable multimodal convolutional networks for brain tumour segmentation. In:

Descoteaux M, Maier-Hein L, Franz A, Jannin P, Collins DL, Duchesne S, editors. Medical Image Computing and Computer Assisted Intervention – MICCAI 2017. Lecture Notes in Computer Science. New York City, New York: Springer International Publishing; 2017. pp. 285-293. DOI: 10.1007/978-3-319-66179-7_33

[119] Pham TX, Siarry P, Oulhadj H. Integrating fuzzy entropy clustering with an improved PSO for MRI brain image segmentation. Applied Soft Computing. 2018;**65**:230-242. DOI: 10.1016/j.asoc.2018.01.003

[120] Pham TX, Siarry P, Oulhadj H. Segmentation of MR brain images through hidden Markov random field and hybrid metaheuristic algorithm. IEEE Transactions on Image Processing. 2020;**29**:6507-6522. DOI: 10.1109/TIP.2020.2990346

[121] Thuy Xuan Pham, Patrick Siarry, Hamouche Oulhadj; A multi objective optimization approach for brain MRI segmentation using fuzzy entropy clustering and region-based active contour methods, Magnetic Resonance Imaging. 2019;61:41-65. Available from: https://www.sciencedirect.com/science/article/pii/S0730725X18301991?via%3Dihub [Accessed: February 26, 2023]

[122] Mishro PK, Agrawal S, Panda R, Abraham A. A novel Type-2 fuzzy C-means clustering for brain MR image segmentation. IEEE Transactions on Cybernetics. 2021;**51**(8):3901-3912. DOI: 10.1109/TCYB.2020.2994235

[123] Caesarendra W, Rahmaniar W, Mathew J, Thien A. Automated cobb angle measurement for adolescent idiopathic scoliosis using convolutional neural network. Diagnostics. 2022;**12**(2):396. DOI: 10.3390/diagnostics12020396

[124] Chockalingam N, Dangerfield PH, Giakas G, Cochrane T, Dorgan JC. Computer-assisted cobb measurement of scoliosis. European Spine Journal. 2002;**11**(4):353-357. DOI: 10.1007/s00586-002-0386-x

[125] Shea KG, Stevens PM, Nelson M, Smith JT, Masters KS, Yandow S. A comparison of manual versus computer-assisted radiographic measurement. Intraobserver measurement variability for cobb angles. Spine. 1998;**23**(5):551-555. DOI: 10.1097/00007632-199803010-00007

[126] Jin C, Wang S, Yang G, Li E, Liang Z. A review of the methods on cobb angle measurements for spinal curvature. Sensors. 2022;**22**(9):3258. DOI: 10.3390/s22093258

[127] Wang J, Zhang J, Xu R, Chen TG, Zhou KS, Zhang HH. Measurement of scoliosis cobb angle by end vertebra tilt angle method. Journal of Orthopaedic Surgery. 2018;**13**(1):223. DOI: 10.1186/s13018-018-0928-5

[128] Sun Y, Xing Y, Zhao Z, Meng X, Xu G, Hai Y. Comparison of manual versus automated measurement of cobb angle in idiopathic scoliosis based on a deep learning keypoint detection technology. European Spine Journal. 2022;**31**(8):1969-1978. DOI: 10.1007/s00586-021-07025-6

[129] Tomita N, Cheung YY, Hassanpour S. Deep neural networks for automatic detection of osteoporotic vertebral fractures on CT scans. Computers in Biology and Medicine. 2018;**98**:8-15. Available from: https://www.sciencedirect.com/science/article/pii/S0010482518301185?via%3Dihub [Accessed: February 26, 2023]

[130] Small JE, Osler P, Paul AB, Kunst M. CT cervical spine fracture detection using a convolutional neural

network. AJNR. American Journal of Neuroradiology. 2021;**42**(7):1341-1347. DOI: 10.3174/ajnr.A7094

[131] Derkatch S, Kirby C, Kimelman D, Jozani MJ, Davidson JM, Leslie WD. Identification of vertebral fractures by convolutional neural networks to predict nonvertebral and hip fractures: A registry-based cohort study of dual X-ray absorptiometry. Radiology. 2019;**293**(2):405-411. DOI: 10.1148/radiol.2019190201

[132] Lehnen NC, Haase R, Faber J, et al. Detection of degenerative changes on MR images of the lumbar spine with a convolutional neural network: A feasibility study. Diagnostics. 2021;**11**(5):902. DOI: 10.3390/diagnostics11050902

[133] Whitehead W, Moran S, Gaonkar B, Macyszyn L, Iyer S. A deep learning approach to spine segmentation using a feed-forward chain of pixel-wise convolutional networks. In: 2018 IEEE 15th International Symposium on Biomedical Imaging (ISBI 2018). New York City, New York, USA; 2018. pp. 868-871. DOI: 10.1109/ISBI.2018.8363709

[134] Huang J, Shen H, Wu J, et al. Spine explorer: A deep learning based fully automated program for efficient and reliable quantifications of the vertebrae and discs on sagittal lumbar spine MR images. The Spine Journal. 2020;**20**(4):590-599. DOI: 10.1016/j.spinee.2019.11.010

[135] Shen H, Huang J, Zheng Q, et al. A deep-learning-based, fully automated program to segment and quantify major spinal components on axial lumbar spine magnetic resonance images. Physical Therapy. 2021;**101**(6):pzab041. DOI: 10.1093/ptj/pzab041

[136] Cheng YK, Lin CL, Huang YC, et al. Automatic segmentation of specific intervertebral discs through a two-stage MultiResUNet model. Journal of Clinical Medicine. 2021;**10**(20):4760. DOI: 10.3390/jcm10204760

[137] Miotto R, Percha BL, Glicksberg BS, et al. Identifying acute low Back pain episodes in primary care practice from clinical notes: Observational study. JMIR Medical Informatics. 2020;**8**(2):e16878. DOI: 10.2196/16878

[138] Meola A, Cutolo F, Carbone M, Cagnazzo F, Ferrari M, Ferrari V. Augmented reality in neurosurgery: A systematic review. Neurosurgical Review. 2017;**40**(4):537-548. DOI: 10.1007/s10143-016-0732-9

[139] Sun GC, Wang F, Chen XL, et al. Impact of virtual and augmented reality based on intraoperative magnetic resonance imaging and functional neuronavigation in glioma surgery involving eloquent areas. World Neurosurgery. 2016;**96**:375-382. DOI: 10.1016/j.wneu.2016.07.107

[140] Bopp MHA, Saß B, Pojskić M, et al. Use of neuronavigation and augmented reality in transsphenoidal pituitary adenoma surgery. Journal of Clinical Medicine. 2022;**11**(19):5590. DOI: 10.3390/jcm11195590

[141] Rychen J, Goldberg J, Raabe A, Bervini D. Augmented reality in superficial temporal artery to middle cerebral artery bypass surgery: Technical note. Operative Neurosurgery. 2020;**18**(4):444. DOI: 10.1093/ons/opz176

[142] Cakmakci D, Karakaslar EO, Ruhland E, et al. Machine learning assisted intraoperative assessment of brain tumor margins using HRMAS NMR spectroscopy. PLoS Computational Biology. 2020;**16**(11):e1008184. DOI: 10.1371/journal.pcbi.1008184

[143] Rashad Jabarkheel, Chi-Sing Ho, Adrian J Rodrigues, Michael C Jin, Jonathon J Parker, Kobina Mensah-Brown, Derek Yecies, Gerald A Grant; Rapid intraoperative diagnosis of pediatric brain tumors using Raman spectroscopy: A machine learning approach, Neuro-Oncology Advances, Oxford Academic. 2022; 4(1):vdac118; https://academic.oup.com/noa/article/4/1/vdac118/6650324 [Accessed: March 6, 2023]

[144] Chang M, Canseco JA, Nicholson KJ, Patel N, Vaccaro AR. The role of machine learning in spine surgery: The future is now. Frontiers in Surgery 2020;7, 54. Available from: https://www.frontiersin.org/articles/10.3389/fsurg.2020.00054 [Accessed: March 6, 2023]

[145] Rasouli JJ, Shao J, Neifert S, et al. Artificial intelligence and robotics in spine surgery. Global Spine Journal. 2021;**11**(4):556-564. DOI: 10.1177/2192568220915718

[146] Arvind V, Kim JS, Oermann EK, Kaji D, Cho SK. Predicting surgical complications in adult patients undergoing anterior cervical discectomy and fusion using machine learning. Neurospine. 2018;**15**(4):329-337. DOI: 10.14245/ns.1836248.124

[147] Kim JS, Merrill RK, Arvind V, et al. Examining the ability of artificial neural networks machine learning models to accurately predict complications following posterior lumbar spine fusion. Spine. 2018;**43**(12):853-860. DOI: 10.1097/BRS.0000000000002442

[148] Jinhua Yu, Zhifeng Shi, Yuxi Lian, Zeju Li, Tongtong Liu, Yuan Gao, Yuanyuan Wang, Liang Chen, Ying Mao; Noninvasive IDH1 mutation estimation based on a quantitative radiomics approach for grade II glioma. European Radiology. 2017; 27(8):3509-3522; Available from: https://pubmed.ncbi.nlm.nih.gov/28004160/ [Accessed: March 6, 2023]

[149] Reider-Demer M, Raja P, Martin N, Schwinger M, Babayan D. Prospective and retrospective study of videoconference telemedicine follow-up after elective neurosurgery: Results of a pilot program. Neurosurgical Review. 2018;**41**(2):497-501. DOI: 10.1007/s10143-017-0878-0

[150] Harrer S. Attention is not all you need: The complicated case of ethically using large language models in healthcare and medicine. eBioMedicine. 2023;**90**:104512. DOI: 10.1016/j.ebiom.2023.104512

[151] Information Blocking. HealthIT.gov. https://www.healthit.gov/topic/information-blocking [Accessed: July 31, 2023]

[152] Khanna NN, Maindarkar MA, Viswanathan V, et al. Economics of artificial intelligence in healthcare: Diagnosis vs. treatment. Healthcare. 2022;**10**(12):2493. DOI: 10.3390/healthcare10122493

[153] Yoon JS, Tang OY, Lawton MT. Volume-cost relationship in neurosurgery: Analysis of 12,129,029 admissions from the National Inpatient Sample. World Neurosurgery. 2019;**129**:e791-e802. DOI: 10.1016/j.wneu.2019.06.034

[154] Wolff J, Pauling J, Keck A, Baumbach J. The economic impact of artificial intelligence in health care: Systematic review. Journal of Medical Internet Research. 2020;**22**(2):e16866. DOI: 10.2196/16866

[155] Sanyal S. How much does artificial intelligence cost in 2021? Analytics Insight. 2021. p. 1. Available from:

https://www.analyticsinsight.net/how-much-does-artificial-intelligence-cost-in-2021/ [Accessed: March 2, 2023]

[156] Luzniak K. Cost of AI in healthcare industry. Neoteric. 2021. pp. 1-11. Available from: https://neoteric.eu/blog/whats-the-cost-of-artificial-intelligence-in-healthcare/ [Accessed: March 2, 2023]

[157] Parikh RB, Helmchen LA. Paying for artificial intelligence in medicine. Npj Digital Medicine. 2022;**5**(1):1-5. DOI: 10.1038/s41746-022-00609-6

[158] Abràmoff MD, Roehrenbeck C, Trujillo S, et al. A reimbursement framework for artificial intelligence in healthcare. Npj Digital Medicine. 2022;**5**(1):1-6. DOI: 10.1038/s41746-022-00621-w

[159] Sallam M. ChatGPT utility in healthcare education, research, and practice: Systematic review on the promising perspectives and valid concerns. Healthcare. 2023;**11**(6):887. DOI: 10.3390/healthcare11060887

[160] Bubeck S, Chandrasekaran V, Eldan R, et al. Sparks of artificial general intelligence: Early experiments with GPT-4. arXiv. 2023;**5**:1-155. DOI: 10.48550/arXiv.2303.12712

[161] Iqbal J, Jahangir K, Mashkoor Y, et al. The future of artificial intelligence in neurosurgery: A narrative review. Surgical Neurology International. 2022;**13**:536. DOI: 10.25259/SNI_877_2022

[162] Kelly CJ, Karthikesalingam A, Suleyman M, Corrado G, King D. Key challenges for delivering clinical impact with artificial intelligence. BMC Medicine. 2019;**17**(1):195. DOI: 10.1186/s12916-019-1426-2

[163] Kamulegeya LH, Okello M, Bwanika JM, et al. Using artificial intelligence on dermatology conditions in Uganda: A case for diversity in training data sets for machine learning. African Health Sciences. 2023;**23**(2):753-763. DOI: 10.1101/826057

[164] Larrazabal AJ, Nieto N, Peterson V, Milone DH, Ferrante E. Gender imbalance in medical imaging datasets produces biased classifiers for computer-aided diagnosis. Proceedings of the National Academy of Sciences. 2020;**117**(23):12592-12594. DOI: 10.1073/pnas.1919012117

[165] Zemmar A, Lozano AM, Nelson BJ. The rise of robots in surgical environments during COVID-19. Nature Machine Intelligence. 2020;**2**(10):566-572. DOI: 10.1038/s42256-020-00238-2

[166] Awuah WA, Kalmanovich J, Mehta A, et al. Harnessing artificial intelligence to bridge the neurosurgery gap in low-income and middle-income countries. Postgraduate Medical Journal. 2023;**99**(1173):651-653. DOI: 10.1136/pmj-2022-141992

[167] Layard Horsfall H, Palmisciano P, Khan DZ, et al. Attitudes of the surgical team toward artificial intelligence in neurosurgery: International 2-stage cross-sectional survey. World Neurosurgery. 2021;**146**:e724-e730. DOI: 10.1016/j.wneu.2020.10.171

[168] Staartjes VE, Stumpo V, Kernbach JM, et al. Machine learning in neurosurgery: A global survey. Acta Neurochirurgica. 2020;**162**(12):3081-3091. DOI: 10.1007/s00701-020-04532-1

[169] Dennler C, Bauer DE, Scheibler AG, et al. Augmented reality in the operating room: A clinical feasibility study. BMC Musculoskeletal Disorders. 2021;**22**(1):451. DOI: 10.1186/s12891-021-04339-w

Chapter 11

AI in Healthcare: Implications for Family Medicine and Primary Care

Thomas Wojda, Carlie Hoffman, Jeffrey Jackson, Traci Conti and John Maier

Abstract

Artificial Intelligence (AI) has begun to transform industries including healthcare. Unfortunately, Primary Care and the discipline of Family Medicine have tended to lag behind in the implementation of this novel technology. Although the relationship between Family Medicine and AI is in its infancy greater engagement from Primary Care Physician's (PCP's) is a must due to the increasing shortage of practitioners. AI has the chance to overturn this problem as well as speed up its development. Considering the vast majority of PCP's utilize Electronic Medical Records (EMR's) the field is ripe for innovation. Regrettably, much of the information available remains unused for practice disruption. Primary Care offers a large data platform that can be leveraged with the use of technology to deliver ground-breaking trails forward to provide better comprehensive care for a wide-variety of patients from various backgrounds. The purpose of this chapter is to provide context to AI implementation as it relates to Primary Care and the practice of Family Medicine.

Keywords: artificial intelligence, machine learning, technology, primary care, family medicine, screening, management, and treatment

1. Introduction

Although Artificial Intelligence (AI) in Healthcare has recently become trendy, the concept is not new. Alan Turning developed the concept of machines that could think around the 1950's [1]. Soon thereafter, John McCarthy proposed the term "Artificial Intelligence" to describe the process of computers that could perform the cognitive functions of humans. Since these early propositions healthcare has seen a monumental increase in data available for interpretation. Consequently, the power and usefulness of computers in data analysis has become paramount to the success of a healthcare organization as it is unrealistic for individuals and even highly organized teams to extrapolate important information. Subsequently, various medical societies and disciplines have invested heavily in AI to meet the growing demands of modern medicine. Alarmingly, Family Medicine appears to lag behind other specialties in advancing its footprint in the AI healthcare space. Specifically, the American Board of Family Medicine performed an extensive literature review in the year 2020 and found no publications for this specialty during that time despite knowledge that Family Medicine scholars were actively pursuing research related to Primary Care and AI [2].

The importance of the discipline of Family Medicine being actively involved in AI research cannot be understated as historically this profession has lagged behind when the adoption of new technology takes place. Subsequently, the discipline and more importantly, the patients have needlessly suffered for it. For example, when the Health Information Technology for Economic and Clinical Health (HITECH) Act was passed, it was widely assumed the introduction of electronic medical records (EMR) would enhance the patient, physician, and organizational experience through the optimization of efficient, equitable, and effective healthcare delivery [3]. Certainly, EMR's have had numerous positive impacts on an individual patient and systems-based perspective [4]. No one would rightly argue for a return to paper charts and hand-written notes. Nevertheless, we cannot ignore the role the implementation of EMR has had on increased physician burnout and decreased face-to-face time with patients. Moreover, because of the lack of Family Medicine involvement in the role-out of EMR's many in our field strongly feel as though its usability, interoperability, and applicability have fallen short of the initial intended goals of EMR. This is likely due to lack of engagement from family physicians in the design, advocacy, and implementation of EMR. Accordingly, there is a rising concern that healthcare technology has grown to suit hospital administrators more than patients and physicians [4].

With the advancement of AI, the specialty of Family Medicine must be an active participant to further influence this transformation. The relationship-oriented nature of Family Medicine will allow for technology to focus on providing value to patients and communities as opposed to administrators and technology companies. Healthcare costs continue to escalate and without FM providers who are focused on providing value AI will likely only exacerbate the sentiment that only those who can afford such advances in healthcare will benefit from it. The ethos of Family Medicine is that the development of the therapeutic relationship optimizes treatment outcomes and positively effects health on a population level. Without this belief AI will only further reduce the patient-physician interaction through increased screen-time. Family Medicine practitioners pride themselves on seeing a diverse patient panel. Consequently, if Family Physicians voices are not heard AI may amplify existing biases. Specifically, algorithms used by recognition programs have demonstrated challenges in recognizing persons of color secondary to limited participation [5].

Computers process information faster, more efficiently, and more systematically than humans. They make judgments more regularly and act in response to variations faster. Currently, computers perform automated repetitive tasks once assigned to humans. Clinical decision support systems alert providers when immunizations are due, automatic American Society for Cardiovascular Disease (ASCVD) risk calculators provide myocardial infarction risk assessment, and advertisements for potential drug–drug or allergic reactions pop up before a medication may be administered or prescribed. Moreover, AI can already complete challenging multifactorial jobs to create an accurate differential diagnosis and evidence-based assessment and plan. Worryingly, machines autonomously managing patients may give administrators pause as to the value of human physicians.

Family Practitioner engagement in AI is a must. Primary care offers the grandest healthcare distribution platform and provides an influential stage for data use [6]. Family Practitioners are operations specialists who may practice approaches for the adoption of scientifically validated AI tools. Family Medicine practitioners focus on patient-oriented outcomes and will publish results that affect the patients [7].

Family Medicine practitioners operate between extensive delivery systems practitioners such as mental health, home health, and public health. The familiarity with various healthcare stakeholders will enhance AI performance tools.

Because the amount of data we will manage will only increase, there needs to be a strategy both for the here-and-now and beyond. Without this, Primary Care risks becoming incapacitated, subjugated to metrics, and more prone to burnout. Ultimately, AI should be used to enhance the time we spend with patients and complement the Family Medicine experience. NLP aids computers to comprehend, deduce, and use an individual's vernacular. Moreover, AI may unearth material from prior visits, images, labs, and health data to composite them into the right documents so providers can focus on the human-connection [8]. AI chatbots can replicate human dialog, assist individuals in receiving the optimal care, utilizing advanced technology through patient surveillance between visits and provider consultations [3]. Patients suffering from congestive heart failure (CHF) may broadcast their weight through internet-enabled scales, have their diuretic doses titrated, or ensure that their worsening symptoms are being examined by their PCP. Patients may be reminded of health maintenance services like breast and colon cancer screening, provided education for shared decision making, create referrals, book appointment, and organize tests that need to be performed [9]. AI may data mine environmental, EMR, claims, and pharmaceutical data and integrate these to identify and treat high risk patients afflicted with asthma, MI's, and opioid overdoses to aid appropriate management. AI may explore massive amount of data, convey measures, close care gaps, and most importantly allow providers to spend more time with patients.

While these tools are fascinating, they are not yet equipped to being put into practice. They necessitate improvement, investigation, and substantiation. Privacy, malpractice, and overtreatment must all be carefully weighed and dealt with. Without consideration of fitting payment models AI will be imperfect to influence healthcare delivery. **Figure 1** provides a guide for Family Medicine providers on how to get better involved in leveraging this technology.

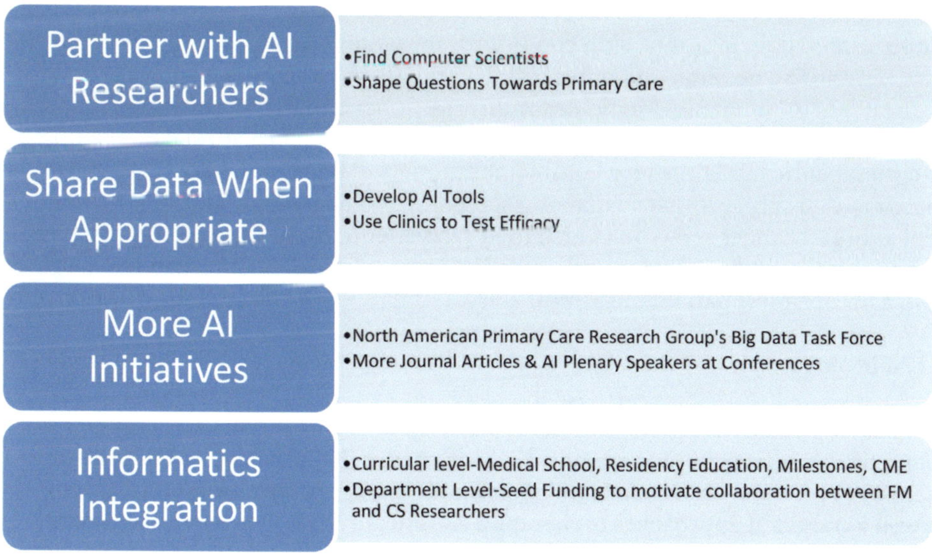

Figure 1.
Steps for family physicians to get involved in artificial intelligence research.

Family physicians pride themselves on the personal relationships they form with their patients. Computers will outdo physicians when it pertains to the performance of complicated undertakings. Nevertheless, creating and upholding strong relationships, recognizing and handling their intricacies, and eliciting and integrating preferences into medical decisions are difficult for technology to replicate. Humans and computers must complement each-other to enable physicians to spend more time with their patients.

2. Methodology

Internet searches using Google Scholar and PubMed was done with the fundamental words "Artificial Intelligence, Machine Learning, Technology, Primary Care, Family Medicine, and screening, management, and treatment." Additional citations were acquired through cross-referencing the main studies. Following the literature review all relevant contributors to the manuscript created an outline that identified the historical context of AI technology in relation to the discipline of Primary Care and Family Medicine, clinical implications for Primary Care and AI technology, and the role of AI technology and Graduate Medical Education as key pieces to include in this chapter. Other studies not pertaining to the aforementioned themes were excluded. The following manuscript includes various purposes employing Artificial Intelligence instruments presently in operation or in progress is portrayed. The names of the articles and their abstracts were vetted by one assessor (T.W). Complete manuscripts were reread for insertion by two authors.

3. AI & Clinical applications for family physicians

The applicability of AI for Family Physicians is vast. A scoping review condensed targeted health conditions that could be aided either through diagnostic or treatment decision support that include: cardiovascular, psychiatric/neurologic/cognitive, diabetic/metabolic/chronic, skin conditions, musculoskeletal, cancer, pulmonary, gastrointestinal, general, and other conditions [10]. A comprehensive breakdown of the use of AI in Family Medicine for diseases is beyond the scope of this chapter. Below, the authors provide a systems-based outline of various AI-related diagnostic and therapeutic modalities for family practitioners to be made aware of as well as more focused sub-sections on diabetes screening, management, and treatment, as well as breast cancer screening given their relevance to PCP's in the outpatient setting and to give the reader a better understanding of the depths to AI research in helping clinicians optimize patient outcomes.

3.1 Neurology

Alzheimer's disease (AD) may account for up to 80% of dementia cases and is a huge cost for society both economically and socially [11]. Although much advancement has been made in the underlying pathophysiological mechanisms of this disease as well as targeted approaches to therapy a significant barrier to any breakthrough occurs in the Identification of patients who will develop AD so that they are able to enroll in clinical trials at the appropriate time to examine the effectiveness of potential disease alternating treatment modalities. To combat this, a study was performed using machine learning (ML) to assess advancement to dementia by two years using data from amyloid positron emission tomography scans [12]. The high accuracy that ML demonstrated relative to standard algorithms holds promise for the development of better individuals to be included in AD clinical trials with the hope that that this will optimize their design and lead to advancement of targeted disease therapies.

3.2 Head, eyes, ears, nose, throat (HEENT)

Glaucoma, an increase of intraocular pressure that results in optic nerve damage and ultimately blindness, can be diagnosed with AI. Through the proliferation of a neural network, retinal images have been mined to aid in in diagnosis of Glaucoma with up to 96% accuracy [13].

Diabetic retinopathy (DR), a common microvascular problem of diabetes, is also a significant source of irreparable loss of sight [14]. This disease and subsequent loss of vision can be averted and assorted therapeutic selections are obtainable. Despite calls for routine screening for DR comprehensive strategies face difficulty with implementation [15]. Implementation issues include: inadequate trained personnel, lack of resources, and inability to cope with an increased disease burden. To combat this concern, a deep-based learning algorithm was created to validate the detection of DR [16]. Retinal images were compared to that of trained ophthalmologists. Results showed high accuracy when compared to current standards of care, which may lead to more efficient and accessible screening for DR.

3.3 Cardiovascular

Cardiovascular disease (CVD), the foremost cause of illness and death globally, consumes extensive preventative measures to curtail risk factors for disease development that center around controlling hypertension, lowering cholesterol, smoking cessation, and optimizing diabetes management. Including age, risk factors for development of CVD are mainly predicted using validated instruments [17–20]. Nevertheless, many people are still at risk for the development of CVD and are unable to be identified with these tools. What's more approximately 50% of myocardial infarctions and strokes will occur in people that do not meet screening criteria and thus are considered to be low risk [21]. Fortunately, machine learning provides a chance to expand precision by taking advantage of multifaceted connections among risk factors. For example, in a prospective cohort study machine learning correctly predicted additional individuals who got CVD versus a standard set of rules [22]. These results show that ML may identify more individuals who might be helped from anticipatory therapy and help others eschew pointless therapy.

3.4 Gastrointestinal (GI)

Gastro-esophageal reflux disease (GERD) is the presence esophageal mucosal interruptions or occurrence of reflux-induced symptoms that significantly impairs quality of life [23]. Symptom evaluation and assessment is vital for disease management. Sadly, symptom evaluation and effects of reflux are currently insufficiently correlated with disease severity. Furthermore, given the ambiguity of these relationships no diagnostic tool remains reliable. A retrospective study of 150 patients compared AI in the form of an artificial neural network (ANN) comprised of 45 clinical variables versus the current standards to esophagoscopy or pH-metry.

The use of ANN to make a diagnosis of GERD demonstrated superior accuracy [24]. Although this work is still in the preliminary stages it shows promise in delivering a non-invasive approach to the diagnosis of GERD.

3.5 Endocrine

Diabetes affects millions of people around the world, accounts for approximately 12% of global health expenditures, and still one in two persons continue to be unaware they have the disease and are sub-optimally treated [25]. Early intensive mediation may prevent onset and decelerates the development of retinopathy, nephropathy, neuropathy, and other difficulties associated with diabetes [26]. Lack of timely, crucial health data is vital for the patient and provider to make well-educated decisions in regards to diabetics care. AI may provide timely information concerning a diabetic patient's health. A review of literature shows that the relationship between AI and diabetes management can be group into four categories that include automated retinal screening that was discussed above, clinical decision support, predictive population risk stratification, and patient self-management support tools [27].

AI-driven extrapolative modeling proactively recognizes diabetics with the greatest risk for needless complications that create avoidable emergency department outings, hospital stays, and readmissions [28]. AI can dig through various patient information to classify and describe diabetes populations [29]. In addition, patients with risk factors for diabetic comorbid conditions may be discovered [30–32]. AI may pinpoint individuals who may benefit from specific diabetes disease management programs [32]. On a molecular level it may aid in the discovery of proteins and genes linked with diabetes [33, 34].

AI can run practice decision-support instruments to aid healthcare professionals tailor diabetes treatments that boosts compliance and maximizes outcomes on a population level [35]. AI-powered devices may even diagnose diabetes noninvasively [36]. Furthermore diabetic neuropathy and diabetic wounds may be more accurately measured and treated [37, 38].

There is ongoing research on a Closed Loop System, which is a synthetic pancreas that blends continuous glucose measurement and an algorithm-run insulin pump to enhance diabetes self-management and lower hypoglycemic episodes [39]. A meta-review of 12 trials compared patient acceptance of Artificial Pancreas Devices (APDs) versus standard of care. Based on the results, the authors surmised that the latest APD were safe and demonstrated high patient satisfaction [40].

More investigations are being done to determine the potential of diabetes apps to support persons in tracing and examining their statistics easily and to convey custom-made evidence-based understandings that diabetic patients may employ every day. For example, all-inclusive dietary databanks can describe nutritional subject matter once a barcode is scanned on a smart device, explore food chain options, common food items, or distinguish food stuffs [41]. Machine Learning and representative analysis can diagnose and enumerate complex happenings and the standard of living of diabetic patients and provide assistance so they are better informed about the decisions they make [42]. AI may possibly quicken wound recovery, avoid unnecessary expenses secondary to commutes, and lower medical expenditures with the use of an AI-based smartphone camera [43]. Pregnant women with gestational diabetes have demonstrated approval of AI supplemented telemedicine appointments to help expedite clinical care via the amalgamation of AI interpreted evidence-based procedures, information obtained from EMR's, and blood sugars, blood pressure readings, and movement sensors [44].

In 2018 Medtronic's Guardian Connect, the first AI-powered continuous glucose monitoring (CGM) system, was approved by the FDA in service of diabetic patients between the ages of 14 and 75 years. A prognostic system signals patients of substantial oscillation in glycaemia up to an hour before the critical event happens. The system has demonstrated accuracy and has been shown to announce around 98.5% of hypoglycemic occurrences; consequently, patients could potentially seize control to stabilize blood sugar [27]. The records can be collectively distributed and supervised by all relevant stakeholders involved in the patient's care.

Several questions persist before technological advancements in diabetes care permeate the health care sector. Practical interoperability, the capacity of two or more structures to interchange and utilize data, remains an obstacle [45]. Cost, overhead, continued expenditures, buy-in from healthcare providers and relevant participants, and the various definitions and involvedness surrounding the term Meaningful Use are all additional barriers to implementation [46]. The ability to replicate outcomes from previous studies remains blurry as well. For various reasons proprietary data such as source codes may be difficult to share. For example A survey of approximately 400 algorithms presented in papers at an Artificial Intelligence conference revealed around 6% of the presenters disseminated an organization's code, a third distributed information utilized to tryout their algorithms, and half provided an abridged of a source code (pseudo-code) [27]. Even if some of this data can be obtained it remains to be seen if the results will end up the same. What's more in machine learning, which stems from mastery of previous encounters, may be influenced by the typology of speech patterns implemented.

Nevertheless, diabetes remains an attractive target from AI research to apply industrial methods to solve the various complexities surrounding this disease. Many technological products have obtained approval from the FDA, are on the market, and have shown promising results. More innovative approaches are being created to challenge the status quo of current diabetic care by the enhancement of reliability, effectiveness, operability, straightforwardness, and patient, family, and provider, satisfaction with applying these products for diabetic management. Ideally, the right mix of monitoring and appropriate feedback will help isolate telling precedents and head to customized understandings that boost patient and provider commitment, conviction, and achievement in optimizing blood sugar control.

3.6 Hematology/oncology

The utilization of artificial intelligence (AI) in cancer screening is becoming increasingly evident in recent studies across multiple types of cancer. This includes lung, breast, colorectal, and cervical [47–50]. Given the overwhelming research across multiple disciplines, the focus of this review will be on the evidence-based application of AI in breast cancer screening. This research can be categorized into two applications: risk assessment and image analysis.

The United States Preventive Services Task Force (USPSTF) guidelines of primary screening for breast cancer with conventional mammography has resulted in a reduction of breast cancer mortality across both randomized trials and screening cohort studies [51]. Outlined in the USPSTF recommendations is screening every 2 years for women aged 50–74 years old, as opposed to individualized decision to start screening between the ages of 40–49 years old [51]. In the latter age group, high-risk individuals who would benefit from starting screening at an earlier age can include those with known underlying genetic mutation (such as BRCA1 or BRCA2 gene mutation) or a history of chest radiation at an early age [51]. There are several risk prediction models for breast cancer. One example is the Breast Cancer Risk Assessment Tool (BCRAT), which can be used to estimate a patient's 5-year and lifetime risk of developing invasive breast cancer. This considers a patient's age, age of menarche, age of first childbirth, number of first-degree relatives with breast cancer, number of previous biopsies, and presence of atypical hyperplasia in a biopsy. Of note, this tool may not be appropriate for assessing risk in patients with a history for certain medical conditions, such as personal history of certain breast cancer types [52]. Considering multiple qualitative and quantitative risk factors can better stratify risk-based screening and maximize the benefit while minimizing the harms of screening [53]. But how can AI advance current tools of risk assessment?

Breast density has been shown to be an independent risk factor for the development of breast cancer [54]. As a result, this has led to updates in prediction models to include this quantitative risk factor, such as the Tyrer Cuzick model, the Breast Cancer Surveillance Consortium Model (BCSCM), and the Breast and Ovarian Analysis of Disease Incidence and Carrier Estimation Algorithm (COADICEA) [52]. In a recent study, the authors created three models to estimate five-year breast cancer risk. One model only considered risk factors. The second model utilized deep/machine learning on mammographic images. The third model was a hybrid of the two. These models were then compared to the Tyrer–Cuzick model, a well-known clinical standard that recently incorporated mammographic breast density into its calculation. They found that their hybrid model had the highest accuracy, followed by the deep/machine learning model, while the Tyrer–Cuzick model had the lowest. These results indicate that a model that considers both traditional risk factors and mammographic data can improve current practices of assessing risk. Future research can aim to identify the imaging features and patterns that are most useful to stratifying risk [52].

Breast density is typically assessed through interpretation of the standard two-view mammogram by a radiologist. A visual estimation of the proportion of glandular and fatty tissue within the breasts is scored and applied to a scale, such as the Breast Imaging Reporting and Data System (BI-RADS). The four BI-RADS categories of breast composition according to breast density are: type 1 fatty breast, type 2 fibroglandular, type 3 heterogeneously dense, and type 4 dense and homogeneous. This subjective quantification of breast density requires certain training and experience to allow for accurate and reproducible scoring. Even so, there is a certain amount of user variation among radiologists that contributes to error [55].

There are 3 potential approaches to applying AI to mammogram image analysis: as a standalone system, for triage, and for reader aid [56]. In a simulation performed by McKinney et al., the findings demonstrated the ability of an AI system to outperform a group of radiologists in accurately interpreting mammograms [57]. Using deep learning-based AI, Balta et al. found that the breast cancer screening workflow, which typically requires double-reading, could be replaced by a single-reading. This was achieved by AI-driven identification of normal-appearing screening mammograms, which were then verified by a single human reader [56]. Similarly, in a retrospective study by Dembrower et al., AI was used to triage mammograms into those requiring no further radiologist assessment and those requiring further radiologist assessment. This system demonstrated potential for detecting a significant number of cases where breast cancer was not identified by human readers, but then diagnosed later [58]. Rodriguez-Ruiz et al. showed that radiologists interpreting mammograms with the support of an AI computer system performed better at diagnosing breast cancer than without [59].

The application of AI in mammogram-based breast cancer screening is by no means limited to the approaches previously discussed. These include more precise stratification of risk assessment, increasing accuracy of detecting breast cancer during image analysis, and potentially decreasing workload burden in breast imaging radiologists. Given the evidence shown across retrospective studies and simulations, AI has the potential to improve current breast cancer screening practices. As studies continue to explore its application in the various aspects of cancer screening, it is likely that AI will become a more prevalent tool in medicine and, hopefully, lead to better patient outcomes.

4. AI and administrative capabilities

The ambulatory clinic is an indispensable feature of patient-centered medical care. Today, many different stakeholders are involved to ensure the patient experience is enhanced and clinical outcomes optimized. Consequently, ensuring a clinic runs smoothly has proven to be labor intensive. Numerous obstacles to realizing a well-organized workflow for pre-visit planning (PVP) exist. These barriers include a lack of workforce shortages as well as limitations on time. The vast majority of time consumed administering care is sandwiched between appointments. PVP improves the possibility that an appointment will flow more easily, require not as much time, and develops a sophisticated and fulfilling patient-provider experience. AI tools may enhance pre-visit planning (PVP) [60, 61]. PVP contains distinct information built on predictable timetables and patient-provider messages that serve modern EMR and AI well. Criticisms of AI implementation include: absence of needs assessments, minimal real world applicability, and ignored complexity of healthcare with subsequent misallocation of investments [10, 62].

Clinicians are interested in automated PVP if it affords them more time with patients and saves them time on administrative duties. Technology already supports clinician work through: advanced solutions such as chat bots that monitor signs and symptoms, rudimentary functions like electronic sticky notes in the EHR, and updated best practices that serve as a reminder for outstanding or upcoming health maintenance. Current technological advancements include: algorithms that pool healthcare data in order to produce a summary of care gaps [63–65], automated patient questionnaires sent through a secure electronic portal [66–70] and programmed schemes that inform providers of requisite activities [65, 71]. The rise of value-based care along with telemedicine secondary to the recent Covid-19 pandemic has moved treatment of patients in the virtual space. This situation means that attention will needed to be further allocated to inter-visit happenings [72].

With the appearance of AI, particular aspect of PVP may be better supported. Unfortunately, there remains of dearth of literature that demonstrates the impartial value of this technology. PVP and its present condition must be further investigated, hindrances to performance examined, and areas for potential automation realized. Technology and AI obviously exhibit an ability to enhances the principally human method for PVP; however unless the structures surrounding value-based care is more refined, than the underestimation and subsequent dearth or compensation for PVP will remain a significant obstruction. Specifically, challenges such as ease of use, confidentiality, safekeeping of patient information, EMR interoperability, and workflow for providers need to be addressed [72].

5. AI and education in family medicine

The final section of this chapter concerns the role of AI and graduate medical education (GME). Family Medicine Residency in the United States is three years. During this time the residents must develop appropriately so that upon completion of their training they may feel confident practicing medicine independently. Although there are many issues that could be addressed concerning GME and AI the two the authors focus on in this chapter include motivational interviewing (MI) and shared decision making (SDM).

5.1 AI & Motivational Interviewing

Motivational Interviewing (MI) is a scientifically validated, short-form interventional style that has been established to positively affect change in chronic disease management. MI is a driving force towards constructive, healthy, patient focused behavior change. MI concentrates on the aims, trepidations, and viewpoint of the patient. Unfortunately, this process often contradicts the directional, instructional, and educational role healthcare providers have undertaken [73, 74]. Therefore providers must unlearn these behaviors to permit a more patient-oriented encounter. Critical skills to master include talking less, listening more, and reflecting on the patient's wishes. Open-ended questions help facilitate this rapport. Instantaneous feedback greatly enhances skill development [75, 76]. Unfortunately, for a variety of reasons insufficient advice is often given during the early stages of instruction. Consequently due to inadequate and unproductive training MI is underdeveloped.

AI may help to apply MI by delivering timely, well-organized feedback in a time and resource-constrained environment. Real-time Assessment of Dialog in Motivational Interviewing (ReadMI), utilizes natural language processing that delivers specific motivational interviewing indicators that helps pinpoint areas for improvement during the patient's visit [77]. The benefits of ReadMI include cost-effectiveness, portability, and immediate valuation and breakdown of the MI process. Advantages include: deep-learning-based speech recognition, NLP, AI-human interaction, and mobile cloud-based computing. The following (**Figures 2** and **3**) demonstrate the architecture, advantages, and encounter process of ReadMI respectively. What's more, the team involved in the patient interview may go over past cases and correlate the trainee's behavior and speech with the AI scores. Afterwards, these sessions generate novel records that make possible auxiliary fine-tuning of the program and the natural language based performance coding designation. Currently, ReadMI constructs comprehensive transcriptions of the discourse with greater than 92% accuracy, displays above 95% accuracy when measuring the amount of time the provider speaks versus the patient, and has over 92% accuracy when determining the amount of open-ended versus close-ended questions [77].

ReadMI has been shown to be as valid and reliable as humans when rating the kinds of questions and assertions that trainees yield when performing motivational interviewing. Physicians who are too loquacious in contrast to the patient are doubtful to produce high-level motivational interviewing techniques. These early results show that AI can produce instantaneously reliable scores to relevant stakeholders to enhance the educational experience. Specifically, if a learner talks too much and does not ask enough open-ended questions then the educator can use this information to promptly fine-tune the interview process. Because of the limitations on time, leveled proficiency improvement through AI based measures is invaluable. Moreover, less

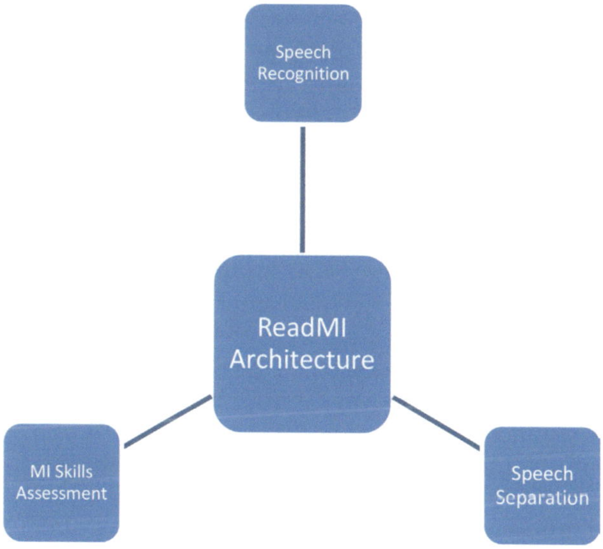

Figure 2.
Framework for ReadMI artificial intelligence.

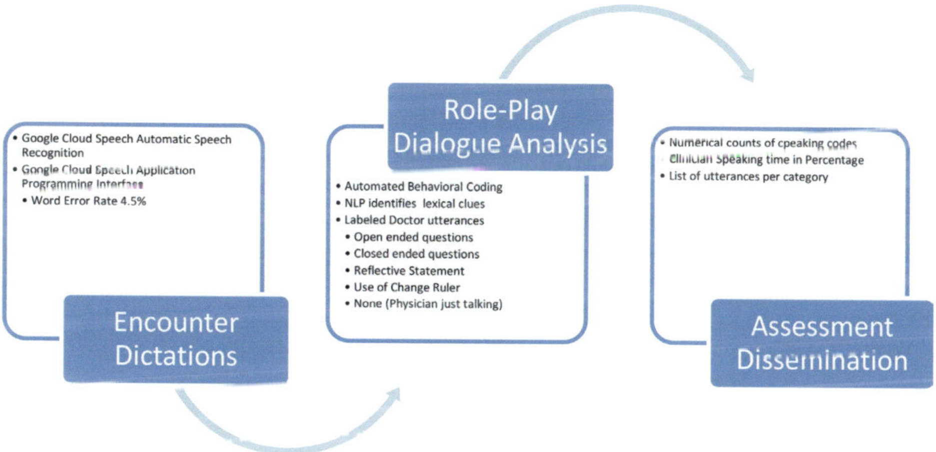

Figure 3.
General flow of the motivational interview process with ReadMI.

skewed criticisms directed towards the learner as well as less onerous video review sessions will advance medical education. Finally as clinicians become better decision support agents they may improve healthcare quality by aiding patients in living healthier lives.

5.2 AI and shared decision making

Shared decision making (SDM) is an approach where the patient and provider work in concert to formulate evidence-based medical choices that align with patient values [78]. Thus, the final choice is based on what matters most to the patient with medical data as an adjunct [79]. Unfortunately, real world applicability is lacking [80–82].

Constraints on time, difficulties with generalizability, and medical circumstances are all obstacles to SDM [83]. AI may advance SDM through better informed decision-making, which allows providers to concentrate their energy on the patient [84]. Furthermore, AI may discover missed correlations by individuals participating in clinical assessments [85]. Nevertheless, bioethical concerns for AI and health decision-making remain [84]. Moreover, AI-based decision aids remain foreign in regards to their patient-centeredness [86]. Lastly, the facilitation of AI and shared decision making remains unknown. A three step scheme has been offered [87, 88]. It is further depicted in (**Figure 4**).

A scoping review showed the range of AI systems applied to SDM [89]. Sadly, few studies concerned primary care. Of the involved studies, three devised AI interventions for primary care involving the support of chronic conditions such as diabetes and stroke [90–92]. These studies focused on the decision-making step of SDM either by launching trials to calculate clinically significant results or for medical advice. Wang et al. aimed to tailor knowledge and choices about medications in type 2 diabetics [92]. SDM is essential secondary to the complexity of diabetics. In this report information from an EHR was compiled to aid clinicians with decision support tools to enable patients to better comprehend their well-being. Over 2500 patients with type 2 diabetes, 77 features, and eight different medications were amassed to generate a prototype for reference. The AI model had a correctness of 0.76. The records just pertained to hospitalized individuals and the result of medication utilization was not accounted for. Still, the intervention exhibited practicability and adaptability, meaning if the scheme did not remain current, the mediation could be fine-tuned without any impact to the interoperability of the hospital EHR. Moreover, the program was created with the patient in mind, which allowed key stakeholders to evaluate an individual's ailment more systematically and modify discussions in an up-to-date manner.

Kökciyan et al. made "CONSULT," a decision-support agent to help stroke survivors in treatment compliance and self-care in partnership with a practioner [90, 91]. It was generated through an argumentation construct, which is beyond the scope of this chapter. However, a brief description is as follows. Health sensors and EHR information as well as medical standards were used as inputs. Proposals and written descriptions for systematized choices were provided as outputs. The program was carried out with a mobile Android app. Six unpaid workers in decent health were

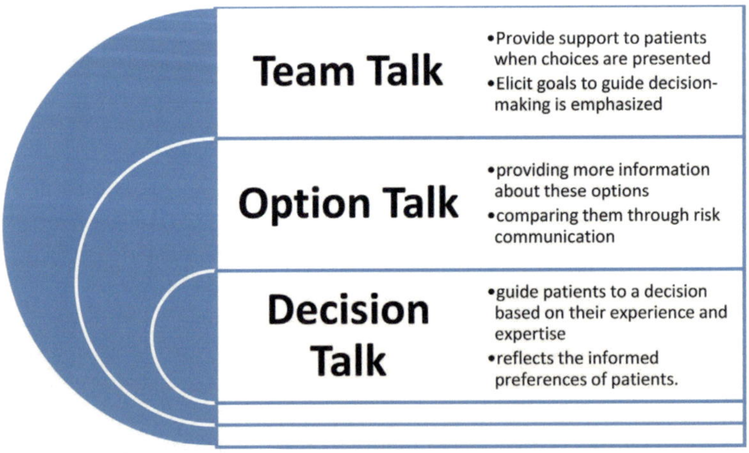

Figure 4.
3-step model of shared decision making (SDM) for clinical practice.

enrolled for one week, used various system features, and were solicited to gather information from wellness sensors and input data. The CONSULT system aided the decision-making point in SDM by showing the latest interpretation of the clinical picture via individualized measurements taken from the health record and wireless sensor input. After, stylistic descriptions of automatic findings supplemented the medical suggestions offered. Overall, the existing, pertinent, concise information plus medication options and proposals helped buoy the patient-provider decision-making moment.

Overall, the relationship between AI and SDM is young. More research is needed to examine, apply, and gage the impact of AI on SDM, standardize its use, and evaluate its impact on choices that effect a population. Importantly, any AI intervention must be human-centered. Lastly, SDM is a stepwise process; therefore research must demonstrate how AI interventions better re-enforce the therapeutic relationship.

6. Discussion

The authors recognized and elaborated on various research studies concerning AI, Family Medicine, and Primary Care and separated this manuscript into three predominant categories. First, on the subject of the history of Family Medicine adoption of technology, an overwhelming trend when contextualizing this issue is the lack of involvement of Family Medicine stakeholders in the literature [10]. Secondly, concerning clinical applicability, there is a wide variety of functions that AI could perform for PCP's. Clinical trials repeatedly established AI to strengthen problem-solving or management of chronic diseases. Still, the results exhibit Artificial Intelligence remains at an initial phase of development for applicability; therefore much remains to be done to measure AI's influence on the primary care system.

7. Future research

To conclude this section of the chapter the authors shed some light on novel research and funding to expand the Family Medicine footprint in the AI realm. Specifically, in 2022 the American Board of Family Medicine (ABFM) established a funding program to support Family Medicine Departments in hiring Artificial Intelligence/Machine Learning (AI/ML) focused research faculty. The initial cohort of funded institutions include: University of Houston, University of Pittsburgh, University of California, San Diego and University of Texas, San Antonio. Each institution is pursuing its own focused work with the shared general aims of establishing a sustained AI/ML research presence, securing further external funding and producing peer-reviewed research publications. This program also includes regular convening of the research teams to share progress and information hosted by the Stanford Healthcare AI Applied Research Team.

8. Conclusion

AI in healthcare has arrived. Nevertheless, many Family Physicians are unaware of its uses and how it will impact their practice. Subsequently, Family Medicine remains constrained by its limitations and the ethical implications remain unclear.

This chapter hopes to act as a guide to front line health care works like Family Physicians. Primary care is essential to the well-being of a population and is unmatched in its ability to interconnect the various parts of a healthcare system. The profound bonds Family Physicians create with both their patients and community makes this discipline inimitably fitting to steer the health care AI revolution. In order to do so it is vital that Family Physicians collaborate with engineers to guarantee that AI use is pertinent and patient-centered, improves health care AI implementations, and acts inclusively and ethically AI that optimize outcomes and reduce inequities.

Author details

Thomas Wojda[1*], Carlie Hoffman[1], Jeffrey Jackson[1], Traci Conti[1] and John Maier[2]

1 UPMC Department of Family Medicine-McKeesport, Mckeesport, United States

2 Department of Family Medicine-Innovation and Strategic Initiatives, Pittsburgh, United States

*Address all correspondence to: wojdatr@upmc.edu

References

[1] Turing AM. Computing machinery and intelligence. In: Parsing the Turing Test. Dordrecht, Netherlands: Springer; 2009. pp. 23-65

[2] Newton W. The American Board of Family Medicine: what's next? American Board of Family Medicine. 2019;**32**:282-284

[3] Liaw W, Kakadiaris I. Artificial intelligence and family medicine: Better together. Family Medicine. 2020;**52**(1):8-10

[4] DeVoe JE et al. The ADVANCE network: Accelerating data value across a national community health center network. Journal of the American Medical Informatics Association. 2014;**21**(4):591-595

[5] Wilson B, Hoffman J, Morgenstern J. Predictive inequity in object detection. arXiv preprint arXiv:1902.11097. 2019

[6] Green LA et al. The Ecology of Medical Care Revisited. Waltham, Massachusetts: Mass Medical Soc; 2001. pp. 2021-2025

[7] Shaughnessy AF, Slawson DC, Bennett JH. Becoming an information master: A guidebook to the medical information jungle. Journal of Family Practice. 1994;**39**(5):489-500

[8] Deliberato RO, Celi LA, Stone DJ. Clinical note creation, binning, and artificial intelligence. JMIR Medical Informatics. 2017;**5**(3):e7627

[9] Nakamura N, Koga T, Iseki H. A meta-analysis of remote patient monitoring for chronic heart failure patients. Journal of Telemedicine and Telecare. 2014;**20**(1):11-17

[10] Kueper JK et al. Artificial intelligence and primary care research: A scoping review. Annals of Family Medicine. 2020;**18**(3):250-258

[11] Pouryamout L et al. Economic evaluation of treatment options in patients with Alzheimer's disease: A systematic review of cost-effectiveness analyses. Drugs. 2012;**72**:789-802

[12] Mathotaarachchi S et al. Identifying incipient dementia individuals using machine learning and amyloid imaging. Neurobiology of Aging. 2017;**59**:80-90

[13] Samanta S et al. Haralick features based automated glaucoma classification using back propagation neural network. In: Proceedings of the 3rd International Conference on Frontiers of Intelligent Computing: Theory and Applications (FICTA), 2014. Bhubaneswar, Odissa, India: Springer; 2015

[14] Yau JW et al. Global prevalence and major risk factors of diabetic retinopathy. Diabetes Care. 2012;**35**(3):556-564

[15] Wang LZ et al. Availability and variability in guidelines on diabetic retinopathy screening in Asian countries. British Journal of Ophthalmology. 2017;**101**(10):1352-1360

[16] Li Z et al. An automated grading system for detection of vision-threatening referable diabetic retinopathy on the basis of color fundus photographs. Diabetes Care. 2018;**41**(12):2509-2516

[17] Goff DC Jr et al. ACC/AHA guideline on the assessment of cardiovascular risk: A report of the American College of Cardiology/ American Heart Association task force

on practice guidelines. Circulation. 2013, 2014;**129**(25_suppl_2):S49-S73

[18] Hippisley-Cox J et al. Predicting cardiovascular risk in England and Wales: Prospective derivation and validation of QRISK2. BMJ. 2008;**336**(7659):1475-1482

[19] D'Agostino RB Sr et al. General cardiovascular risk profile for use in primary care: The Framingham heart study. Circulation. 2008;**117**(6):743-753

[20] Ridker PM et al. Development and validation of improved algorithms for the assessment of global cardiovascular risk in women: The Reynolds risk score. JAMA. 2007;**297**(6):611-619

[21] Ridker PM et al. Rosuvastatin to prevent vascular events in men and women with elevated C-reactive protein. New England Journal of Medicine. 2008;**359**(21):2195-2207

[22] Weng SF et al. Can machine-learning improve cardiovascular risk prediction using routine clinical data? PLoS One. 2017;**12**(4):e0174944

[23] Dent J et al. An evidence-based appraisal of reflux disease management—The Genval workshop report. Gut. 1998;**44**(suppl. 2):S1-S16

[24] Pace F et al. Artificial neural networks are able to recognize gastro-oesophageal reflux disease patients solely on the basis of clinical data. European Journal of Gastroenterology & Hepatology. 2005;**17**(6):605-610

[25] Atlas D, International diabetes federation. IDF Diabetes Atlas. 7th ed. Vol. 33. Brussels, Belgium: International Diabetes Federation; 2015. p. 2

[26] Control, D. and C.T.R. Group. The effect of intensive treatment of diabetes on the development and progression of long-term complications in insulin-dependent diabetes mellitus. New England Journal of Medicine. 1993;**329**(14):977-986

[27] Dankwa-Mullan I et al. Transforming diabetes care through artificial intelligence: The future is here. Population Health Management. 2019;**22**(3):229-242

[28] Han L et al. Rule extraction from support vector machines using ensemble learning approach: An application for diagnosis of diabetes. IEEE Journal of Biomedical and Health Informatics. 2014;**19**(2):728-734

[29] Wei W-Q et al. A high throughput semantic concept frequency based approach for patient identification: A case study using type 2 diabetes mellitus clinical notes. In: AMIA Annual Symposium Proceedings. Washington, DC: American Medical Informatics Association; 2010

[30] Corey KE et al. Development and validation of an algorithm to identify nonalcoholic fatty liver disease in the electronic medical record. Digestive Diseases and Sciences. 2016;**61**:913-919

[31] Neves J et al. A soft computing approach to kidney diseases evaluation. Journal of Medical Systems. 2015;**39**:1-9

[32] Rau H-H et al. Development of a web-based liver cancer prediction model for type II diabetes patients by using an artificial neural network. Computer Methods and Programs in Biomedicine. 2016;**125**:58-65

[33] Vyas R et al. Building and analysis of protein-protein interactions related to diabetes mellitus using support vector machine, biomedical text mining and network analysis. Computational Biology and Chemistry. 2016;**65**:37-44

[34] López B et al. Single nucleotide polymorphism relevance learning with random forests for type 2 diabetes risk prediction. Artificial Intelligence in Medicine. 2018;**85**:43-49

[35] Lo-Ciganic W-H et al. Using machine learning to examine medication adherence thresholds and risk of hospitalization. Medical Care. 2015;**53**(8):720

[36] Shu T, Zhang B, Tang YY. An extensive analysis of various texture feature extractors to detect diabetes mellitus using facial specific regions. Computers in Biology and Medicine. 2017;**83**:69-83

[37] Katigari MR et al. Fuzzy expert system for diagnosing diabetic neuropathy. World Journal of Diabetes. 2017;**8**(2):80

[38] Wang L et al. Area determination of diabetic foot ulcer images using a cascaded two-stage SVM-based classification. IEEE Transactions on Biomedical Engineering. 2016;**64**(9):2098-2109

[39] DeJournett L, DeJournett J. In silico testing of an artificial-intelligence-based artificial pancreas designed for use in the intensive care unit setting. Journal of Diabetes Science and Technology. 2016;**10**(6):1360-1371

[40] Thabit H et al. Home use of an artificial beta cell in type 1 diabetes. New England Journal of Medicine. 2015;**373**(22):2129-2140

[41] Zhang W et al. "Snap-n-eat" food recognition and nutrition estimation on a smartphone. Journal of Diabetes Science and Technology. 2015;**9**(3):525-533

[42] Cvetković B et al. Activity recognition for diabetic patients using a smartphone. Journal of Medical Systems. 2016;**40**:1-8

[43] Wang L et al. Smartphone-based wound assessment system for patients with diabetes. IEEE Transactions on Biomedical Engineering. 2014;**62**(2):477-488

[44] Rigla M et al. Gestational diabetes management using smart mobile telemedicine. Journal of Diabetes Science and Technology. 2018;**12**(2):260-264

[45] Benson T. Principles of Health Interoperability HL7 and SNOMED. London, UK: Springer Science & Business Media; 2012

[46] Adler-Milstein J et al. Electronic health record adoption in US hospitals: Progress continues, but challenges persist. Health Affairs. 2015;**34**(12):2174-2180

[47] Espinoza JL, Dong LT. Artificial intelligence tools for refining lung cancer screening. Journal of Clinical Medicine. 2020;**9**(12):3860

[48] Gräwingholt A. The role of artificial intelligence in breast cancer screening: How can it improve detection? Expert Review of Molecular Diagnostics. 2020;**20**(12):1161-1162

[49] Mitsala A et al. Artificial intelligence in colorectal cancer screening, diagnosis and treatment. A new era. Current Oncology. 2021;**28**(3):1581-1607

[50] Xue P, Ng MTA, Qiao Y. The challenges of colposcopy for cervical cancer screening in LMICs and solutions by artificial intelligence. BMC Medicine. 2020;**18**:1-7

[51] Nelson HD et al. Screening for Breast Cancer: A Systematic Review to Update the 2009 US Preventive Services Task

Force Recommendation. Rockville (MD), USA: Agency for Healthcare Research and Quality; 2016

[52] Kim G, Bahl M. Assessing risk of breast cancer: A review of risk prediction models. Journal of Breast Imaging. 2021;**3**(2):144-155

[53] Houssami N, Kerlikowske K. AI as a new paradigm for risk-based screening for breast cancer. Nature Medicine. 2022;**28**(1):29-30

[54] Ekpo EU et al. Assessment of interradiologist agreement regarding mammographic breast density classification using the fifth edition of the BI-RADS atlas. American Journal of Roentgenology. 2016;**206**(5):1119-1123

[55] Martin KE et al. Mammographic density measured with quantitative computer-aided method: Comparison with radiologists' estimates and BI-RADS categories. Radiology. 2006;**240**(3):656-665

[56] Freeman K et al. Use of artificial intelligence for image analysis in breast cancer screening programmes: Systematic review of test accuracy. BMJ. 2021;**1872**:374

[57] McKinney SM et al. Reply to: Transparency and reproducibility in artificial intelligence. Nature. 2020;**586**(7829):E17-E18

[58] Dembrower K et al. Effect of artificial intelligence-based triaging of breast cancer screening mammograms on cancer detection and radiologist workload: A retrospective simulation study. The Lancet Digital Health. 2020;**2**(9):e468-e474

[59] Rodríguez-Ruiz A et al. Detection of breast cancer with mammography: Effect of an artificial intelligence support system. Radiology. 2019;**290**(2):305-314

[60] Lin SY, Mahoney MR, Sinsky CA. Ten ways artificial intelligence will transform primary care. Journal of General Internal Medicine. 2019;**34**(8):1626-1630

[61] Esteva A et al. A guide to deep learning in healthcare. Nature Medicine. 2019;**25**(1):24-29

[62] Smith M et al. From code to bedside: Implementing artificial intelligence using quality improvement methods. Journal of General Internal Medicine. 2021;**36**(4):1061-1066

[63] Wilkinson C, Champion JD, Sabharwal K. Promoting preventive health screening through the use of a clinical reminder tool: An accountable care organization quality improvement initiative. Journal for Healthcare Quality. 2013;**35**(5):7-19

[64] Kawamoto K et al. Long-term impact of an electronic health record-enabled, team-based, and scalable population health strategy based on the chronic care model. In: AMIA Annual Symposium Proceedings. Chicago, Illinois: American Medical Informatics Association; 2016

[65] Savarino JR et al. Improving clinical remission rates in pediatric inflammatory bowel disease with previsit planning. BMJ Open Quality. 2016;**5**(1):u211063.w4361

[66] Bose-Brill S et al. Validation of a novel electronic health record patient portal advance care planning delivery system. Journal of Medical Internet Research. 2018;**20**(6):e9203

[67] Wald JS et al. Implementing practice-linked pre-visit electronic journals in primary care: Patient and physician use and satisfaction. Journal of the American Medical Informatics Association. 2010;**17**(5):502-506

[68] Grant RW et al. Pre-visit prioritization for complex patients with diabetes: Randomized trial design and implementation within an integrated health care system. Contemporary Clinical Trials. 2016;**47**:196-201

[69] Vo MT et al. Prompting patients with poorly controlled diabetes to identify visit priorities before primary care visits: A pragmatic cluster randomized trial. Journal of General Internal Medicine. 2019;**34**(6):831-838

[70] Howard BJ, Sturner R. Use of an online clinical process support system as an aid to identification and Management of Developmental and Mental Health Problems. Current Developmental Disorders Reports. 2017;**4**(4):108-117

[71] Contratto E et al. Physician order entry clerical support improves physician satisfaction and productivity. Southern Medical Journal. 2017;**110**(5):363-368

[72] Lin S, Sattler A, Smith M. Retooling primary care in the COVID-19 era. In: Mayo Clinic Proceedings. Rochester, Minnesota: Elsevier; 2020

[73] Noordman J, van der Weijden T, van Dulmen S. Communication-related behavior change techniques used in face-to-face lifestyle interventions in primary care: A systematic review of the literature. Patient Education and Counseling. 2012;**89**(2):227-244

[74] Werner JJ et al. Comparing primary care physicians' smoking cessation counseling techniques to motivational interviewing. Journal of Addiction Medicine. 2013;**7**(2):139

[75] Vickers NJ. Animal communication: When i'm calling you, will you answer too? Current Biology. 2017;**27**(14):R713-R715

[76] Barwick MA et al. Training health and mental health professionals in motivational interviewing: A systematic review. Children and Youth Services Review. 2012;**34**(9):1786-1795

[77] Vasoya MM et al. Read MI: An innovative app to support training in motivational interviewing. Journal of Graduate Medical Education. 2019;**11**(3):344-346

[78] Charles C, Gafni A, Whelan T. Shared decision-making in the medical encounter: What does it mean? (or it takes at least two to tango). Social Science & Medicine. 1997;**44**(5):681-692

[79] Barry MJ, Edgman-Levitan S. Shared decision making—The pinnacle patient-centered care. The New England Journal of Medicine. 2012;**366**(9):780-781

[80] Couët N et al. Assessments of the extent to which health-care providers involve patients in decision making: A systematic review of studies using the OPTION instrument. Health Expectations. 2015;**18**(4):542-561

[81] Edwards M, Davies M, Edwards A. What are the external influences on information exchange and shared decision-making in healthcare consultations: A meta-synthesis of the literature. Patient Education and Counseling. 2009;**75**(1):37-52

[82] Holmes-Rovner M et al. Implementing shared decision-making in routine practice: Barriers and opportunities. Health Expectations. 2000;**3**(3):182-191

[83] Légaré F et al. Barriers and facilitators to implementing shared decision-making in clinical practice: Update of a systematic review of

health professionals' perceptions. Patient Education and Counseling. 2008;**73**(3):526-535

[84] Triberti S, Durosini I, Pravettoni G. A "third wheel" effect in health decision making involving artificial entities: A psychological perspective. Frontiers in Public Health. 2020;**8**:117

[85] Braun M et al. Primer on an ethics of AI-based decision support systems in the clinic. Journal of Medical Ethics. 2021;**47**(12):e3-e3

[86] Hassan N et al. Clinicians' and patients' perceptions of the use of artificial intelligence decision aids to inform shared decision making: A systematic review. The Lancet. 2021;**398**:S80

[87] Elwyn G et al. Shared decision making: A model for clinical practice. Journal of General Internal Medicine. 2012;**27**:1361-1367

[88] Elwyn G et al. A three-talk model for shared decision making: Multistage consultation process. BMJ. 2017;**359**:j4891

[89] Abbasgholizadeh Rahimi S et al. Application of artificial intelligence in shared decision making: Scoping review. JMIR Medical Informatics. 2022;**10**(8):e36199

[90] Kokciyan N et al. A collaborative decision support tool for managing chronic conditions. In: The 17th World Congress of Medical and Health Informatics. London, UK: King's College Open Access; 2019

[91] Kökciyan N et al. Applying metalevel argumentation frameworks to support medical decision making. IEEE Intelligent Systems. 2021;**36**(2):64-71

[92] Wang Y et al. A shared decision-making system for diabetes medication choice utilizing electronic health record data. IEEE Journal of Biomedical and Health Informatics. 2016;**21**(5):1280-1287

Chapter 12

Artificial Intelligence in Musculoskeletal Conditions

Juan Manuel Román-Belmonte, Hortensia De la Corte-Rodríguez, Beatriz Adriana Rodríguez-Damiani and Emérito Carlos Rodríguez-Merchán

Abstract

Artificial intelligence (AI) refers to computer capabilities that resemble human intelligence. AI implies the ability to learn and perform tasks that have not been specifically programmed. Moreover, it is an iterative process involving the ability of computerized systems to capture information, transform it into knowledge, and process it to produce adaptive changes in the environment. A large labeled database is needed to train the AI system and generate a robust algorithm. Otherwise, the algorithm cannot be applied in a generalized way. AI can facilitate the interpretation and acquisition of radiological images. In addition, it can facilitate the detection of trauma injuries and assist in orthopedic and rehabilitative processes. The applications of AI in musculoskeletal conditions are promising and are likely to have a significant impact on the future management of these patients.

Keywords: artificial intelligence, musculoskeletal conditions, musculoskeletal radiology, skeletal trauma, physical and rehabilitation medicine, orthopedic surgery, sports medicine

1. Introduction

The term "artificial intelligence" (AI) was proposed by John McCarthy in 1956 [1]. It refers to computer capabilities that resemble human intelligence. It is a broad concept, involving both virtual (computing) and physical (robotics) elements [2], and this chapter is going to focus on the virtual aspects.

The term "AI" has been mistakenly used to refer to automated digital systems or probabilistic algorithms. It implies the ability to learn, for example, to perform tasks that have not been specifically programmed. An AI can analyze data and make decisions much like a person [3].

It is thought that AI could help change the mechanistic model of current medicine. Health being the result of a complex system based on multiple nonlinear interactions, it could help to better understand its functioning [4].

Nowadays, AI is deeply established in today's society. They are used in personal assistants (Alexa, Siri), music platforms to display recommendations (Spotify), or graphical applications (FaceApp). Although there are promising results, the application of AI in musculoskeletal medicine is just starting its way [5]. However, it is likely that AI will be part of our routine clinical practice in a few years.

2. Methodology

On 30 January 2023, a bibliographic search was carried out in PubMed and the Cochrane Library (Cochrane Reviews) using "artificial intelligence musculoskeletal" as keywords. We found 957 articles in PubMed and 18 in the Cochrane Library (of which 10 were repeated in PubMed). In other words, we used a total of 965 article abstracts, of which we finally analyzed 51 because we subjectively considered them to be the best and most closely related to the chapter title. The remaining 914 articles were excluded (**Figure 1**). This way of including and excluding articles and the fact that we did not use other bibliographic search engines (Web of Science, Google Scholar, and Embase) can be considered as two limitations of this chapter, as some important publications were probably not included in it. In addition, due to the novelty of the topic studied, we have included one book and three websites because of their relevance and the topicality of their content. However, we would like to mention that the bibliographical references are so abundant (thousands) that one way or another, there could always be something important left out, even if a systematic review and meta-analysis is carried out.

3. Types of AI

An AI is an iterative process involving the ability of computerized systems to capture information, transform it into knowledge, and process it to produce adaptive

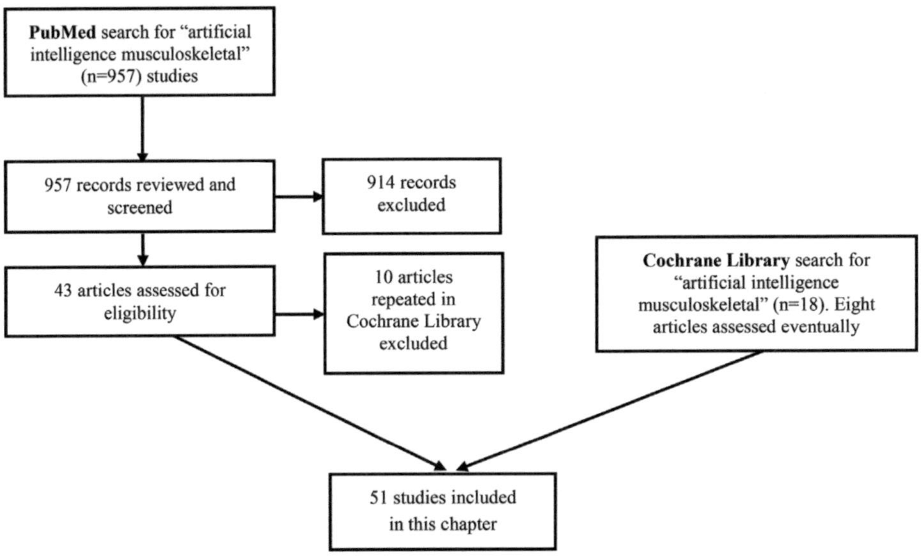

Figure 1.
Flow chart of our search strategy regarding artificial intelligence (AI) in musculoskeletal conditions.

changes in the environment. AI is capable of surpassing the speed of human analysis in many cases. Within this broad framework, there are different systems with their own characteristics.

Machine learning (ML) is a branch of artificial intelligence that refers to systems and algorithms capable of learning and improving through data analysis. Unsupervised ML does not require a labeled database to perform its training. Instead, it can identify nonapparent or hidden relationships in different data patterns. Supervised ML requires a labeled database in order to perform training. This database contains information in which the input and output are linked. This is what the computer uses to perform the correct matching.

Deep Learning (DL) is a type of ML capable of learning complex tasks through the analysis of large amounts of information with which it is trained [6]. An artificial neural network composed of nodes arranged in a hierarchy of levels is used in the DL. The network is able to process basic information at the initial level and forward it to the next level. There it is integrated with data from other nodes and passed to the next level. This process is done iteratively until the system learns the task, such as identifying a particular pattern. For example, DL techniques can be applied to radiologic studies to develop computer algorithms capable of analyzing images, classifying, and segmenting them [7].

Convolutional neural networks (CNN) are a subtype of DL especially used in image processing. They use learnable layers and filters through which data are passed and processed in a complex way, until they are completely transformed to the final layer or output layer. CNNs take advantage of the position of pixels in the images to reduce the processing complexity and parameter requirements per layer.

One of the great advantages of DL and CNN is their ability to be trained end-to-end. This means that the training model only needs input data, for example, knee magnetic resonance imaging (MRI) and a set of gold standard labels, medial meniscal lesion, and no medial meniscal lesion. The algorithm is capable of self-learning, considering by itself which elements are most relevant to perform a process. Since training a CNN is an iterative process, a larger volume of information usually yields better performance of the algorithm. In addition, although the computational power required to train DL algorithms is high, subsequent analysis of new data is faster and easier than in other AI systems.

4. How to generate AI in musculoskeletal medicine?

To generate an AI, a large volume of labeled data are needed to train the AI system and generate a robust algorithm. Otherwise, the algorithm can only be applied in a limited way. In the case of radiology, 49% of the papers using DL use databases of 101 to 1000 cases, 25% less than 100 cases, and only 6% use more than 10,000 cases [7]. It seems necessary that centers could coordinate to increase the size of their databases. In this regard, there are de-identified public databases that can be used to train AI algorithms, such as musculoskeletal radiographs (MURA), with almost 41,000 images of the upper extremity labeled as fracture or nonfracture by radiologists [8].

Many times, images processed by AI systems are manually selected, which is very time-consuming. It is vital that the database that is going to train the AI is appropriate to what is to be analyzed and has no flaws. In addition, it is recommended for the data to be homogeneous and of a volume proportional to the complexity of the computational task.

Unsupervised learning is likely to be critical in the future for building new AI systems. However, most successful AIs currently use supervised learning that may actually hinder their development [9].

One element used in some algorithms is heat maps in DL systems. Their use allows us to find out the part of the image that contributes the most within the analysis and reduce the impact of incorrect data. For example, if the heat map points out that a part of the image is being analyzed while the lesion is in a different one, it can be discovered that the algorithm is not processing the correct data.

5. Applications of AI in musculoskeletal medicine

5.1 Application in image interpretation

Errors in image interpretation in trauma radiology can increase morbidity and mortality, and it has been estimated that there can be up to a 4% error rate even by a trained radiologist [10]. There is an increasing pressure on physicians to interpret radiological images due to their growing use. It has been estimated that the greatest number of undiagnosed fractures occur in patients assessed between 8:00 p.m. and 2:00 a.m. This is probably because physicians who can assess these images may not be available in certain facilities or at certain times of the day [11].

The application of an AI in the world of radiology is the natural consequence of history and discipline, which has been characterized by incorporating technological innovation into clinical practice [12]. However, most existing algorithms used to identify fractures usually provide performance similar to, but not superior to, the capabilities of an expert radiologist. Therefore, it is possible that physicians who are not specialists in musculoskeletal radiology may benefit the most from using these AI tools. For example, CNNs have been used to detect fractures on radiographs in different anatomic locations, including the upper extremity, lower extremity, hip, and spine [13].

On the other hand, AI-based imaging systems are usually used in specific anatomical locations, so they should be integrated with each other to have an impact on clinical practice. An example of this would be a study in which 715,343 radiographs from 16 anatomical sites and 10 CNNs were used to detect fractures with promising results [14]. Another example would be the use of DL on computed tomography (CT) images to detect osteoporotic femoral neck, calcaneal, and vertebral fractures with an acceptable result [15]. An interesting aspect is the ability of the AI to detect fractures that are inconspicuous to the human eye. An algorithm with the ability to detect subtle lesions might not be able to discover radiographically obvious fractures [16].

Algorithms have also been used to detect anterior cruciate ligament tears, finding no difference in sensitivity or specificity versus expert radiologists [17]. AI has also shown good results for diagnosing meniscal tears [18]. DL has also been used to evaluate acute and chronic cartilage lesions [19].

5.2 Application in orthopedic surgery and orthopedic trauma

The incorporation of AI to assist in the surgical procedure has aroused great interest at present. For example, AI has been used as an assistant for image segmentation. The algorithm is able to differentiate the image fragment that is a healthy tissue from the mass to be studied or removed. This facilitates a time-consuming task in a fast and automated way [20].

AI has also been used in algorithms for predicting outcomes or costs associated with the surgical procedure. The DL is able to process a large amount of input data (age, comorbidities, and gender) and generate a certain outcome with predictive capacity (cost of hospitalization). For example, one paper analyzed 175,042 patients undergoing primary total knee replacement surgery with 15 preoperative variables, being able to estimate length of hospital stay and hospital costs, adjusting certain comorbidities [21].

Furthermore, AI has been used to help decide on the appropriateness of performing a surgical intervention, for example, to preoperatively assess the risk of death or complication. This would serve to provide the surgeon and patient with better information when deciding on the optimal management option [22].

5.3 Clinical workflow

In general, AI systems have the potential to assist physicians in certain tasks by improving the ability to diagnose and treat accurately despite the increased workload. Within the radiological practice, AI could improve two very important aspects such as effectiveness and efficiency. Effectiveness implies accuracy in interpreting radiological images and taking optimal clinical action. On the other hand, efficiency implies the optimization of workflows to make the best use of available resources and avoid clinical errors. These benefits would be achieved even considering the increased care pressure on physicians nowadays and the enormous workload involved in imaging on modern musculoskeletal radiology machines [12].

AI can be used to optimize clinical workflow and prioritize the tasks to be performed by clinicians. For example, an algorithm would be able to analyze a queue of images pending assessment and determine those that should be reviewed earlier because they are more likely to be pathological. This could be a critical advance in emergency situations, such as reviewing brain scan images to rule out intracranial hemorrhage [23].

Furthermore, it could accelerate image acquisition. Algorithms have been used to obtain MRI scans in five minutes that have higher image quality than other conventional MRI scans and can be optimally assessed by specialist radiologists [24].

5.4 Clinical decision-making

AI has been used as a decision support tool [25]. For example, in the field of rehabilitation, a DL algorithm has been developed to recommend to patients with low back pain, and according to clinical aspects whether they should go to their primary care physician, a physical therapist, or whether they can perform self-management [26].

DL has also been used to develop pain phenotypes based on resonance imaging findings. However, due to the complexity of pain, the role of this classification in daily care is unclear [27].

One aspect that AI could enhance would be biomarkers. In many cases, certain biomarkers cannot be used because they are too costly to obtain in terms of time or money. For example, in frailty, DL has been used to analyze body composition (bone mass, muscle mass, and fat distribution) in a CT slice at third lumbar vertebra (L3) to assess frailty and sarcopenia [28]. This would allow obtaining important data that would allow prescribing rehabilitation programs more appropriately.

AI has also been used to classify fractures. There are algorithms that have shown 72% accuracy in calcaneal fracture classification using CT [29], with similar or superior effectiveness to orthopedic surgeons for classification of proximal humerus fractures [30], good performance in hip fractures [31], femur [32], and ankle [33].

AI systems that combine clinical data in rib fractures with imaging test results have been published to improve sensitivity and reduce diagnostic time compared with expert radiologists [34].

DL has also been used to discover hidden fractures by combining clinical and radiological data. For example, an algorithm could predict the likelihood of posterior malleolar fracture in patients with tibial shaft fractures by analyzing the image along with other clinical, demographic, and injury data of the patient such as age, mechanism of injury, and fracture type [35].

5.5 Prediction and risk of musculoskeletal injuries

A growing field for the use of AI is sports medicine, although not only for the purpose of predicting whether an athlete is going to suffer an injury during a match or training but also about measuring the risk of injury to the athlete by analyzing all intrinsic and extrinsic factors and their relationship to each other, since injuries occur because of these. For example, in basketball, extrinsic factors could include the ball, the type of floor, the playing field, the temperature, or the time at which the game is played. Within intrinsic factors, we would have previous injuries, age, or gender [36].

In addition to the sport, the predictive factors are probably related to biological variables of the athletes, although no clear relationship has been established. Static traits such as flexibility, strength, or balance have usually been considered to predict injury. However, the dynamic and changing aspect of these characteristics, as well as their mutual influence, have not been taken into account [37]. AI could help manage this data.

5.6 Application to improve health literacy

Literacy is a heterogeneous and multidimensional concept that implies the ability to understand, evaluate, use, and interact with written texts in order to participate in society, achieve one's goals and develop one's potential. Health literacy involves the ability to enable individuals to obtain, understand, appreciate, and use information to make decisions and take actions that have a significant impact on their health status [38].

To improve health literacy, one tool that could be used within AI would be the use of chatbots. A chatbot is a computer system that mimics a human conversation by text or voice. Despite its potential, users of these systems often abandon them after the first or second encounter with it [39]. AI has been incorporated to achieve more empathetic and human interfaces that more realistically simulate user interaction [40].

Chatbots could facilitate health literacy, improve disease self-management, stimulate treatment adherence, or improve administrative services, such as medical appointment management [41].

These systems are also used to facilitate adherence to a home rehabilitation exercise program at hospital discharge. The role of algorithms here would be to enhance exercise adherence, achieving improved patient motivation and involvement [42]. In addition, AI could solve the fact that resources to assist patients in home-based Rehabilitation are often generic and not well adapted to individual needs and preferences [43]. For that reason, AI has been used to improve the performance of home exercise programs [44].

5.7 Data management and wearable devices

A fundamental aspect of data management today is big data. Big data involves a set of tools that analyzes data too large or too complex to be processed by traditional statistical systems. This complexity has led to the use of AI systems to analyze Big Data. For example, it has been successfully employed to coordinate the results of massive multicenter studies in the field of drug discovery [45].

In the field of musculoskeletal diseases, a large volume of data are being recorded through imaging, electronic medical records, sensors in wearable devices, and in genome sequencing. Major advances are also being made in analysis and processing systems. Thus, analyzing in detail the multidimensional information in a patient's electronic health record would provide a powerful tool to facilitate individualized health management [46].

Fuzzy logic-based AI systems that are capable of analyzing questionable, incomplete, or inconsistent clinical information have been employed and still facilitate the diagnostic management of certain pathologies [47].

Wearable devices are ubiquitous today. These devices are equipped with different sensors (accelerometers, global positioning system, gyroscopes. ..) that can record a large number of biological parameters and also have permanent connectivity. Internet of Things (IoT) refers to the set of physical objects with sensors and programs connected to other devices and systems through a network. One of the practical applications of this type of technology would be to extract a high volume of data from lifestyles, training, and sport events [48]. AI could use all this data and integrate it with other sources of information to generate algorithms to make clinical decisions or predict adverse events.

In addition to sports activity, wearables are used by users to record sleep quality, general physical activity, and walking (speed, distance traveled, and number of steps). However, it has not yet been possible to leverage this information to optimize healthcare or decrease healthcare costs [49]. It is thought that AI may be the solution to harness the performance of all this data and improve patient health.

5.8 Bioethics

By facilitating the acquisition and analysis of images, AI could improve equity in healthcare. This would facilitate access to optimal radiological assessments in areas where specialists are not available such as developing countries or rural areas [50].

It has been proposed to use AI-based systems to facilitate the entry of clinical information to reduce the time and cognitive load required to perform such a task. However, from an ethical and human point of view, there are controversies, since the doctor–patient relationship is based on trust and close treatment, and these are not assumable by a computer [51]. Clinical care remains a human process. It should never be reduced to applying more or less complex diagnostic or treatment algorithms. A patient's health should not be limited to a mere statistical concept [52]. It seems unreasonable and unethical to make clinical decisions based solely on computerized processes.

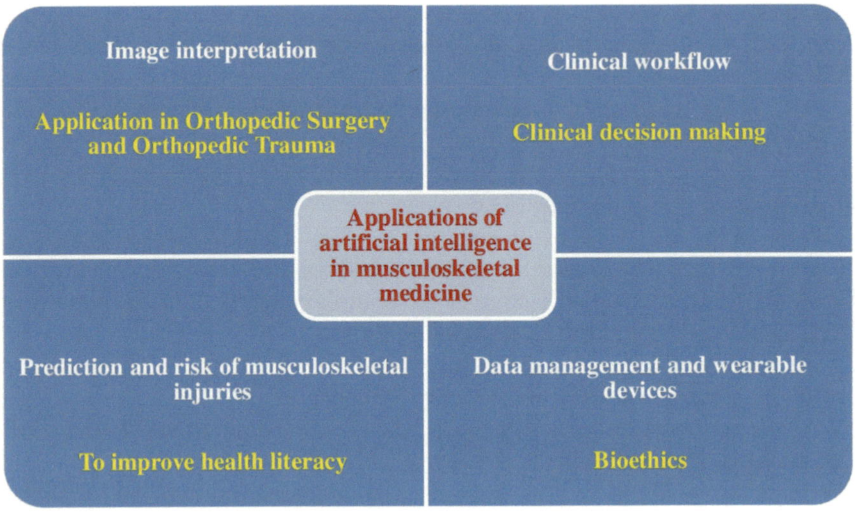

Figure 2.
Current applications of artificial intelligence (AI) in musculoskeletal medicine.

Another aspect of ethical interest is related to the costs associated with surgical procedures in which the use of algorithms to adjust the payment models per procedure has been evaluated. Although the price of interventions is usually fixed, patient comorbidities are known to increase the number of perioperative complications and produce worse outcomes [53]. This could result in some centers selecting lower-risk patients to extract a higher financial return, creating an ethical issue that must be resolved before recommending widespread use of these algorithms [54].

When interpreting radiological evidence, the physician not only classifies and analyzes the images but also interprets them within a broad clinical context. This clinical reasoning ability is acquired through the clinician's professional experience and even during the undergraduate years [55]. In fact, not all clinical decisions are made based on objective aspects. Sometimes, an experienced clinician may make clinical decisions based on experience or intuition. Even the clinician cannot explain why he or she makes this decision, and yet, in many instances, these decisions are accurate. An AI, devoid of feelings and emotions, can hardly make up for this aspect [52]. It is controversial to think what will happen in the case where an algorithm recommends one course of action and the clinician thinks that another clinical action should be taken.

On the other hand, clinical decision-making based on the use of AI algorithms, and the possible errors in diagnosis and treatment that this may cause, implies an important liability issue. And it is not clear who should assume this responsibility: the clinician, the health center or the company that has designed the algorithm. **Figure 2** summarizes current applications of AI in musculoskeletal medicine.

6. Limitations of artificial intelligence

AI is far from being able to solve all the problems that exist in musculoskeletal disease management today. To train AI systems, large, appropriately labeled databases are needed, which are expensive to build. In addition, if there are many correlated variables, AI can establish false correlations.

In radiological image interpretation, two parameters must be taken into account: accuracy and recall. An algorithm that has a high recall will classify all images with lesions as positive, but will have a low accuracy. However, an algorithm that only classifies a lesion when it is completely certain will have high accuracy but low recall. There is still great difficulty in achieving AI systems that are effective in both capabilities, so algorithms should be used depending on the clinical task to be performed: confirmation or screening [18].

On the other hand, many algorithms can only be applied in common pathologies. This makes them not applicable across the board. In addition, different AI systems may analyze the same data differently.

7. Conclusions

AI is an emerging reality that could produce a paradigm shift in the management of musculoskeletal diseases, from mechanistic to predictive medicine. The different algorithms may also facilitate the acquisition and interpretation of radiological images, provide information related to surgical processes, facilitate the decision-making process by clinicians, or enhance patient health education. However, they still have many limitations and raise important ethical issues. An algorithm cannot replace the role of clinicians, as they must bring their knowledge, experiences, skill, and humanity to patient care. Finally, AI systems must be integrated sensibly and moderately within care processes.

Author details

Juan Manuel Román-Belmonte[1], Hortensia De la Corte-Rodríguez[2],
Beatriz Adriana Rodríguez-Damiani[1] and Emérito Carlos Rodríguez-Merchán[3]*

1 Department of Physical and Rehabilitation Medicine, "Cruz Roja San José y Santa Adela" University Hospital, Madrid, Spain

2 Department of Physical and Rehabilitation Medicine, "La Paz" University Hospital-IdiPaz, Madrid, Spain

3 Department of Orthopedic Surgery, "La Paz" University Hospital-IdiPaz, Madrid, Spain

*Address all correspondence to: ecrmerchan@hotmail.com

References

[1] McCorduck P. Machines Who Think. 2nd ed. Natick, MA: A. K. Peters; 2004

[2] Anderson D. Artificial intelligence and applications in PM&R. American Journal of Physical Medicine & Rehabilitation. 2019;**98**(11):e128-e129. DOI: 10.1097/PHM.0000000000001171

[3] Liew C. The future of radiology augmented with artificial intelligence: A strategy for success. European Journal of Radiology. 2018;**102**:152-156. DOI: 10.1016/j.ejrad.2018.03.019. Epub 2018 Mar 14

[4] Goldenfeld N, Kadanoff LP. Simple lessons from complexity. Science. 1999;**284**(5411):87-89. DOI: 10.1126/science.284.5411.87

[5] Cabitza F, Locoro A, Banfi G. Machine learning in orthopedics: A literature review. Frontiers in Bioengineering and Biotechnology. 2018;**6**:75. DOI: 10.3389/fbioe.2018.00075

[6] Suzuki K. Overview of deep learning in medical imaging. Radiological Physics and Technology. 2017;**10**(3):257-273. DOI: 10.1007/s12194-017-0406-5. Epub 2017 Jul 8

[7] Soffer S, Ben-Cohen A, Shimon O, Amitai MM, Greenspan H, Klang E. Convolutional neural networks for radiologic images: A Radiologist's guide. Radiology. 2019;**290**(3):590-606. DOI: 10.1148/radiol.2018180547. Epub 2019 Jan 29

[8] Rajpurkar P, Irvin J, Bagul A, et al. MURA: Large dataset for abnormality detection in musculoskeletal radiographs. 2018; arXiv:1712.06957v4 [physics.med-ph]. DOI: 10.48550/arXiv.1712.06957

[9] Brownlee J. Supervised and Unsupervised Machine Learning Algorithms. Online Machine Learning Mastery; 2016. Available from: https://sciarium.com/file/195809/ [Accessed: March 21, 2023]

[10] Bruno MA, Walker EA, Abujudeh HH. Understanding and confronting our mistakes: The epidemiology of error in radiology and strategies for error reduction. Radiographics. 2015;**35**(6):1668-1676. DOI: 10.1148/rg.2015150023

[11] Hallas P, Ellingsen T. Errors in fracture diagnoses in the emergency department--characteristics of patients and diurnal variation. BMC Emergency Medicine. 2006;**6**:4. DOI: 10.1186/1471-227X-6-4

[12] Gore JC. Artificial intelligence in medical imaging. Magnetic Resonance Imaging. 2020;**68**:A1-A4. DOI: 10.1016/j.mri.2019.12.006. Epub 2019 Dec 16

[13] Kalmet PHS, Sanduleanu S, Primakov S, Wu G, Jochems A, Refaee T, et al. Deep learning in fracture detection: A narrative review. Acta Orthopaedica. 2020;**91**(2):215-220. DOI: 10.1080/17453674.2019.1711323 Epub 2020 Jan 13. Update in: Acta Orthop. 2020;91(3):362

[14] Jones RM, Sharma A, Hotchkiss R, Sperling JW, Hamburger J, Ledig C, et al. Assessment of a deep-learning system for fracture detection in musculoskeletal radiographs. NPJ Digital Medicine. 2020;**3**:144. DOI: 10.1038/s41746-020-00352-w

[15] Laur O, Wang B. Musculoskeletal trauma and artificial intelligence: Current trends and projections. Skeletal Radiology. 2022;**51**(2):257-269. DOI: 10.1007/s00256-021-03824-6. Epub 2021 Jun 5

[16] Langerhuizen DWG, Bulstra AEJ, Janssen SJ, Ring D, Kerkhoffs GMMJ, Jaarsma RL, et al. Is deep learning on par with human observers for detection of radiographically visible and occult fractures of the scaphoid? Clinical Orthopaedics and Related Research. 2020;**478**(11):2653-2659. DOI: 10.1097/CORR.0000000000001318

[17] Liu F, Guan B, Zhou Z, Samsonov A, Rosas H, Lian K, et al. Fully automated diagnosis of anterior cruciate ligament tears on knee MR images by using deep learning. Radiology: Artificial Intelligence. 2019;**1**(3):180091. DOI: 10.1148/ryai.2019180091

[18] Roblot V, Giret Y, Bou Antoun M, Morillot C, Chassin X, Cotten A, et al. Artificial intelligence to diagnose meniscus tears on MRI. Diagnostic and Interventional Imaging. 2019;**100**(4): 243-249. DOI: 10.1016/j.diii.2019.02.007. Epub 2019 Mar 28

[19] Liu F, Zhou Z, Samsonov A, Blankenbaker D, Larison W, Kanarek A, et al. Deep learning approach for evaluating knee MR images: Achieving high diagnostic performance for cartilage lesion detection. Radiology. 2018;**289**(1):160-169. DOI: 10.1148/radiol.2018172986. Epub 2018 Jul 31

[20] Dreizin D, Zhou Y, Chen T, Li G, Yuille AL, McLenithan A, et al. Deep learning-based quantitative visualization and measurement of extraperitoneal hematoma volumes in patients with pelvic fractures: Potential role in personalized forecasting and decision support. Journal of Trauma and Acute Care Surgery. 2020;**88**(3):425-433. DOI: 10.1097/TA.0000000000002566

[21] Ramkumar PN, Karnuta JM, Navarro SM, Haeberle HS, Iorio R, Mont MA, et al. Preoperative prediction of value metrics and a patient-specific payment model for primary Total hip arthroplasty: Development and validation of a deep learning model. The Journal of Arthroplasty. 2019;**34**(10):2228-2234.e1. DOI: 10.1016/j.arth.2019.04.055. Epub 2019 May 2

[22] Loftus TJ, Tighe PJ, Filiberto AC, Efron PA, Brakenridge SC, Mohr AM, et al. Artificial intelligence and surgical decision-making. JAMA Surgery. 2020;**155**(2):148-158. DOI: 10.1001/jamasurg.2019.4917

[23] O'Neill TJ, Xi Y, Stehel E, Browning T, Ng YS, Baker C, et al. Active reprioritization of the Reading worklist using artificial intelligence has a beneficial effect on the turnaround time for interpretation of head CT with intracranial hemorrhage. Radiology: Artificial Intelligence. 2020;**3**(2):e200024. DOI: 10.1148/ryai.2020200024

[24] Recht MP, Zbontar J, Sodickson DK, Knoll F, Yakubova N, Sriram A, et al. Using deep learning to accelerate knee MRI at 3 T: Results of an interchangeability study. AJR. American Journal of Roentgenology. 2020;**215**(6):1421-1429. DOI: 10.2214/AJR.20.23313. Epub 2020 Oct 14

[25] Tack C. Artificial intelligence and machine learning | applications in musculoskeletal physiotherapy. Musculoskeletal Science & Practice. 2019;**39**:164-169. DOI: 10.1016/j.msksp.2018.11.012. Epub 2018 Nov 23

[26] Oude Nijeweme-d'Hollosy W, van Velsen L, Poel M, Groothuis-Oudshoorn CGM, Soer R, Hermens H. Evaluation of three machine learning models for self-referral decision support on low back pain in primary care. International Journal of Medical Informatics. 2018;**110**:31-41.

DOI: 10.1016/j.ijmedinf.2017.11.010. Epub 2017 Nov 23

[27] Lötsch J, Ultsch A. Machine learning in pain research. Pain. 2018;**159**(4):623-630. DOI: 10.1097/j.pain.0000000000001118

[28] Weston AD, Korfiatis P, Kline TL, Philbrick KA, Kostandy P, Sakinis T, et al. Automated abdominal segmentation of CT scans for body composition analysis using deep learning. Radiology. 2019;**290**(3):669-679. DOI: 10.1148/radiol.2018181432. Epub 2018 Dec 11

[29] Aghnia Farda N, Lai JY, Wang JC, Lee PY, Liu JW, Hsieh IH. Sanders classification of calcaneal fractures in CT images with deep learning and differential data augmentation techniques. Injury. 2021;**52**(3):616-624. DOI: 10.1016/j.injury.2020.09.010. Epub 2020 Sep 16

[30] Chung SW, Han SS, Lee JW, Oh KS, Kim NR, Yoon JP, et al. Automated detection and classification of the proximal humerus fracture by using deep learning algorithm. Acta Orthopaedica. 2018;**89**(4):468-473. DOI: 10.1080/17453674.2018.1453714. Epub 2018 Mar 26

[31] Krogue JD, Cheng KV, Hwang KM, Toogood P, Meinberg EG, Geiger EJ, et al. Automatic hip fracture identification and functional subclassification with deep learning. Radiology: Artificial Intelligence. 2020;**2**(2):e190023. DOI: 10.1148/ryai.2020190023

[32] Tanzi L, Vezzetti E, Moreno R, Aprato A, Audisio A, Massè A. Hierarchical fracture classification of proximal femur X-ray images using a multistage deep learning approach. European Journal of Radiology. 2020;**133**:109373. DOI: 10.1016/j.ejrad.2020.109373. Epub 2020 Oct 23

[33] Olczak J, Emilson F, Razavian A, Antonsson T, Stark A, Gordon M. Ankle fracture classification using deep learning: Automating detailed AO Foundation/orthopedic trauma association (AO/OTA) 2018 malleolar fracture identification reaches a high degree of correct classification. Acta Orthopaedica. 2021;**92**(1):102-108. DOI: 10.1080/17453674.2020.1837420. Epub 2020 Oct 26

[34] Zhou QQ, Tang W, Wang J, Hu ZC, Xia ZY, Zhang R, et al. Automatic detection and classification of rib fractures based on patients' CT images and clinical information via convolutional neural network. European Radiology. 2021;**31**(6):3815-3825. DOI: 10.1007/s00330-020-07418-z. Epub 2020 Nov 17

[35] Hendrickx LAM, Sobol GL, Langerhuizen DWG, Bulstra AEJ, Hreha J, Sprague S, et al. A machine learning algorithm to predict the probability of (occult) posterior malleolar fractures associated with Tibial shaft fractures to guide "malleolus first" fixation. Journal of Orthopaedic Trauma. 2020;**34**(3):131-138. DOI: 10.1097/BOT.0000000000001663

[36] López-Valenciano A, Ayala F, Puerta JM, MBA DESC, Vera-Garcia FJ, Hernández-Sánchez S, et al. A preventive model for muscle injuries: A novel approach based on learning algorithms. Medicine and Science in Sports and Exercise. 2018;**50**(5):915-927. DOI: 10.1249/MSS.0000000000001535

[37] Kakavas G, Malliaropoulos N, Pruna R, Maffulli N. Artificial intelligence: A tool for sports trauma prediction. Injury. 2020;**51**(Suppl 3):S63-S65. DOI: 10.1016/j.injury.2019.08.033. Epub 2019 Aug 19

[38] Nutbeam D, Lloyd JE. Understanding and responding to health literacy

as a social determinant of health. Annual Review of Public Health. 2021;**42**:159-173. DOI: 10.1146/annurev-publhealth-090419-102529. Epub 2021 Oct 9

[39] Fadhil A. Can a chatbot determine my diet? Addressing challenges of chatbot application for meal recommendation. Computer Science, Medicine ArXiv. 2018. Available from: https://arxiv.org/ftp/arxiv/papers/1802/1802.09100.pdf [Accessed: March 21, 2023]

[40] Hernandez JPT. Network diffusion and technology acceptance of a nurse Chatbot for chronic disease self-management support : A theoretical perspective. The Journal of Medical Investigation. 2019;**66**(1.2):24-30. DOI: 10.2152/jmi.66.24

[41] Gabarron E, Larbi D, Denecke K, Årsand E. What do we know about the use of Chatbots for public health? Studies in Health Technology and Informatics. 2020;**270**:796-800. DOI: 10.3233/SHTI200270

[42] Vourganas I, Stankovic V, Stankovic L. Individualised responsible artificial intelligence for home-based rehabilitation. Sensors (Basel). 2020;**21**(1):2. DOI: 10.3390/s21010002

[43] Vourganas I, Stankovic V, Stankovic L. Kerr a factors that contribute to the use of stroke self-rehabilitation technologies: A review JMIR. Biomedical Engineering. 2019;**4**(1):e13732. DOI: 10.2196/13732

[44] Simonov M, Delconte G. Humanoid assessing rehabilitative exercises. Methods of Information in Medicine. 2015;**54**(2):114-121. DOI: 10.3414/ME13-02-0054. Epub 2014 Jul 1

[45] Zhu H. Big data and artificial intelligence modeling for drug discovery. Annual Review of Pharmacology and Toxicology. 2020;**60**:573-589. DOI: 10.1146/annurev-pharmtox-010919-023324 Epub 2019 Sep 13

[46] Bates DW, Saria S, Ohno-Machado L, Shah A, Escobar G. Big data in health care: Using analytics to identify and manage high-risk and high-cost patients. Health Affairs (Millwood). 2014;**33**(7):1123-1131. DOI: 10.1377/hlthaff.2014.0041

[47] Richter AN, Khoshgoftaar TM. A review of statistical and machine learning methods for modeling cancer risk using structured clinical data. Artificial Intelligence in Medicine. 2018;**90**:1-14. DOI: 10.1016/j.artmed.2018.06.002 Epub 2018 Jul 14

[48] Ehrmann FE, Duncan CS, Sindhusake D, Franzsen WN, Greene DA. GPS and injury prevention in professional soccer. Journal of Strength and Conditioning Research. 2016;**30**(2):360-367. DOI: 10.1519/JSC.0000000000001093

[49] Piwek L, Ellis DA, Andrews S, Joinson A. The rise of consumer health wearables: Promises and barriers. PLoS Medicine. 2016;**13**(2):e1001953. DOI: 10.1371/journal.pmed.1001953

[50] Shen YT, Chen L, Yue WW, Xu HX. Artificial intelligence in ultrasound. European Journal of Radiology. 2021;**139**:109717. DOI: 10.1016/j.ejrad.2021.109717. Epub 2021 Apr 12

[51] Pellegrini CA. Trust: The keystone of the patient-physician relationship. Journal of the American College of Surgeons. 2017;**224**(2):95-102. DOI: 10.1016/j.jamcollsurg.2016.10.032. Epub 2016 Oct 20

[52] El-Hassoun O, Maruscakova L, Valaskova Z, Bucova M, Polak S,

Hulin I. Artificial intelligence in service of medicine. Bratislavské Lekárske Listy. 2019;**120**(3):218-222. DOI: 10.4149/BLL_2019_028

[53] Navarro SM, Wang EY, Haeberle HS, Mont MA, Krebs VE, Patterson BM, et al. Machine learning and primary Total knee arthroplasty: Patient forecasting for a patient-specific payment model. The Journal of Arthroplasty. 2018;**33**(12):3617-3623. DOI: 10.1016/j.arth.2018.08.028. Epub 2018 Sep 5

[54] Humbyrd CJ. The ethics of bundled payments in Total joint replacement: "cherry picking" and "lemon dropping". The Journal of Clinical Ethics. 2018;**29**(1):62-68

[55] Popkin G. Is it foolish to model nature's complexity with equations? 2015. Online WIRED. Available from: https: //www.wired.com/2015/10/ is-it-foolish-to-model-natures-complexity-with-equations/ [Accessed: March 21, 2023]

Section 4

Artificial Intelligence and Machine Learning: Applications in Healthcare Diagnostics Monitoring and Clinical Workflow Management

Chapter 13

The New Landscape of Diagnostic Imaging with the Incorporation of Computer Vision

Manuel Cossio

Abstract

Diagnostic medical imaging is a key tool in medical care. In recent years, thanks to advances in computer vision research, a subfield of artificial intelligence, it has become possible to use medical imaging to train and test machine learning models. Among the algorithms investigated, there has been a boom in the use of neural networks since they allow a higher level of automation in the learning process. The areas of medical imaging that have developed the most applications are X-rays, computed tomography, positron emission tomography, magnetic resonance imaging, ultrasonography and pathology. In fact, the COVID-19 pandemic has reshaped the research landscape, especially for radiological and resonance imaging. Notwithstanding the great progress that has been observed in the field, obstacles have also arisen that had to be overcome to continue to improve applications. These obstacles include data protection and the expansion of available datasets, which involves a large investment of resources, time and academically trained manpower.

Keywords: artificial intelligence, computer vision, healthcare, deep learning, diagnostic imaging

1. Introduction

A large part of diagnosis in various specialties of medical care relies heavily on image analysis. Depending on the type of technique used, more or less detail of the structures of interest can be obtained. It will also depend on the type of technique, whether the image is in two dimensions or if there are several slices that then can form a three dimensional reconstruction [1]. Some specific techniques can also produce video output [2]. All of these different formats can be adapted for use as training and testing material for computer vision models. Computer vision, a subfield of artificial intelligence (AI), comprises all those techniques that allow a computer system to understand an image or a set of images and produce as a result a numerical or symbolic output. This output can be used to make a decision about the image [3]. When these models are applied to healthcare images, the output can be used to make a clinical decision [4]. Within computer vision algorithms, we have those that are handcrafted, where a person analyzes the set of images to be classified and chooses the features to be extracted from those images. For example, if we want to classify cardboard boxes in a scene, the person will probably choose to detect the edges of the box and the texture of the cardboard, as a first step [3]. Now, thanks to advances in research in this area, neural networks can also be used. A neural network is a computational algorithm composed of a set of interconnected nodes called artificial neurons, which are similar in function to neurons in the human nervous system. A neuron in this network receives information from the preceding neuron, processes it, and transmits it to other neurons. Networks can be simple, with very few layers of neurons, or complex, with many layers and many interconnections [5]. These models have the advantage that the determination of the features is automatic and does not need to be handcrafted. However, neural networks require a large amount of data to be able to perform accurate feature extraction with minimal error. In addition, as the number of connections between its different neurons is very high, it becomes complex to elucidate which features have been selected to produce an output from an initial image [3, 5, 6]. In the following chapter, we will discuss the most common AI applications of neural networks as computer vision models in the clinical medical field. In addition, we will analyze the different obstacles that the field of AI has encountered in its development along with the advancement that these vision applications have brought to the medical field.

2. Methods

A targeted review of the literature was carried out using the criteria "AI," "Computer Vision," and "Medical Imaging." The databases consulted were PUBMED and Google Scholar until January 2022, selecting only articles in English. Our initial search revealed 860 articles of which a subgroup of 130 was selected. The inclusion criteria focused on the quality of the research, the robustness of the models, the transfer to the clinical setting, and the optimization of the parameters for the rational use of resources.

3. Computer vision with neural networks

Computer vision (CV) and AI research have several decades of steady progress. Specifically, the part of this discipline that uses convolutional neural networks (CNN) for image processing had its first boom with handwritten digit identification in 1989. This application was developed by Yann LeCun using some of the insights previously proposed by Kunihiko Fukushima [5]. Since computational capabilities at that time were scarce, there was little research in this area between 1990 and 2000. Thanks to the progressive increase in processing and storage capacities, in 2012 the AlexNet model was tested in competition with great success and from then on, the field of computer vision began to be populated with numerous applications [7]. The applications varied according to the type of task required and the type of dataset used. Also at this time, several authors began to investigate further the structure of the different published models and started to work on their taxonomy. Thus, we have articles that examined the components of various CNNs and their interconnection [8] and others that analyzed the different architectures, their engineering challenges, and their possible future applications [4, 9].

4. Healthcare computer vision

The advancement of computer vision in the field of medical imaging awakened in the late 2000s [4]. As partially mentioned earlier, the advances were made possible by advances in deep learning (DL) research, increased local processing capabilities with graphic processing units (GPUs), and the creation of medical image datasets [10]. The creation of larger and more complete datasets was mainly due to the increasing digitization of medical records in several countries. These electronic health records (EHR) are able to store, in addition to the images that will constitute the raw material, the labels that will be used to guide the training of the models [11]. These EHRs started out as a tool to generate billing codes for different medical practices. Then they changed their use, becoming digital support for clinical practice [12]. This change allowed its adoption not only in institutions or networks of institutions but also in entire regions and countries [12, 13]. The extension of the coverage territory allowed to expand even more the image datasets and included more patient variability, which is key to obtain models with wide generalization power.

5. Operation of computer vision algorithms

When applying AI models, specifically computer vision models to different types of medical images, we can perform different tasks. According to Huo et al., these tasks can be classified into four categories [14]. The first one is classification, in which the input is an image and the output is a label. The label can be numerical (e.g., 1, 2) or it can be text (e.g., cancerous, noncancerous) [14, 15]. The second is detection, which consists of the identification of an object in the image by means of a bounding box. This task offers an extra degree of information since in addition to locating the object it can inform about its position by means of coordinates in the input image [14, 16, 17]. The third is segmentation, which provides the highest degree of information about an image. In this task, each pixel receives a label, and the final result is a mask that groups several pixels. This enables the segmentation of precise structures within medical images, such as glomeruli or metastatic zones in pathology slides, or entire organs, such as the bladder in CT images [14, 18–20]. The last task is synthesis. It consists of generating images from noise or other images. For this, two different models work antagonistically, one generates the images *de novo* from available data and the other model tries to discriminate this artificially generated image from a real image. With each iteration of the process, both the generator and the discriminator become more efficient, which produces images with high similarity to the real ones [14, 21]. This task allows for example to generate of more training samples to populate datasets and thus, to achieve models with more generalization power [22, 23].

6. Transfer learning and data augmentation

As neural networks increase their number of layers and the connections between them, their complexity increases. Neural networks with many layers have demonstrated more than satisfactory performance in several tasks, many of them superior to human performance [24]. However, when working with these complex networks it is necessary to have a large amount of data for training, to avoid overfitting, and to expand the power of generalization. The use of networks with few layers trained on small datasets has also been researched, which has shown that there is a tendency to overfitting or underfitting [25]. In the AI medical field, it is very difficult to have very large datasets, as this demands a lot of specialized manpower. Specialized manpower (doctors, biologists, geneticists, etc.) is the one that analyzes the data and aggregates the labels to train the algorithms [25, 26]. Therefore, two solutions have been found to deal with this problem of small datasets. The first one consists of data augmentation. This group of techniques creates images in virtual form from the original images of the dataset. For example, you can alter the position of the images, rotate them on their axis, and change the contrast and brightness, just to mention a few [25, 27]. The second solution is transfer learning. This technique consists of training a complex network on a massive dataset (ImageNet) usually of common images (dogs, cats, etc.), and then performing a finetuning. The finetunning is the training with the specific medical dataset, which only alters the weights of the last layers of the neural network. This helps to obtain better results than training the network from scratch on the specific dataset [25, 28].

7. Model performance evaluation

Being able to measure the performance of our models is crucial to be able to evaluate their suitability for different tasks. Also, when performing finetunning, it is important to be able to have performance measures to know which parameters promote the best results. First of all, every time we test a model, we will have part of a dataset (in this particular case, images) that already has the labels assigned to it. The assignment of labels is done by the medical professionals specialized in the pathology being worked on. When the model processes the samples and predicts the new labels, these are compared with the original ones (called ground truth). With the result of the comparison, what is called a confusion matrix is constructed [29, 30]. This structure contains the true positives (TP) and true negatives (TN) and false positives (FP) and false negatives (FN). A TP or TN is established when the prediction and the ground truth are the same for a given sample (e.g., is a TN when the model predicted negative and the image was negative). On the contrary, a FP or FN is established when there is no coincidence between the model and the ground truth (e.g., the model predicted negative and the ground truth indicated a positive sample, therefore, the sample is a FN) [29]. Almost all the other global metrics that are usually reported in the different publications are derived from the four previous metrics. For example, the accuracy of a model corresponds to the number of samples correctly predicted by the model over the total number of samples. Then, considering the previous metrics, the correctly predicted samples would be included in the sum of the TP and TN. Additionally, the total number of samples would not be more than the sum of the TP, TN, FP, and FN [29].

8. Healthcare applications of AI and computer vision

8.1 X-ray imaging

Medical X-ray imaging consists of the emission of these rays by a transmitter that passes through the area of the patient. According to the radiographic density (depending on the density of the tissue and the atomic number of its components), the structures in the area will absorb the rays differentially, which will result in lights and shadows [31]. In the AI field of computer vision applied to X-ray, there is a preponderance of work in the area of the thoracic cavity [32]. Thus, we found work focused on the detection of pulmonary nodules with models trained on images from one pool of patients and tested in a different pool. We also found longitudinal work, where the model was trained and tested on images from the same patients, with images separated by a time window [32–34]. Another large part of the work focused on the detection of pneumonia. Several models were trained on datasets from different hospitals, which showed variations in various image features between hospitals. As expected, the models showed better metrics when trained and tested on data from the same hospital [32, 35–37]. With the advent of COVID-19, there was an explosion of research in the detection of this pathology in X-ray images. Thus, numerous models were created that attempted to distinguish COVID-19 pneumonia from viral or bacterial pneumonia. These developments were key since they allowed screening and managing patients automatically and to avoid spreading the contagion of COVID-19 patients [32, 38–41]. Work was also carried out to contribute to the detection of tuberculosis in chest images. These models demonstrated satisfactory performance in screening tuberculosis images with respect to normal lungs or other pulmonary pathologies. However, the models did not show the ability to distinguish between active and quiescent disease [32, 42, 43]. Additionally, part of the research was also directed to the detection of pneumothorax. This part of the development was of important value in patient triaging, especially in determining the size and position of the pneumothorax and its changes over time in the same patient. Several of these models have already received FDA clearance as assistive devices in the emergency unit [32, 44–46]. As a final part of this section, to a lesser extent than the previous ones, models were also built for the detection of other types of pulmonary involvement, such as consolidation, edema, emphysema, fibrosis, and pleural effusion [32, 47].

8.2 Computed tomography

Computed tomography (CT) integrates many X-ray images taken from different angles thanks to the high-speed rotating platform that rotates on the same axis where the patient lies. The type of images it produces is cross-sectional [1]. Using AI computer vision techniques, it is possible to operate directly on a fixed plane (one section) or to use complete volumes (several consecutive sections). Most of the research in this area is classification (about 36%), followed by segmentation (27%), detection (22%), and others (15%) [30]. Broadly speaking we can list the works in this area in the identification of organs (kidney [48], liver [49, 50], lungs [51, 52], and heart [53, 54]) and in the identification of substructures or lesions (artery calcification [55], nodules [56], polyps [57, 58], and lymph nodes [59–61]). Among the most commonly used measures to report the performance of the different models are accuracy, sensitivity, specificity, AUC-ROC, and F1 score [1]. The processing of the images as input is also diverse. It is possible to use 3-dimensional inputs, that is, several consecutive slices that form a volume. Projection methods, such as maximum intensity projection, can also be used to transform a 3-dimensional input into a 2-dimensional one [1, 62].

8.3 Positron emission tomography

Positron emission tomography (PET) is a technique that allows the observation of metabolic processes in different tissues of the patient's body. Radiolabeled compounds that follow a specific metabolic pathway are injected, the radiation is detected by sensors and then the complete image is reconstructed with the areas of highest activity [1]. 18F-fluorodeoxyglucose (FDG) is one of the most widely used radioactive substrates as a marker in PET [1, 63]. Among the applications of AI computer vision to this medical imaging modality, we have the segmentation of tumor areas in the brain [64], heart [65], head and neck [66], and nasopharynx [67] to adjust the dose and position of the radiotherapy intervention. With respect to classification tasks, work has been published on esophageal cancer [68], Alzheimer's disease typing [69], and Hodgkin's lymphoma [1, 70].

8.4 Magnetic resonance imaging

Magnetic resonance imaging (MRI) is a technique that uses high-intensity electromagnetic fields and radiofrequency waves to detect changes in the rotational axis of protons, mostly in water molecules. Water makes up almost all the tissues in the body and the difference in the percentage of water influences the axis changes. Deep learning applications in the field of MRI can be grouped into two broad categories. The first is related to the physical aspects and the generation of images on the device. In this category, you can find works that focus on image restoration, image reconstruction, and multimodal image registration [71]. The second category emphasizes applications for medical purposes, in which the determination of pathology or its progress is the main purpose [71–74]. Focusing on the second category, we find works on brain aging [75], brain vascular lesions [76], Alzheimer's disease [77], multiple sclerosis [78], glioma [79], and meningioma [80]. In the abdominal cavity, we find works of identification and segmentation of organs [81], polycystic kidneys [82], and renal transplantation [83]. Finally, isolating the spine as the focus of the study, we found works on labeling and separation of vertebrae [84], spinal stenosis grading [85], and identification and segmentation of spinal metastasis [86]. It is important to mention that organ segmentation is a very important focus in deep learning applications for MRI images. With the definition of organ contours in each plane (slice), the determination of the organ coordinates and the addition of consecutive areas, volumes can be calculated. The calculation of volumes is of crucial importance since they can be used to determine the dilation of organs (e.g., splenomegaly). The measurement of dilation is not only an important initial measurement. Thanks to the volumetric determination, it is possible to follow up on patients to observe the efficiency of treatments [81].

8.5 Ultrasonography

Ultrasonography (US) consists of the use of ultrasound (usually at a frequency greater than 20,000 hz) to form images of the inner regions of the organism. To do this, a probe emits waves and they bounce back at different speeds according to the type of tissue [87]. From this technique, we can count on two different outputs. One is an image (frame) where the structure of medical interest is located. The other is a complete video where we can visualize, for example, blood flow or muscle contraction. Within the research in AI computer vision applied to US, most of the works include the analysis of individual frames. In this way, frames can be produced directly from the device or they can be extracted from ultrasound videos. When extracting frames from videos, the regions of interest for the specific task is usually timely located and the rest are discarded [88]. Other less common and more integrative methodologies can use videos directly as input. They produce the division into frames, use a model (CNN) to extract features from each frame, and then integrate all the extracted features with a recurrent model (e.g., long short-term memory network) following a timeline [2]. Focusing on applications, in those works that performed classification we found the study of breast lesions [88–90], thyroid nodules [88, 91], liver fibrosis [88, 92], and focal liver disease [88, 93]. Regarding the detection of lesions, some works focused on papillary thyroid carcinoma [94] and breast cancer [95]. Continuing in the detection task, but moving from lesions to the detection of the fetal standard plan, several papers proposed different methodologies [88, 96, 97]. These works constituted important pillars for the improvement of automatic guidance tools in the fetal US that could be embedded in image production software. Finally, in the segmentation task, several works have been registered with approaches in areas similar to those mentioned above, such as breast lesions [88, 98] and lymph node contouring [88, 99, 100]. However, in this part, there is also an application that has several works and that has an important diagnostic value in the clinical setting. This application is the detection of atheroma plaques in the carotid artery and the automation of this process would allow screening and prevention in a faster and more cost-effective way [101, 102]. In fact, a multicenter clinical study has already been published to evaluate the feasibility of the technique [102].

8.6 Computational pathology

Classical pathology consists, very briefly, of the preservation, treatment, and staining of very small portions of tissue in slides. Stains can be standard ones, which highlight general structures, such as nuclei or cytoplasm, or immunohistochemical stains, in which specific cellular markers are targeted [103]. Thanks to advances in storage capabilities and the availability of cloud computing, the last few years have seen a migration from direct microscopic observation of stained tissues to the digitization of slides. Digital slides are stored in a specific file type called whole slide image (WSI), where it is possible to store the different magnification planes with very high compression. The scanning of the slides and the production of WSI for different uses, such as telepathology, constitute a branch of pathology called digital pathology [30, 104]. In addition, the increasing production and cataloging of WSIs for the diagnosis of different diseases made it possible to use them as training and testing materials for computer vision algorithms. This application of algorithms in WSIs has been called computational pathology and most of the published works use deep learning as a basis for different tasks. In a very general manner, one could describe the process of creating a computational pathology pipeline for any disease. Once the WSIs of the pathology to be studied are available, the final magnification to work with must be selected (20×, 40×) and consecutive patches of the different zones (disease and healthy tissue) must be generated [30]. The patches are generated due to the large size of the WSIs (the highest magnification can exceed 3e10 pixels). Consequently, the patches are used as input to the model and the model will learn, according to the task, to identify tumor and non-tumor zones [30]. In test WSIs, the same technique can be used to generate patches, process them with the model and then reconstruct the final image with a heat map. The heat map will identify the regions with the highest probability of belonging to a class (healthy or tumor). Jiang et al. categorize the implementation of computational pathology in oncology into five purposes, which are tumor diagnosis, subtyping, grading, staging, and prognosis [30]. Thus, we can find applications of these five purposes for breast cancer [30, 105–108], lung cancer [30, 109–111], colorectal cancer [30, 112–115], gastric cancer [30, 116, 117], prostate cancer [30, 118, 119], and thyroid cancer [30, 120, 121]. Another set of applications of computational pathology lies in the automatic analysis for the identification of rejection in organ transplantation. Several papers have been published for kidney [122, 123] and heart [124] transplantation.

9. COVID-19 research landscape remodeling

The COVID-19 pandemic created a compelling need for innovation in testing to generate solutions that were cheap, easy to use, fast, and ubiquitous. Since lung imaging is a useful diagnostic tool, during the pandemic many research groups began to look for solutions using AI and computer vision [125]. As lung imaging is an important resource in emergency medicine for optimal triage of patients with suspected COVID-19 infection, computer vision solutions aimed to be a rapid analysis element that could speed up patient management times. From 2019 to 2020, a nearly two-fold increase in the number of publications on the artificial intelligence applied to medical imaging was observed. Moreover, starting from zero publications in 2019, by 2020 about 15% of all deep learning research associated with medical imaging was on COVID-19. With respect to the focus on the type of medical imaging, it was observed that of all the proposed computer vision solutions, almost half (49.7%) were focused only on X-rays. The remaining modalities were CT (38.7%), multimodality (10.2%), and ultrasonography (1.5%) [125]. As the research progressed, the usefulness of ultrasound as a tool for the diagnosis and management of COVID-19 was also observed. The ease of maintaining sterility, the possibility of performing bedside operations, the reduced time to obtain the image, and the possibility of using only one operator for the procedure have made this imaging modality highly suitable for this pandemic. The group of Born et al. opened the door to the use of deep learning with ultrasound for COVID-19 screening [126, 127]. Several groups followed with different proposals and today, the field has grown considerably by extending applications to other pathologies [128, 129].

10. Challenges for the field

As we briefly mentioned in one of the previous sections, one of the biggest challenges facing the field of AI and computer vision applied to medicine is the availability of datasets. Generating general datasets, although it is a task that requires time, can be done in a more laborsaving way. For instance, it does not require a high degree of training to classify common images. In fact, some search engines ask their users when they access specific content to first select from a group of images those that have a traffic light in it. That generates labels and in this way very large datasets are built. As we also mentioned before, in order to generate medical image datasets, trained doctors are needed to perform the same activity. That requirement makes the process complex, time-consuming, and expensive [25, 26]. Another problem facing the field is the variability between different hospital centers' samples. As we have already explained before, the greater the amount of data that the algorithm trains with, the higher its generalization power. However, when the data comes from different hospitals, even if they are in the same city, samples of the same medical condition may suffer variations in color, brightness, contrast, and position, to mention just a few. These variations respond to the different equipment used by hospitals and the different sample preparation techniques that different laboratories may have. This variability is manifested in its maximum expression in computational pathology. Moreover, the most current works usually include studies with different scanners and from different hospitals to analyze the robustness of the model [124]. Another challenge that specifically affects computational pathology is the weight of each sample. As we mentioned before, the WSI of the pathology samples contains a considerable amount of pixels, especially at their highest magnification level. This makes it challenging to be able to share the images and store complete datasets. It is worth mentioning that also operating digitally with these images raises the hardware requirements to high levels. For this reason, parallelization tasks or image batch processing can become complex, which also increases processing times [130]. Finally, a crucial aspect must be addressed. Operating with medical images requires a high degree of data protection and the use of anonymization techniques. In order to use hospital data, an ethics committee must first review the scope of the project. The ethics committee will determine the degree of consent that patients must provide in order to use their data. In many retrospective studies, depending on the amount of private data being used, committees may approve the waiving of informed consent (IC). For example, if patients have already consented to the original study and no further identifying data will be added to the project, this may be a favorable setting for not requiring additional IC. However, that decision rests solely with the committee and this entity will decide the constraints of the project. Ethics committees may be slow to grant project approval, especially if the scope of the project is extensive. Also, should new ICs be required, this can also add cost and time to the project [131].

11. Innovating through challenges

The challenges that have crossed the field of AI and computer vision in healthcare have also promoted the search for solutions. This search has sparked ideas and achieved some interesting proposals that are slowly being incorporated into daily practice. To begin with, the problem of generating labels in WSIs gave rise to a new technique called multiple instance learning (MIL). This technique uses as labels only the diagnosis of the patient (which is usually available in EHRs). Thanks to this new approach, a group managed to analyze 44,732 WSIs without any kind of data curation, incredibly speeding up project times [132]. As we also mentioned, the variability between samples from different hospitals is a problem that threatens the creation of large datasets. One of the solutions to this problem was the creation of stain normalization. This is a method that in one of its variants uses autoencoders and allows to standardize of the color distribution in the images, using another image as a template [133]. Thanks to this method, it is possible to have more homogeneous images, even if they come from different laboratories. Regarding the weight of the WSIs, generally, only a small part of the image is used by the deep learning models for the task they perform. For example, as the image passes through the successive layers of a CNN, the information is reduced. In the last layers, only the essential information remains that will complete the task with the least possible error. Using this principle, one group created the concept of neural compression. Basically what this group proposed is to create abstract representations of the WSI images after passing through successive steps in a convolutional network. In this way, noise is removed at each step and only a small, compressed representation remains [134]. This concept would help store WSIs more efficiently with only the information needed for the task. Finally, to provide the greatest privacy protection to patients and also speed up data exchange processes, blockchain networks and interplanetary file system (IPFS) can be used. In this way, the information is decentralized, which reduces the risk of data leakage. In addition, the different hospitals participating in the study can provide the files, which can be fragmented and hashed according to IFPS. The entire process would be governed by one or several smart contracts, which would ensure that only authorized nodes contribute data or extract data. Smart contracts may also contain portions of sensitive information, which would eliminate the need for human interaction and the possible breach of confidentiality [135–137].

12. Conclusions

The use of AI and computer vision algorithms, especially neural networks, has advanced greatly in recent years. The various applications with different types of medical images have made numerous diagnostic and prognostic applications available to the medical field. The field of oncology has seen the greatest number of developments. Particularly, computational pathology applied to oncology has developed a high degree of diversification in vision tasks, achieving models that could perform diagnosis, subtyping, grading, staging, and prognosis. However, just as innovative applications have emerged, the field has also had to overcome obstacles, which are still complex to analyze for some conditions today. The difficulty of constructing medical datasets, the variability of samples between different institutions, and the mandatory data protection are some of them. However, these obstacles have promoted the creation of ideas to overcome them and that is how we have neural compression and stain normalization that can be great allies to exponentially expand the datasets. Finally, the COVID-19 pandemic was a major trigger for research in AI and computer vision applied to the field of medical imaging, specifically lung imaging. It could be seen that a modeler of the research landscape was the feasibility in the clinical field. In fact, the ease of use, the short operating time, and the possibility of maintaining sterility were part of the parameters that promoted the use of ultrasonography expanding the research with deep learning in this imaging modality. Despite these great advances, more studies must be done to further refine computer vision models to ensure that patients receive the best quality of medical care.

Author details

Manuel Cossio
Department of Mathematics and Computer Science, Universitat de Barcelona, Barcelona, Spain

*Address all correspondence to: manuel.cossio@ub.edu

References

[1] Domingues I, Pereira G, Martins P, Duarte H, Santos J, Abreu PH. Using deep learning techniques in medical imaging: A systematic review of applications on ct and pet. Artificial Intelligence Review. 2020;**53**(6):4093-4160

[2] Barros B, Lacerda P, Albuquerque C, Conci A. Pulmonary covid-19: Learning spatiotemporal features combining cnn and lstm networks for lung ultrasound video classification. Sensors. 2021;**21**(16): 5486

[3] Szeliski R. Computer Vision: Algorithms and Applications. Switzerland AG: Springer Nature; 2022

[4] Bhatt D et al. Cnn variants for computer vision: History, architecture, application, challenges and future scope. Electronics. 2021;**10**(20):2470

[5] LeCun Y et al. Handwritten digit recognition with a back-propagation network. Advances in Neural Information Processing Systems. 1989;**2**

[6] Lauzon FQ. An introduction to deep learning. In: 2012 11th International Conference on Information Science, Signal Processing and their Applications (ISSPA). Institute of Electrical and Electronics Engineers; 2012. pp. 1438-1439

[7] Krizhevsky A, Sutskever I, Hinton GE. Imagenet classification with deep convolutional neural networks. Communications of the ACM. 2017; **60**(6):84-90

[8] Khan A, Sohail A, Zahoora U, Qureshi AS. A survey of the recent architectures of deep convolutional neural networks. Artificial Intelligence Review. 2020;**53**(8):5455-5516

[9] Alzubaidi L et al. Review of deep learning: Concepts, cnn architectures, challenges, applications, future directions. Journal of Big Data. 2021; **8**(1):1-74

[10] Esteva A et al. Deep learning-enabled medical computer vision. NPJ Digital Medicine. 2021;**4**(1):1-9

[11] Datta S, Bernstam EV, Roberts K. A frame semantic overview of nlp-based information extraction for cancer-related ehr notes. Journal of Biomedical Informatics. 2019;**100**:103301

[12] Evans RS. Electronic health records: Then, now, and in the future. Yearbook of Medical Informatics. 2016;**25**(S 01): S48-S61

[13] Lehmann CU, Altuwaijri M, Li Y, Ball M, Haux R. Translational research in medical informatics or from theory to practice. Methods of Information in Medicine. 2008;**47**(01):1-3

[14] Huo Y, Deng R, Liu Q, Fogo AB, Yang H. Ai applications in renal pathology. Kidney International. 2021; **99**(6):1309-1320

[15] Goodfellow I, Bengio Y, Courville A. Deep Learning. Massachusetts Institute of Technology Press; 2016

[16] Temerinac-Ott M et al. Detection of glomeruli in renal pathology by mutual comparison of multiple staining modalities. In: Proceedings of the 10th International Symposium on Image and Signal Processing and Analysis. Institute of Electrical and Electronics Engineers; 2017. pp. 19-24

[17] George J, Skaria S, Varun V, et al. Using yolo based deep learning network for real time detection and localization of

lung nodules from low dose ct scans. In: Medical Imaging 2018: Computer-Aided Diagnosis. Vol. 10575. SPIE; 2018. pp. 347-355

[18] Ginley B et al. Computational segmentation and classification of diabetic glomerulosclerosis. Journal of the American Society of Nephrology. 2019;**30**(10):1953-1967

[19] Gibson E et al. Automatic multi-organ segmentation on abdominal ct with dense v-networks. IEEE Transactions on Medical Imaging. 2018; **37**(8):1822-1834

[20] Cha KH, Hadjiiski L, Samala RK, Chan H-P, Caoili EM, Cohan RH. Urinary bladder segmentation in ct urography using deep-learning convolutional neural network and level sets. Medical Physics. 2016;**43**(4):1882-1896

[21] Suganthi K et al. Review of medical image synthesis using gan techniques. In: ITM Web of Conferences. Vol. 37. Édition Diffusion Presse Sciences; 2021. p. 01005

[22] Brock A, Donahue J, Simonyan K. Large scale gan training for high fidelity natural image synthesis. arXiv preprint arXiv:1809.11096. 2018

[23] Cossio M. Computational pathology in renal disease: A comprehensive perspective. arXiv preprint arXiv: 2210.10162. 2022

[24] He K, Zhang X, Ren S, Sun J. Deep residual learning for image recognition. In: Proceedings of the Institute of Electrical and Electronics Engineers Conference on Computer Vision and Pattern Recognition. 2016. pp. 770-778

[25] Alzubaidi L et al. Towards a better understanding of transfer learning for medical imaging: A case study. Applied Sciences. 2020;**10**(13):4523

[26] Tan C, Sun F, Kong T, Zhang W, Yang C, Liu C. A survey on deep transfer learning. In: International Conference on Artificial Neural Networks. Springer; 2018. pp. 270-279

[27] Shorten C, Khoshgoftaar TM. A survey on image data augmentation for deep learning. Journal of Big Data. 2019; **6**(1):1-48

[28] Alzubaidi L, Al-Shamma O, Fadhel MA, Farhan L, Zhang J, Duan Y. Optimizing the performance of breast cancer classification by employing the same domain transfer learning from hybrid deep convolutional neural network model. Electronics. 2020;**9**(3):445

[29] Samsir S, Sitorus JHP, Ritonga Z, Nasution FA, Watrianthos R, et al. Comparison of machine learning algorithms for chest x-ray image covid-19 classification. In: Journal of Physics: Conference Series. Vol. 2021. Institute of Physics Publishing; 1933. p. 012040

[30] Jiang Y, Yang M, Wang S, Li X, Sun Y. Emerging role of deep learning-based artificial intelligence in tumor pathology. Cancer Communications. 2020;**40**(4):154-166

[31] Corne J, Au-Yong I. Chest X-Ray Made Easy E-Book. 5th ed. Elsevier Health Sciences; 2022. p. 202. ISBN: 9780702082344, ISBN: 9780702082368

[32] Moses DA. Deep learning applied to automatic disease detection using chest x-rays. Journal of Medical Imaging and Radiation Oncology. 2021;**65**(5):498-517

[33] Pesce E, Withey SJ, Ypsilantis P-P, Bakewell R, Goh V, Montana G. Learning to detect chest radiographs containing pulmonary lesions using

visual attention networks. Medical Image Analysis. 2019;**53**:26-38

[34] Kim Y-G et al. Short-term reproducibility of pulmonary nodule and mass detection in chest radiographs: Comparison among radiologists and four different computer-aided detections with convolutional neural net. Scientific Reports. 2019;**9**(1):1-9

[35] Zech JR, Badgeley MA, Liu M, Costa AB, Titano JJ, Oermann EK. Variable generalization performance of a deep learning model to detect pneumonia in chest radio-graphs: A cross-sectional study. PLoS Medicine. 2018;**15**(11):e1002683

[36] Stephen O, Sain M, Maduh UJ, Jeong D-U. An efficient deep learning approach to pneumonia classification in healthcare. Journal of Healthcare Engineering. 2019;**2019**:2040-2295

[37] Ravi V, Narasimhan H, Pham TD. A cost-sensitive deep learning-based meta-classifier for pediatric pneumonia classification using chest x-rays. Expert Systems. 2022;**39**(1):e12966

[38] Khan AI, Shah JL, Bhat MM. Coronet: A deep neural network for detection and diagnosis of covid-19 from chest x-ray images. Computer Methods and Programs in Biomedicine. 2020;**196**:105581

[39] Apostolopoulos ID, Mpesiana TA. Covid-19: Automatic detection from x-ray images utilizing transfer learning with convolutional neural networks. Physical and Engineering Sciences in Medicine. 2020;**43**(2):635-640

[40] Vogado L, Araújo F, Neto PS, Almeida J, Tavares JMR, Veras R. A ensemble methodology for automatic classification of chest x-rays using deep learning. Computers in Biology and Medicine. 2022;**145**:105442

[41] Asif S, Zhao M, Tang F, Zhu Y. A deep learning-based framework for detecting covid-19 patients using chest x-rays. Multimedia Systems. 2022;**28**(13):1-19

[42] Lopes U, Valiati JF. Pre-trained convolutional neural networks as feature extractors for tuberculosis detection. Computers in Biology and Medicine. 2017;**89**:135-143

[43] Lakhani P, Sundaram B. Deep learning at chest radiography: Automated classification of pulmonary tuberculosis by using convolutional neural networks. Radiology. 2017; **284**(2):574-582

[44] Taylor AG, Mielke C, Mongan J. Automated detection of moderate and large pneumothorax on frontal chest x-rays using deep convolutional neural networks: A retrospective study. PLoS Medicine. 2018;**15**(11):e1002697

[45] Jun TJ, Kim D, Kim D. Automated diagnosis of pneumothorax using an ensemble of convolutional neural networks with multi-sized chest radiography images. arXiv preprint arXiv:1804.06821. 2018

[46] Feng S, Liu Q, Patel A, Bazai SU, Jin CK, Kim JS, et al. Automated pneumothorax triaging in chest X-rays in the New Zealand population using deep-learning algorithms. Journal of medical imaging and radiation oncology. 2022;**66**(8):1035-1043. DOI: 10.1111/1754-9485.13393

[47] Wang X, Peng Y, Lu L, Lu Z, Bagheri M, Summers RM. Chestx-ray8: Hospitalscale chest x-ray database and benchmarks on weakly-supervised classification and localization of common thorax diseases. In: Proceedings of the Institute of Electrical and Electronics Engineers Conference on

Computer Vision and Pattern Recognition. 2017. pp. 2097-2106

[48] Liu J, Wang S, Linguraru MG, Yao J, Summers RM. Computer-aided detection of exophytic renal lesions on non-contrast ct images. Medical Image Analysis. 2015;**19**(1):15-29

[49] Vivanti R, Szeskin A, Lev-Cohain N, Sosna J, Joskowicz L. Automatic detection of new tumors and tumor burden evaluation in longitudinal liver ct scan studies. International Journal of Computer Assisted Radiology and Surgery. 2017;**12**(11):1945-1957

[50] Perez AA et al. Deep learning ct-based quantitative visualization tool for liver volume estimation: Defining normal and hepatomegaly. Radiology. 2022;**302**(2):336-342

[51] Gerard SE, Patton TJ, Christensen GE, Bayouth JE, Reinhardt JM. Fissurenet: A deep learning approach for pulmonary fissure detection in ct images. IEEE Transactions on Medical Imaging. 2018; **38**(1):156-166

[52] Choe J et al. Content-based image retrieval by using deep learning for interstitial lung disease diagnosis with chest ct. Radiology. 2022;**302**(1):187-197

[53] Dormer JD, Halicek M, Ma L, Reilly CM, Schreibmann E, Fei B. Convolutional neural networks for the detection of diseased hearts using ct images and left atrium patches. In: Medical Imaging 2018: Computer-Aided Diagnosis. Vol. 10575. Society for Optics and Photonics; 2018. pp. 671-677

[54] Hoori A, Hu T, Lee J, Al-Kindi S, Rajagopalan S, Wilson DL. Deep learning segmentation and quantification method for assessing epicardial adipose tissue in ct calcium score scans. Scientific Reports. 2022;**12**(1):1-10

[55] Liu J, Lu L, Yao J, Bagheri M, Summers RM. Pelvic artery calcification detection on ct scans using convolutional neural networks. In: Medical Imaging 2017: Computer-Aided Diagnosis. Vol. 10134. Society for Optics and Photonics; 2017. pp. 319-325

[56] Lyu J, Ling SH. Using multi-level convolutional neural network for classification of lung nodules on ct images. In: 2018 40th Annual International Conference of the IEEE Engineering in Medicine and Biology Society (EMBC). Vol. 2018. Institute of Electrical and Electronics Engineers. pp. 686-689

[57] Näppi JJ, Pickhardt P, Kim DH, Hironaka T, Yoshida H. Deep learning of contrast-coated serrated polyps for computer-aided detection in ct colonography. In: Medical Imaging 2017: Computer-Aided Diagnosis. Vol. 10134. Society for Optics and Photonics; 2017. pp. 114-120

[58] Wesp P et al. Deep learning in ct colonography: Differentiating premalignant from benign colorectal polyps. European Radiology. 2022;**32**(7): 1-11

[59] Oda H et al. Dense volumetric detection and segmentation of mediastinal lymph nodes in chest ct images. In: Medical Imaging 2018: Computer-Aided Diagnosis. Vol. 10575. Society for Optics and Photonics; 2018. p. 1057502

[60] Murugesan M, Kaliannan K, Balraj S, Singaram K, Kaliannan T, Albert JR. A hybrid deep learning model for effective segmentation and classification of lung nodules from ct images. Journal of Intelligent & Fuzzy Systems. 2022; **Preprint**:1-13

[61] Sourlos N, Wang J, Nagaraj Y, van Ooijen P, Vliegenthart R. Possible bias in

supervised deep learning algorithms for ct lung nodule detection and classification. Cancers. 2022;**14**(16):3867

[62] Belharbi S et al. Spotting l3 slice in ct scans using deep convolutional network and transfer learning. Computers in Biology and Medicine. 2017;**87**:95-103

[63] Vaquero JJ, Kinahan P. Positron emission tomography: Current challenges and opportunities for technological advances in clinical and preclinical imaging systems. Annual Review of Biomedical Engineering. 2015; **17**:385-414

[64] Blanc-Durand P, Van Der Gucht A, Schaefer N, Itti E, Prior JO. Automatic lesion detection and segmentation of 18f-fet pet in gliomas: A full 3d u-net convolutional neural network study. PLoS One. 2018;**13**(4):e0195798

[65] Wang X et al. Heart and bladder detection and segmentation on fdg pet/ct by deep learning. BMC Medical Imaging. 2022;**22**(1):1-13

[66] Huang B, Chen Z, Wu PM, Ye Y, Feng ST, Wong CO, et al. Fully Automated Delineation of Gross Tumor Volume for Head and Neck Cancer on PET-CT Using Deep Learning: A Dual-Center Study. Contrast Media & Molecular Imaging, 2018:8923028. DOI: 10.1155/2018/8923028

[67] Zhao L, Lu Z, Jiang J, Zhou Y, Wu Y, Feng Q. Automatic nasopharyngeal carcinoma segmentation using fully convolutional networks with auxiliary paths on dual-modality pet-ctimages. Journal of Digital Imaging. 2019;**32**(3): 462-470

[68] Ypsilantis P-P et al. Predicting response to neoadjuvant chemotherapy with pet imaging using convolutional neural networks. PLoS One. 2015;**10**(9): e0137036

[69] Cheng D, Liu M. Combining convolutional and recurrent neural networks for alzheimer's disease diagnosis using pet images. In: 2017 IEEE International Conference on Imaging Systems and Techniques (IST). Institute of Electrical and Electronics Engineers; 2017. pp. 1-5

[70] Pereira G. Deep learning techniques for the evaluation of response to treatment in hogdkin lymphoma [Ph.D. dissertation]. Universidade of Coimbra Publishing Registry; 2018

[71] Lundervold AS, Lundervold A. An overview of deep learning in medical imaging focusing on mri. Zeitschrift für Medizinische Physik. 2019;**29**(2):102-127

[72] Fritz B, Fritz J. Artificial intelligence for mri diagnosis of joints: A scoping review of the current state-of-the-art of deep learning-based approaches. Skeletal Radiology. 2022;**51**(2):315-329

[73] Turkbey B, Haider MA. Deep learning-based artificial intelligence applications in prostate mri: Brief summary. The British Journal of Radiology. 2022;**95**(1131):20210563

[74] Verburg E et al. Deep learning for automated triaging of 4581 breast mri examinations from the dense trial. Radiology. 2022;**302**(1):29-36

[75] Cole JH et al. Predicting brain age with deep learning from raw imaging data results in a reliable and heritable biomarker. NeuroImage. 2017;**163**: 115-124

[76] Moeskops P et al. Evaluation of a deep learning approach for the segmentation of brain tissues and white

matter hyperintensities of presumed vascular origin in mri. NeuroImage: Clinical. 2018;**17**:251-262

[77] Liu M, Zhang J, Adeli E, Shen D. Landmark-based deep multi-instance learning for brain disease diagnosis. Medical Image Analysis. 2018;**43**:157-168

[78] Yoo Y et al. Deep learning of joint myelin and t1w mri features in normal-appearing brain tissue to distinguish between multiple sclerosis patients and healthy controls. NeuroImage: Clinical. 2018;**17**:169-178

[79] Perkuhn M et al. Clinical evaluation of a multiparametric deep learning model for glioblastoma segmentation using heterogeneous magnetic resonance imaging data from clinical routine. Investigative Radiology. 2018;**53**(11):647

[80] Laukamp KR et al. Fully automated detection and segmentation of meningiomas using deep learning on routine multiparametric mri. European Radiology. 2019;**29**(1):124-132

[81] Bobo MF et al. "Fully convolutional neural networks improve abdominal organ segmentation," in Medical Imaging 2018: Image Processing, Society for Optics and Photonics. vol. 10574. 2018. pp. 750-757

[82] Kline TL et al. Performance of an artificial multi-observer deep neural network for fully automated segmentation of polycystic kidneys. Journal of Digital Imaging. 2017;**30**(4): 442-448

[83] Shehata M et al. Computer-aided diagnostic system for early detection of acute renal transplant rejection using diffusion-weighted mri. Institute of Electrical and Electronics Engineers Transactions on Biomedical Engineering. 2018;**66**(2):539-552

[84] Forsberg D, Sjöblom E, Sunshine JL. Detection and labeling of vertebrae in mr images using deep learning with clinical annotations as training data. Journal of Digital Imaging. 2017;**30**(4):406-412

[85] Lu J-T et al. Deep spine: Automated lumbar vertebral segmentation, disc-level designation, and spinal stenosis grading using deep learning. In: Machine Learning for Healthcare Conference, PMLR. 2018. pp. 403-419

[86] Wang X et al. Searching for prostate cancer by fully automated magnetic resonance imaging classification: Deep learning versus non-deep learning. Scientific Reports. 2017;7(1):1-8

[87] Callen PW. Ultrasonography in Obstetrics and Gynecology E-Book. Elsevier Health Sciences; 2011

[88] Wang Y, Ge X, Ma H, Qi S, Zhang G, Yao Y. Deep learning in medical ultrasound image analysis: A review. Institute of Electrical and Electronics Engineers Access. 2021;**9**:54310-54324

[89] Zhu Y-C et al. A generic deep learning framework to classify thyroid and breast lesions in ultrasound images. Ultrasonics. 2021;**110**:106300

[90] Jabeen K et al. Breast cancer classification from ultrasound images using probability-based optimal deep learning feature fusion. Sensors. 2022; **22**(3):807

[91] Pavithra S, Vanithamani R, Justin J. Classification of stages of thyroid nodules in ultrasound images using transfer learning methods. In: International Conference on Image Processing and Capsule Networks. Springer; 2021. pp. 241-253

[92] Nonsakhoo W, Saiyod S, Sirisawat P, Suwanwerakamtorn R, Chamadol N,

Khuntikeo N. Liver ultrasound image classification of periductal fibrosis based on transfer learning and fcnet for liver ultrasound images analysis system. In: in 2021 International Conference on Computing, Communication, and Intelligent Systems (ICCCIS). Institute of Electrical and Electronics Engineers; 2021. pp. 569-575

[93] Căleanu CD, Sırbu CL, Simion G. Deep neural architectures for contrast enhanced ultrasound (ceus) focal liver lesions automated diagnosis. Sensors. 2021;**21**(12):4126

[94] Zhou H, Liu B, Liu Y, Huang Q, Yan W. Ultrasonic Intelligent Diagnosis of Papillary Thyroid Carcinoma Based on Machine Learning. Journal of Healthcare Engineering. 2022:6428796. DOI: 10.1155/2022/6428796

[95] Yap MH et al. Breast ultrasound region of interest detection and lesion localisation. Artificial Intelligence in Medicine. 2020;**107**:101880

[96] Ni D. et al. Selective Search and Sequential Detection for Standard Plane Localization in Ultrasound. In: Yoshida H, Warfield S, Vannier MW, editors. Abdominal Imaging. Computation and Clinical Applications. ABD-MICCAI 2013. Lecture Notes in Computer Science. Vol. 8198. Berlin, Heidelberg: Springer; 2013. DOI: 10.1007/978-3-642-41083-3_23

[97] Wu L, Cheng J-Z, Li S, Lei B, Wang T, Ni D. Fuiqa: Fetal ultrasound image quality assessment with deep convolutional networks. Institute of Electrical and Electronics Engineers Transactions on Cybernetics. 2017;**47**(5): 1336-1349

[98] Kumar V et al. Automated and real-time segmentation of suspicious breast masses using convolutional neural network. PLoS One. 2018;**13**(5):e0195816

[99] Zhang Y, Ying MT, Yang L, Ahuja AT, Chen DZ. Coarse-to-fine stacked fully convolutional nets for lymph node segmentation in ultrasound images. In: 2016 Institute of Electrical and Electronics Engineers International Conference on Bioinformatics and Biomedicine (BIBM). IEEE; 2016. pp. 443-448

[100] Sun S et al. Deep learning prediction of axillary lymph node status using ultrasound images. Computers in Biology and Medicine. 2022;**143**:105250

[101] Jain PK, Sharma N, Giannopoulos AA, Saba L, Nicolaides A, Suri JS. Hybrid deep learning segmentation models for atherosclerotic plaque in internal carotid artery b-mode ultrasound. Computers in Biology and Medicine. 2021;**136**:104721

[102] Jain PK et al. Unseen artificial intelligence—Deep learning paradigm for segmentation of low atherosclerotic plaque in carotid ultrasound: A multicenter cardiovascular study. Diagnostics. 2021;**11**(12):2257

[103] Feldman AT, Wolfe D. Tissue processing and hematoxylin and eosin staining. Methods Mol Biol. 2014;**1180**: 31-43. DOI: 10.1007/978-1-4939-1050-2_3. PMID: 25015141

[104] Jain RK et al. Atypical ductal hyperplasia: Interobserver and intraobserver variability. Modern Pathology. 2011;**24**(7):917-923

[105] Araújo T et al. Classification of breast cancer histology images using convolutional neural networks. PLoS One. 2017;**12**(6):e0177544

[106] Jiang Y, Chen L, Zhang H, Xiao X. Breast cancer histopathological image

classification using convolutional neural networks with small se-resnet module. PLoS One. 2019;**14**(3):e0214587

[107] Ragab M, Albukhari A, Alyami J, Mansour RF. Ensemble deep-learning-enabled clinical decision support system for breast cancer diagnosis and classification on ultrasound images. Biology. 2022;**11**(3):439

[108] Balaha HM, Saif M, Tamer A, Abdelhay EH. Hybrid deep learning and genetic algorithms approach (hmb-dlgaha) for the early ultrasound diagnoses of breast cancer. Neural Computing and Applications. 2022; **34**(11):8671-8695

[109] Teramoto A, Tsukamoto T, Kiriyama Y, Fujita H. Automated Classification of Lung Cancer Types from Cytological Images Using Deep Convolutional Neural Networks. BioMed Research International. 2017:4067832. DOI: 10.1155/2017/4067832

[110] Wang S et al. Comprehensive analysis of lung cancer pathology images to discover tumor shape and boundary features that predict survival outcome. Scientific Reports. 2018;**8**(1): 1-9

[111] Chen Y et al. A whole-slide image (wsi)-based immunohistochemical feature prediction system improves the subtyping of lung cancer. Lung Cancer. 2022;**165**:18-27

[112] Korbar B et al. Deep learning for classification of colorectal polyps on whole-slide images. Journal of Pathology Informatics. 2017;**8**(1):30

[113] Kather JN et al. Deep learning can predict microsatellite instability directly from histology in gastrointestinal cancer. Nature Medicine. 2019;**25**(7):1054-1056

[114] Song JH, Hong Y, Kim ER, Kim S-H, Sohn I. Utility of artificial intelligence with deep learning of hematoxylin and eosin-stained whole slide images to predict lymph node metastasis in t1 colorectal cancer using endoscopically resected specimens; prediction of lymph node metastasis in t1 colorectal cancer. Journal of Gastroenterology. 2022;**57**(9):654-666

[115] Soldatov SA, Pashkov DM, Guda SA, Karnaukhov NS, Guda AA, Soldatov AV. Deep learning classification of colorectal lesions based on whole slide images. Algorithms. 2022;**15**(11):398

[116] Wang S et al. Rmdl: Recalibrated multi-instance deep learning for whole slide gastric image classification. Medical Image Analysis. 2019;**58**:101549

[117] Sharma H, Zerbe N, Klempert I, Hellwich O, Hufnagl P. Deep convolutional neural networks for automatic classification of gastric carcinoma using whole slide images in digital histopathology. Computerized Medical Imaging and Graphics. 2017;**61**:2-13

[118] Schaumberg AJ, Rubin MA, Fuchs TJ. H&e-stained whole slide image deep learning predicts spop mutation state in prostate cancer. BioRxiv. 2018:064279

[119] Singhal N et al. A deep learning system for prostate cancer diagnosis and grading in whole slide images of core needle biopsies. Scientific Reports. 2022; **12**(1):1-11

[120] Guan Q et al. Deep convolutional neural network vgg-16 model for differential diagnosing of papillary thyroid carcinomas in cytological images: A pilot study. Journal of Cancer. 2019;**10**(20):4876

[121] Wang Y et al. Using deep convolutional neural networks for multi-

classification of thyroid tumor by histopathology: A large-scale pilot study. Annals of Translational Medicine. 2019;7 (18):468-468

[122] Yi Z et al. Deep learning identified pathological abnormalities predictive of graft loss in kidney transplant biopsies. Kidney International. 2022;**101**(2): 288-298

[123] Hermsen M et al. Convolutional neural networks for the evaluation of chronic and inflammatory lesions in kidney transplant biopsies. The American Journal of Pathology. 2022;**192**(10): 1418-1432

[124] Lipkova J et al. Deep learning-enabled assessment of cardiac allograft rejection from endomyocardial biopsies. Nature Medicine. 2022;**28**(3): 575-582

[125] Born J et al. On the role of artificial intelligence in medical imaging of covid-19. Patterns. 2021;**2**(6):100269

[126] Born J et al. Pocovid-net: Automatic detection of covid-19 from a new lung ultrasound imaging dataset (pocus). arXiv preprint arXiv:2004.12084. 2020

[127] Born J et al. Accelerating detection of lung pathologies with explainable ultrasound image analysis. Applied Sciences. 2021;**11**(2):672

[128] Wang J et al. Review of machine learning in lung ultrasound in covid-19 pandemic. Journal of Imaging. 2022; **8**(3):65

[129] Zhao L, Lediju Bell MA. A review of deep learning applications in lung ultrasound imaging of covid-19 patients. BME Frontiers. 2022;**2022**

[130] Hemati S. Learning Compact Representations for Efficient Whole Slide Image Search in Computational Pathology. UWSpace. 2022. Available from: http://hdl.handle.net/10012/18637

[131] Astromskė K, Peičius E, Astromskis P. Ethical and legal challenges of informed consent applying artificial intelligence in medical diagnostic consultations. AI & Society. 2021;**36**(2):509-520

[132] Campanella G et al. Clinical-grade computational pathology using weakly supervised deep learning on whole slide images. Nature Medicine. 2019;**25**(8): 1301-1309

[133] Janowczyk A, Basavanhally A, Madabhushi A. Stain normalization using sparse autoencoders (stanosa): Application to digital pathology. Computerized Medical Imaging and Graphics. 2017;**57**:50-61

[134] Tellez D, Litjens G, van der Laak J, Ciompi F. Neural image compression for gigapixel histopathology image analysis. IEEE Transactions on Pattern Analysis and Machine Intelligence. 2019;**43**(2): 567-578

[135] Sun J, Yao X, Wang S, Wu Y. Blockchain-based secure storage and access scheme for electronic medical records in ipfs. IEEE Access. 2020;**8**: 59389-59401

[136] Kumar S, Bharti AK, Amin R. Decentralized secure storage of medical records using blockchain and ipfs: A comparative analysis with future directions. Security and Privacy. 2021; **4**(5):e162

[137] Cossio M. Ethereum, Ipfs and Neural Compression to Decentralize and Protect Patient Data in Computational Pathology. Camrbigde Open Engage. 2022. Preprint

Chapter 14

Developing and Deploying a Sepsis Deterioration Machine Learning Algorithm

Rohith Mohan, Alexandra King, Sarma Velamuri and Andrew Hudson

Abstract

A sepsis deterioration index is a numerical value predicting the chance of a patient become septic by a predictive model. This model usually has pre-specified input variables that have a high likelihood of predicting the output variable of sepsis. For the purposes of predicting sepsis deterioration, we will primarily be using regression to determine the association between variables (also known as features) to eventually predict an outcome variable which in this case is sepsis. Among the cohort examined in our model at Cedars Sinai, we found patients who met or exceeded the set threshold of 68.8 had an 87% probability of deterioration to sepsis during their hospitalization with sensitivity of 39% and a median lead time of 24 hours from when the threshold was first exceeded. There is no easy way to determine an intervention point of the deterioration predictive model. The author's recommendation is to continually modify this inflection point guided by data from near-misses and mis-categorized patients. Collecting real-time feedback from end-users on alert accuracy is also crucial for a model to survive. An ML deterioration model to predict sepsis produces ample value in a healthcare organization if deployed in conjunction with human intervention and continuous prospective re-assessment.

Keywords: sepsis, deterioration, ML, AI in medicine, deterioration index, algorithm deployment

1. Introduction to sepsis

1.1 Defining sepsis

Sepsis is the body's exaggerated response to an infection where a cascade of inflammation can potentially lead to multiorgan failure or death [1]. It is a condition that could impact patients across the healthcare continuum whether they are well-appearing neonates or geriatric patients with an abundance of medical problems. It is pervasive in its ability to affect nearly every organ system requiring comprehensive multi-specialty care. Healthcare providers have been grappling with treatment of sepsis for as long as medicine has been practiced. As a field, we have made great strides in the ability to identify and treat sepsis, but it still kills nearly 270,000 people annually in the United States. We have a variety of therapeutics to treat the source of infection but one area that remains elusive is the ability to predict sepsis prior to onset.

1.2 Financial burden of sepsis

"Septicemia" is the most common diagnosis treated in US hospitals, having surpassed osteoarthritis in 2011. The number of aggregate sepsis-related hospitalizations has grown exponentially, with the numbers of additional hospitalizations having tripled when comparing 1997–2011 averaging 48,650 hospitalizations/year to 2011–2018 averaging 160,700 hospitalizations/year [2]. In 2018, the US spent more than $41.5 billion on hospital care for patients with sepsis, accounting for a disproportionate amount of total hospital costs (10.3%). Of the top 10 most common diagnoses, it ranks as the second most costly, averaging $18,700/stay, after acute myocardial infarction [2]. Hospitalizations with sepsis as the principal diagnosis also claim the highest 30-day re-admission rate with 8.3% patients getting re-admitted, and the highest average readmission costs at $19,800 per re-admission [2].

2. Current sepsis evaluation and scoring

In the landmark Sepsis-1 paper, the authors stressed the importance of having a specific definition for sepsis to identify where along the sepsis continuum a patient presents [3]. Since the formalized definitions of SIRS and sepsis were published in 1991, a multitude of different scoring systems have been proposed, tested, and validated to predict deterioration and/or risk of mortality. Each system offers a distinct group of variables with weighted sums or point systems attempting to optimally determine which patients are at the highest risk of deterioration.

Variables used as criteria for scoring have transformed with the evolution of sepsis' definition. The pivot in sepsis' definition from SIRS with concomitant infection to focusing more on the spectrum of end-organ dysfunction resulted in an increased reliance on laboratory values in diagnosis of sepsis. Inclusion or exclusion of each variable in a scoring system was the result of iterative assessments of the variable's ability to predict the risk of an adverse outcome (deterioration and/or death) and its sensitivity in allowing for timely intervention (**Figure 1**).

2.1 Systemic inflammatory response syndrome (SIRS)

The presence of SIRS is defined by derangements in temperature, ventilation, increased heart rate, or leukocytes—all markers of systemic inflammation. The authors of Sepsis-1 specified that SIRS was more for the recognition of sepsis rather than a tool for grading severity of sepsis. Despite this, studies have validated SIRS to have prognostic value. Higher SIRS scores correlate with more rapid progression to sepsis and are positively correlated with mortality rates [4, 5]. Higher SIRS scores also showed stepwise increases in mortality as sepsis severity increased comparing patients with SIRS, sepsis, severe sepsis, and septic shock [4]. However, SIRS scores

	Year published	Scoring System	Location	Population	Intended Use	Age	HR	RR	temp	BP	O2 Sat/supp O2/FiO2	Mental Status	Med History/exam	CBC/diff	BMP	LFTs	Urine Output	ABG	other late variables
adults	1985	Acute physiology and chronic health evaluation (APACHE II)	ICU	all	prognosis/mortality	✓	✓	✓	✓	✓		✓	✓	✓	✓		○	✓	
adults	1992	Systemic inflammatory response syndrome (SIRS)	non-ICU	sepsis	diagnosis of sepsis		✓	○	✓					✓				○	
adults	1993	Simplified Acute Physiology Score (SAPS II)	ICU	all	prognosis/mortality		✓		✓	✓	✓	✓			✓	✓	✓	✓	
adults	1994	sequential organ failure assessment (SOFA)	ICU	all	describe/evaluate for organ dysfunction					✓	✓	✓		✓	○	✓	○	○	
adults	1997	Modified Early Warning Score (MEWS)	Inpatient	all	deterioration		✓	✓	✓	✓		✓					✓		
adults	2006	Standardized Early Warning Score (SEWS)	Inpatient	all	deterioration	✓	✓	✓	✓	✓	✓								
adults	2012	National Early Warning Score (NEWS)	Inpatient	all	deterioration		✓	✓	✓	✓	✓	✓							
adults	2016	quick sequential organ failure assessment (qSOFA)	non-ICU	sepsis	prognosis/mortality			✓		✓		✓							
pediatrics	1992	Systemic inflammatory response syndrome (SIRS)	non-ICU	sepsis	diagnosis of sepsis		✓	○	✓					✓				○	
pediatrics	2011	bedside pediatric early warning system (PEWS)	non-ICU	all	deterioration		✓	✓		✓	✓		✓						
pediatrics	2013	pediatric index of mortality (PIMS III)	ICU	all	prognosis/mortality					✓	✓			✓	✓			✓	✓
pediatrics	2013	pediatric logistic organ dysfunction (PELOD-2)	ICU		prognosis/mortality						✓	✓	✓	✓	✓			✓	✓
pediatrics	2017	pediatric sequential organ failure assessment (pSOFA)	ICU	all	prognosis/mortality						✓	✓		✓	✓	✓		✓	
pediatrics	2017	pediatric sepsis score (PSS)	ICU	sepsis	prognosis/mortality					✓	✓		✓					✓	✓

adapted from: Usman, Omar et al, Amer J of Emerg Med, 2019.

✓ required
○ optional/alternative
■ not available at triage

increasing clinical time →

Figure 1.
Included variables in sepsis scoring systems.

were found to be overly sensitive and poorly specific in predicting mortality leading to overdiagnosis and treatment of sepsis.

2.2 Sequential organ failure assessment (SOFA)

Recognizing sepsis' dependence on SIRS and its inherent limitations in characterizing end-organ damage, Sepsis-3 re-defined sepsis as a "life threatening organ dysfunction caused by a dysregulated host response to infection" and endorsed the sequential organ failure assessment (SOFA) score as a scoring system for mortality [6]. SOFA's summative score of multiple organ systems reflects PaO2/FiO2 (respiratory), platelet count (coagulation), bilirubin (liver), hypotension (cardiovascular), Glasgow coma score (GCS-neurologic), and creatinine or urine output (renal). The creators of SOFA aimed to keep it simple to allow for repeated assessments over time. The worst daily value is used to trend the risk of mortality in patients who are admitted to the intensive care unit. SOFA only uses variables that are obtained routinely and implemented a scoring system from zero to four to stratify a patient's risk rather than using binary categorization.

Key limitations to SOFA include its simplicity in characterizing only six organ systems as detailed above. It is unclear if bilirubin is the best biomarker for the hepatic system given hyperbilirubinemia takes days to manifest and is also the most frequently missing variable if the lab is not ordered [7]. GCS as a measure of neurologic function is at risk of being uninterpretable in hospitalized patients, a patient population in whom sedatives are frequently used.

2.3 Early warning systems (EWS): modified EWS (MEWS) and national early warning score (NEWS)

Compared with mortality risk scores, early warning systems (EWS) monitor a patient's vital signs at shorter intervals and screen for early indications of clinical decline. The first EWS described was the modified Early Warning Score (MEWS) in 1997 and it was the first to gain wide acceptance in the United States. MEWS was later modified and then adopted as the United Kingdom's National Early Warning Score (NEWS). There are over 100 EWS but we will only discuss two here [8]. **Figure 2** compares several well-known scoring systems.

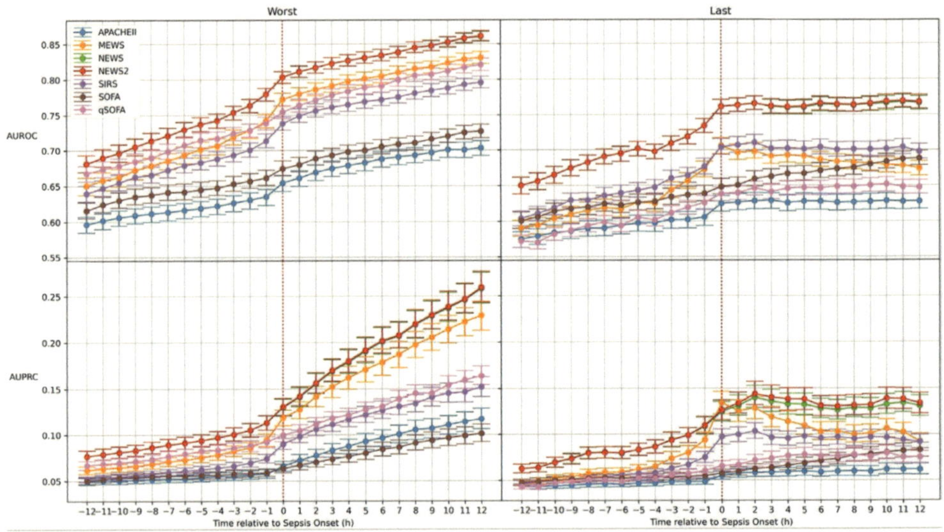

Figure 2.
Early warning score performance for sepsis discrimination.

2.4 Modified early warning score (MEWS)

The modified early warning score (MEWS) evaluates temperature, pulse, respiratory rate, systolic blood pressure, and level of consciousness by the AVPU score (Alert, Reacting to Voice, Reacting to Pain, or Unresponsive). Each parameter is assigned a score from zero to three based on the degree of abnormality and then parameters are aggregated as a MEWS score. Different scoring thresholds trigger pre-determined interventions. For example, a score of 3 may recommend increasing frequency of patient assessment to every 8 hours. MEWS has been validated for use in all hospitalized patients with its parameters easily attainable at bedside allowing for generalized use [9]. MEWS at a cut-point of 4 demonstrated higher sensitivity when utilized with a clinician's input compared with using MEWS with a cutoff score of 4 alone (56.6% vs. 72.4%) [10]. This highlights the need for clinical context when utilizing a deterioration score for decision-making.

2.5 National early warning score (NEWS)

The national early warning score (NEWS) was adapted from MEWS and encompasses all the same variables – temperature, pulse, respiratory rate, systolic blood pressure, AVPU score—while adding oxygen saturation, shown to be a strong independent predictor of mortality [11] and considers the need for respiratory support. It has been validated for use in all admitted patients for predicting deterioration, escalation of care, or death within 24 hours. When compared with thirty-three other EWS, NEWS, based on AUROC (Area Under Receiver Operator Curve), outperformed the others in predicting adverse events and in predicting sepsis prior to onset. The thirty-three EWS compared to NEWS all included the following common variables: heart rate, respiratory rate, systolic blood pressure, temperature, AVPU score for consciousness, oxygen saturation, urine output and age. Each had specific weighted scores and thresholds assigned for triggering specific response [12].

2.6 Key variables

Urine Output: The three EWS that shared the same variables as NEWS that incorporated urine output into their score had minor increases in AUROC, particularly for predicting mortality within 24 hours, but not for clinical deterioration [13–15]. Oliguria and anuria are signs of organ dysfunction and are therefore logically associated with predicting pending mortality.

Age: Age showed statistical significance in predicting the following adverse outcomes:, ICU (Intensive Care Unit) admission, attendance of the cardiac arrest team at a cardiorespiratory emergency, or death at 60 days with a small increase in AUROC from 0.67 to 0.72 [9]. This contradicts a subsequent study that compared multiple EWS and revealed that only the EWS that included age as co-variable did not outperform those excluding age in predicting deterioration [16].

2.7 Pediatric early warning score (PEWS)

Although sepsis is less common in the pediatric population compared with adults, it is more challenging to detect because symptoms like fever and tachycardia, heralding signs in adults, frequently accompany mild illness in pediatric patients. Thus, the ability to detect and differentiate patients at risk for deterioration is even more crucial.

The bedside pediatric early warning score (PEWS) includes seven variables determined by expert consensus: heart rate (HR), capillary refill time (CRT), respiratory rate (RR), respiratory effort, systolic blood pressure (sBP), transcutaneous oxygen saturation, and oxygen therapy [17]. Each variable's ability to discriminate between control and case patients was assessed by logistic regression. HR, RR, respiratory effort, and oxygen therapy had AUROC > 0.75 while CRT, oxygen saturation, sBP, and temperature had intermediate AUROC scores between 0.65 and 0.74 [17]. Temperature was ultimately excluded as a variable due to little added value. Bedside PEWS' AUCROC was 0.91 with a sensitivity of 82% and specificity 93% at a threshold score of eight [17]. Bedside PEWS is sensitive in detecting deterioration with scores increasing 24 hours prior to urgent escalation of care and can identify patients at risk within at least 1 hour's notice of sepsis [18].

2.8 Sepsis deterioration index

A sepsis deterioration index is a numerical value predicting the chance of a patient becoming septic by a predictive model. This model usually has pre-specified input variables that have a high likelihood of predicting the output variable of sepsis. With the proliferation of healthcare data in the last two decades due to the mandated use of electronic health records, we are now approaching an era where there is enough data to train machine learning models to predict sepsis. The electronic health record (EHR) system Epic is estimated to have approximately 30,000 data points per patient [19]. While large volumes of data are now becoming available, the data must be formatted in a way that can be processed by machine learning models. Healthcare data within EHR repositories tends to be heterogenous and require extensive cleansing before becoming usable for this purpose. Clinical data is rarely standardized and is entered into the EHR without the intention of being utilized for back-end data analysis. Prior studies of de-identified Epic-derived data have characterized these issues and encouraged standardized data entry by clinical staff on the front-end [20].

This is a lofty goal which may be attained at some point in the future. For now, data can be entered into machine learning models through feature extraction followed by creative cleansing and wrangling methods to be discussed. We will first describe in detail the derivation of our institution's sepsis deterioration index. Afterwards we will discuss how our model was trained and compare it to existing models.

3. Methodology: creating a sepsis deterioration machine learning model

The dataset to create our Cedars- Sinai Deterioration Index (CS-DI) consisted of 1521 hospital admitted patients from June 1st, 2021– September 1st, 2021, and is a representation of a standard medical/surgical unit patient population, containing 157,845 encounters. We used 70% (110,492) encounters for training, and 30% (47,353) encounters for testing. The average age of patients in the dataset is 63.22 years. 95,844 of patients identified as male, 61,203 of patients identified as female, and 798 of patients identified as other. 89,517 patients identified as Caucasian, 13,430 patients identified as Asian, 23,568 patients identified as Black or African American, 401 patients identified as American Indian or Alaska Native, and 29,624 patients identified as Other/Unknown. The dataset includes lab results, nursing assessments, vital signs, and a predictor for an event, which is a binary indicator for an escalation of care, classified as a transfer to an Intensive Care Unit (ICU), Respiratory or Cardiac Arrest (Code Blue), or Death (Mortality).

3.1 Key variables for the CS-DI

In our model, the CS-DI, our patient cohort was extracted based on meeting the following inclusion criteria:

1. Inpatient Hospital Admission

2. Inpatient Admission Date between 6/1/2021-9/1/2021

3. Hospital Problem List ICD-10 Diagnosis including the following:

A41.2 Sepsis due to unspecified staphylococcus.

A41.51 Sepsis due to *Escherichia coli* [*E. coli*].

A41.52 Sepsis due to Pseudomonas.

A41.59 Other Gram-negative sepsis.

A41.81 Sepsis due to Enterococcus.

A41.9 Sepsis, unspecified organism.

R65.10 SIRS of noninfectious origin w/o acute organ dysfunction.

R65.11 SIRS of non-infectious origin w acute organ dysfunction.

R65.20 Severe sepsis without septic shock.

R65.21 Severe sepsis with septic shock.

Based on these inclusion criteria, our annual patient cohort ranged from approximately from 4462 to 5729 patients per year. The following variables were extracted from our database to be used as features in the CS-DI:

3.2 Demographics

- Patient MRN/Patient ID
- Age

3.3 Admission encounters—Diagnosis, ICU LOS

- Discharge Diagnosis
- Admission Source
- Discharge Disposition
- LOS
- ICU LOS
- 30 day readmission (Y/N)

3.4 Clinical variables

- Respiratory Rate (breaths per minute)
- Oxygen Saturation SpO2 (%)
- Temperature (F)
- Systolic Blood Pressure (mmHg)
- Heart Rate/Pulse Rate (bpm)
- Partial Pressure Co2 (mmHg)
- PaO2
- Urine Output
- Consciousness Level/Mental Status
- A,V,P,U Scale

- White Blood Cells (mm^3)
- Bands (%)
- Bilirubin (Liver Function)
- Platelet Count (Coagulation Function)
- Serum Creatinine (Renal Function)

3.5 Data wrangling

There are numerous EHR systems within the United States but to train a machine learning model with reasonable predictive power, it requires a large enough volume of data and a wide variety of features. Epic is one of the largest EHR systems in the United States and had the most data available from its back-end Caboodle warehouse making it an ideal choice as the data source for our model. Our model was developed at Cedars Sinai which uses Epic as its EHR. Our data was trained with patient data from Cedars Sinai, but our methodologies could be used by other health systems using Epic-derived data if features are defined in a similar fashion to our methodology.

Most machine learning algorithms require data to be converted into numerical values before entry into the model. Clinical data, particularly for lab values, can be extremely noisy with values documented in non-standardized formats in flowsheets. For example, when reporting the results of white blood cell counts in a urine sample, the data could be reported as 0, 1+, 2+, 3+, 4+ or none, or as some, few, many white blood cells with variations in how the text is entered by each technician. A data analyst must go through each data element entered in the algorithm and use code to replace text data or strings into numerical values. This is a painstaking process requiring meticulous data review. Afterwards, a clinician, preferably a clinical informaticist should comb through the data to identify outliers or mis-entered data that would not fit in the dataset with an understanding of the data from a clinical perspective.

Once individual data elements have been cleansed, data elements from different tables will be converted to a format allowing tables to be joined. When extracted from the Epic Caboodle Data Warehouse, data is often stored in rows for each encounter. To merge with data from another table such as vital signs, each lab value needs to be converted to a column for interpretation by the machine learning model. We utilize a pivot function to reformat this data from rows into columns using the common identifiers of medical record number, encounter identifier, measurement value, measurement time, and measurement unit. We then used a merge function to combine data elements from different tables to create a usable dataset. Please refer to the following link for details on our code:

https://github.com/rohith-mohan/caboodledatacleanse/commit/7d17c05fc3eeb043d22cb97e454701d2fbe81075

4. Choice of machine learning (ML) model

In the realm of data science, the choice of the appropriate machine learning model is critical in gaining the most information out of the data extracted while also being mindful of the computing resources needed to run the model (**Figure 3**).

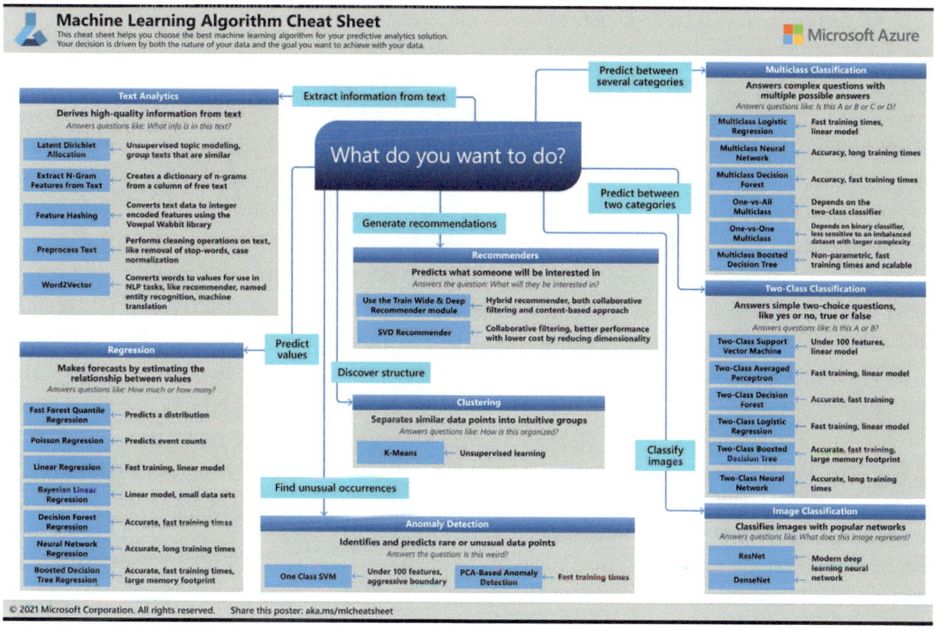

Figure 3.
Rationale for selecting a machine learning algorithm.

For the purposes of predicting sepsis deterioration, we will primarily be using regression to determine the association between variables (also known as features) to eventually predict an outcome variable of sepsis. As seen in our section above regarding validated sepsis scoring methodologies, all of our features are numerical making regression a reasonable choice for our model. The mathematics behind most forms of regression are complex but we will go through the basic premise of a few common types of regression.

- Linear regression is the simplest form of regression which most people are familiar with. It simply uses a set of dependent variables with coefficients that dictate the strength of association with an independent variable (y = mx + b).

- Bayesian linear regression is useful for small datasets since its features are based on a weighted sum of other variables to reduce dependence on the output a single point of data [21].

- Decision forest regression use a set of binary decision branch points to eventually reach a decision node. This is a very popular choice of model given its efficiency in use of computing power, accuracy even when presented with heterogenous data, and speed to train [22].

- Neural network regression determines the relationship between features and output variables through use of "neurons" in "layers" that associate weights to features in the model. They can be used for structured and unstructured data to create highly accurate models but are slow to train and require high amounts of computational power [23].

4.1 Epic deterioration index (EDI)

The epic deterioration index (EDI) is a proprietary prediction model implemented in over 100 U.S. hospitals to support clinical-decision support in diagnosis of sepsis [24]. The EDI aims to detect patients who are deteriorate and require higher levels of care. Its score ranges from 0 to 100, in which the higher numbers denote a greater risk of experiencing a composite adverse outcome of requiring rapid response, resuscitation, ICU-level care, or death in the next 12–38 hours. The EDI uses a cumulative link model, a specific type of ordinal logistic regression model, that uses two parallel linear combinations of clinical inputs drawing two decision boundaries in the space of prediction using proportional odds assumptions. The details of the implementation are proprietary, and Epic has not shared this information publicly or described it in their published literature, but the accuracy of this model is 47.4% [24].

4.2 Cedars Sinai deterioration index (CS-DI)

After evaluating the accuracy of the EDI model, and other early warning systems, a decision was made at our organization to create a Cedars-Sinai deterioration index (CS-DI) machine learning algorithm that uses data from the patient's electronic medical record and calculates a percentage value that predicts the likelihood of a patient deterioration with an escalation of care. The predefined intervention point would automatically be activated if the calculated deterioration percentage value is reached and generate an alert notifying care providers to intervene sooner and possibly prevent further deterioration. Once trained, the CS-DI was deployed as a clinical decision support application to identify patients at risk for sepsis in real-time. Seventy percent of the cohort was used as the training set for the model while the other 30% was used as the test set. We used the CS-DI percentage value calculated to predict a composite outcome of further deterioration, intensive care unit-level care, mechanical ventilation, or hospital death.

Among the cohort examined, we found patients who met or exceeded the set threshold of 68.8 had an 87% probability of a composite outcome during their hospitalization with sensitivity of 39% and a median lead time of 24 hours from when the threshold was first exceeded. Among the patients hospitalized for at least 48 hours who had not experienced a composite outcome, 13% never exceeded 37.9 with a negative predictive value of 90% and a sensitivity above the threshold of 92%. When run against the MEWS early warning system, NEWS early warning system, and the EDI, the CS-DI predicted deterioration on average a full hour ahead of the other deterioration index models.

4.3 Unstructured data in ML models

Recent studies have shown that incorporating non-numerical data including key words from clinical documentation and diagnostic imaging can increase the accuracy of models [25]. This data is first converted to a format usable by machine learning algorithms via natural language processing (NLP). NLP uses sophisticated methods of text analytics to convert text into numerical data usable by an algorithm [26]. Goh et al. use a method of text analytics known as latent Direchlet allocation to group texts that are similar into topics. They identified 100 common text topics that were grouped into one of the following seven categories: (1) clinical status, (2) communication, (3) laboratory tests, (4) non-clinical status, (5) social relationships, (6) symptom, and (7) treatment. The numerical values derived from this text data were combined with structured numerical data like those used in the numerical regression models such as patient demographics, vitals data and laboratory data. By adding text data into the mix, the AUC of their Sepsis early risk assessment (SERA) model was as high as 0.87 with a lead time of 48 hours before the onset of sepsis.

Unstructured data in these models increases the accuracy and lead time as expected. Healthcare professionals rely on a multitude of unstructured data including all the data above and a physical assessment of the patient. The more of these features we can incorporate into models, the more accurate they can become. Humans cannot be omniscient to continuously monitor all the data they are presented and make real-time assessments on every patient in the hospital. If we can train a machine to think like an astute healthcare professional with the processing power of a supercomputer, we can ideally reduce the incidence of sepsis in our healthcare systems before it occurs.

5. Deployment of the CS-DI model

5.1 Prospective scaling of CS-DI

Our model has been used utilized prospectively to determine the risk of patients deteriorating into sepsis. The data was extracted from the Epic Caboodle Data Warehouse and pushed every 15 minutes to an S3 datastore and then to an Amazon Redshift Cloud Data Warehouse. The code to cleanse the data and run the features through our model was stored on docker containers to allow the data to be analyzed prospectively and at scale. The algorithm would calculate a percentage value from 0 to 100% and visually display a near-real time swim lane on an intuitive user interface in our command center. If patients neared a predefined intervention point, a protocol for escalation by the triaging Rapid Response Team (RRT) was initiated.

A crucial step in realizing the potential of ML algorithms is to work closely with the facility's IT department to integrate them into the clinical workflow while minimizing alert-fatigue. Ultimately, the successful integration of ML algorithms should aim to enhance the productivity of clinical teams while avoiding any attempt to replace them entirely.

5.2 Institutional considerations for deployment of sepsis model at cedars-sinai

The deployment of sepsis AI alerting systems can be categorized into two approaches - passive and active, each with distinct staffing models. The passive approach involves a central hub of trained personnel monitoring sepsis alerts at one location such as a command center.

Despite claims of successful implementation at some institutions, this approach has huge dependency on a small group of people and is much more expensive than the second approach which we will cover shortly.

Effective staffing of this passive model requires careful consideration of the number and distribution of generated alerts. The distribution of alerts over time must also be considered. Due to the workflow of data collection that feeds the alert, the distribution of alerts may be bimodal or trimodal. Most alerts may occur during specific times of the day such as when labs are reported, vital signs are entered by nursing or during changes of shift. To adequately manage the expected volume and timing of alerts, staffing requirements should be calculated. Specifically, the team should be capable of handling 30–40 alerts within a 3-hour period, with occasional alerts occurring during off-peak times. In practice, this will likely require the hiring of an additional three full-time equivalent (FTE) nurses for the day shift and 2

FTE nurses for the night shift, with float coverage provided during weekends and vacations. The active approach or the fractal-behavior model is one in which humans work collaboratively with the AI model. In this approach each nurse is responsible for managing their own 4 or 5 patients assigned to them during the shift. There are two phases to the management of a patient based on whether they have sepsis or not.

Phase 1—When the sepsis alert is prevented from firing because the nurse has proactively screened the patient for sepsis using a standardized rule-based ML algorithm that uses a multivariate decision tree—i.e., non-linear decision making. In this case each nurse is consistently evaluating every patient at shift change, or when they first have the patient assigned to them. This method captures data before it is readily available in the EHR (e.g., patient's mental status, clinical appearance, and subjective judgment around source of infection). If a patient screens positive for infection—more action can be taken at that time to implement a diagnostic or treatment workflow.

Phase 2—When the sepsis alert fires—the bedside provider activates a workflow that allows them to perform a secondary clinical evaluation (SCE) to evaluate the alert in the context of the patient's clinical status. Frequently the decentralized active approach is criticized for failing because bedside nurses and providers fail to respond to alerts due to alert fatigue [26–28]. However, this approach only fails when the institution is relying solely on the EHR to mobilize the alert.

Hospital systems should consider adopting a user-centered design (UCD) instead of relying on traditional EHR interfaces. UCD involves the development of an interface that is tailored to clinical workflows thereby maximizing efficiency. Ruminski et al. found that displaying a visual monitor significantly reduced the rate of sepsis [27]. Furthermore, studies have shown that color coding and screen positioning in the user's visual field can improve provider satisfaction and reduce sepsis rates by over 50%. It is vital to align clinical end-users with the facility's IT department to ensure that the product meets clinical expectations while remaining compatible with the EHR.

This approach establishes a highly reliable two-step method that when repeated by hundreds of nurses daily resembles a fractal that is made of repeated behaviors. It is independent of staffing and nursing ratios, does not require additional FTE hires and is more economically feasible the cost of several million dollars a year less in staff salaries to implement than the passive model.

5.3 Model surveillance

Machine learning (ML) models for sepsis are notorious for creating alerts that are not actionable. In addition, these models' predictive performance degrades over time especially when deployed on populations not resembling their training sets. Concept drift, or the change in the underlying data distribution over time, is often not considered in the deployment of ML models. Many companies that provide sepsis ML detection systems fail to account for new data or changes in patient demographics.

For example, let us examine the following example (**Figure 4**) [28]. Models built in states with low death rates will perform poorly when being deployed in states with high death rates and vice versa due to overfitting to a particular population/dataset. Both data drift and concept drift can occur at the same time, leading to inaccurate predictions and reduced model efficacy. It is crucial to incorporate methods that can handle data drift, concept drift and population drift in the maintenance and deployment of ML models, especially in the clinical setting where predictions have an impact on patient outcomes. One solution to these issues is continuously incorporating prospective data to re-calibrate the model. In the case of the CS-DI, if the

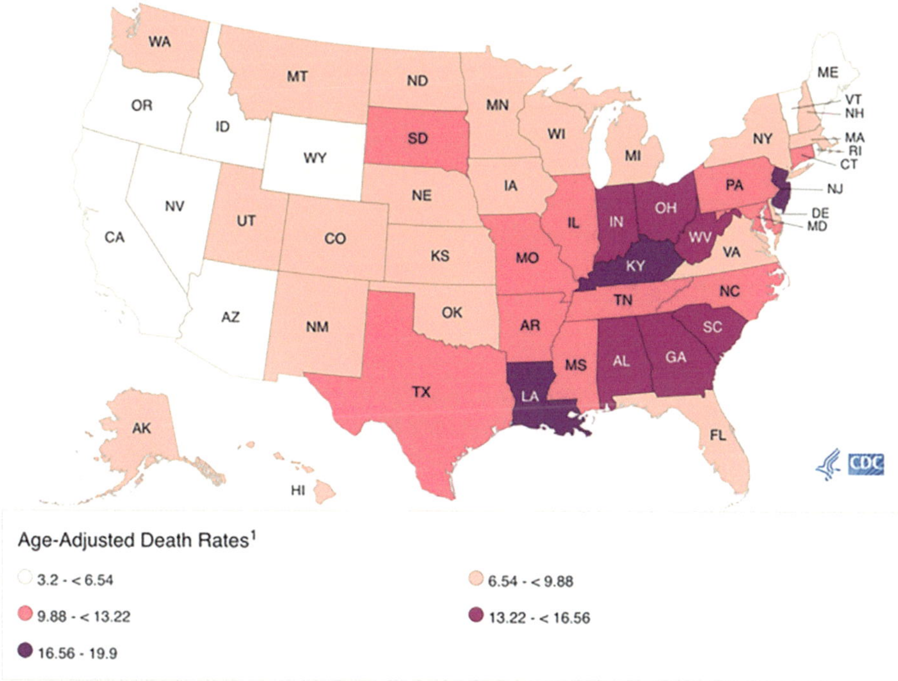

https://www.cdc.gov/nchs/pressroom/sosmap/septicemia_mortality/septicemia.htm

Figure 4.
Septicemia mortality by state.

model predicted sepsis when a patient was not septic, the model should eventually be retrained to correctly categorize that patient.

5.4 Governance of the model

Given patient safety concerns, the governance of a sepsis deterioration model falls under the jurisdiction of a medical executive committee (MEC). Additionally, hospitals now have sepsis steering sub-committees and patient safety committees in advisory roles. Patient risk—especially with respect to false negatives—should be presented and all non-treatment decisions that lead to poor patient outcomes should be examined on a quarterly basis at minimum to ensure patient safety.

Machine learning is how a computer learns to predict a particular outcome based on prior data. Artificial intelligence (AI) is the ability to take the information and translate it into an actionable insight. There remains weariness of AI and fear that it will replace human decision-making capacity. As shown in the development of the model above, AI takes human-derived knowledge but augments the ability to act on that knowledge via computing power. AI is a good servant but a terrible master—all treatment and non-treatment decisions remain with a licensed independent practitioner.

5.5 Determining an intervention point

There is no easy way to determine an intervention point based on the predictive model. The beauty of deploying an ML model based on the active method described above is that one will be able to set an intervention point on when to alert an end user (theoretically at 90% sensitivity and 90% specificity) and leave the decision to intervene with the clinical end user. The author's recommendation is to continually modify this inflection point guided by data from near-misses and mis-categorized patients. Collecting real-time feedback from end-users on alert accuracy is also crucial for a model to survive. In conclusion, an ML deterioration model to predict sepsis produces ample value in a healthcare organization if deployed in conjunction with human intervention and continuous prospective re-assessment.

6. Conclusion

Sepsis is a ubiquitous condition across healthcare continuum causing millions of deaths annually and incurring high costs on the healthcare system. We have made great strides in the ability to identify and treat sepsis, but it still kills nearly 270,000 people annually in the U.S. A sepsis deterioration index is a numerical value predicting the chance of a patient becoming septic by a predictive model. This model usually has pre-specified input variables that have a high likelihood of predicting the output variable of sepsis. For the purposes of predicting sepsis deterioration, we used regression to determine the association between variables (also known as features) to eventually predict sepsis. Among the cohort examined in our model at Cedars Sinai, we found patients who met or exceeded the set threshold of 68.8 had an 87% probability of deterioration to sepsis during their hospitalization and a median lead time of 24 hours from when the threshold was first exceeded. Another model incorporating unstructured text into their deterioration model, had an AUROC (Area Under Receiver Operator Curve) as high as 0.87 with a lead time of 48 hours before the onset of sepsis. There is no easy way to determine an intervention point of the deterioration predictive model. The author's recommendation is to continually modify this inflection point guided by data from near-misses and mis-categorized patients. Collecting real-time feedback from end-users on alert accuracy is also crucial for a model to survive. An ML deterioration model to predict sepsis produces ample value in a healthcare organization if deployed in conjunction with human intervention and continuous prospective re-assessment.

Acronyms and abbreviations

SIRS	systemic inflammatory response syndrome
SOFA	sequential organ failure assessment (formally sepsis organ failure assessment)
PaO2	partial pressure of oxygen
FiO2	fraction of inspired oxygen
GCS	Glasgow Coma Score
EWS	early warning system
MEWS	Modified Early Warning Score
HR, bpm	heart rate, beats per minute
RR	respiratory rate
sBP	systolic blood pressure
NEWS	National Early Warning Score
AVPU	alert, reacting to voice, reacting to pain, unresponsive
AUROC	area under the receiver operator curve

ICU	intensive care unit
PEWS	bedside Pediatric Early Warning Score
CRT	capillary refill time
EHR	electronic health record
CS-DI	Cedars sinai deterioration index
ICD-10	International Classification of Disease, 10th revision
ML	machine learning
EDI	epic deterioration index
NLP	natural language processing
AUC	area under the curve
SERA	sepsis early risk assessment
RRT	rapid response team
IT	information technology
AI	artificial intelligence
FTE	full-time equivalent

Author details

Rohith Mohan*, Alexandra King, Sarma Velamuri and Andrew Hudson
Cedars Sinai Medical Center, Los Angeles, CA, United States

*Address all correspondence to: rmohan1992@gmail.com

References

[1] What is Sepsis? Available from: https://www.cdc.gov/sepsis/what-is-sepsis.html

[2] Healthcare Cost and Utilization Project (HCUP) Statistical Briefs [Internet]. Rockville (MD): Agency for Healthcare Research and Quality (US); Feb 2006. Available from: https://www.ncbi.nlm.nih.gov/books/NBK52651/

[3] Bone RC, Sprung CL, Sibbald WJ. Definitions for sepsis and organ failure. Critical Care Medicine. 1992;**20**(6):724-726

[4] Rangel-Frausto MS et al. The natural history of the systemic inflammatory response syndrome (SIRS). A prospective study. JAMA. 1995;**273**(2):117-123

[5] Jones GR, Lowes JA. The systemic inflammatory response syndrome as a predictor of bacteraemia and outcome from sepsis. QJM: An International Journal of Medicine. 1996;**89**(7):515-522

[6] Singer M et al. The third international consensus definitions for sepsis and septic shock (Sepsis-3). JAMA. 2016;**315**(8):801-810

[7] Moreno R et al. The sequential organ failure assessment (SOFA) score: Has the time come for an update? Critical Care. 2023;**27**(1):15

[8] Kramer AA, Sebat F, Lissauer M. A review of early warning systems for prompt detection of patients at risk for clinical decline. Journal of Trauma and Acute Care Surgery. 2019;**87**(1S Suppl 1): S67-S73

[9] Subbe CP et al. Validation of a modified Early Warning Score in medical admissions. QJM: An International Journal of Medicine. 2001;**94**(10):521-526

[10] Fullerton JN et al. Is the Modified Early Warning Score (MEWS) superior to clinician judgement in detecting critical illness in the pre-hospital environment? Resuscitation. 2012;**83**(5):557-562

[11] Buist M, Bernard S, Anderson J. Epidemiology and prevention of unexpected in-hospital deaths. The Surgeon. 2003;**1**(5):265-268

[12] Smith MEB, Chiovaro JC, O'Neil M, et al. Early Warning System Scores: A Systematic Review [Internet]. Washington (DC): Department of Veterans Affairs (US); Jan 2014. Available from: https://www.ncbi.nlm.nih.gov/books/NBK259026/

[13] Goldhill DR, McNarry AF. Physiological abnormalities in early warning scores are related to mortality in adult inpatients. British Journal of Anaesthesia. 2004;**92**(6):882-884

[14] Barlow GD, Nathwani D, Davey PG. Standardised early warning scoring system. Clinical Medicine (London, England). 2006;**6**(4):422-423. author reply 423-4

[15] von Lilienfeld-Toal M et al. Observation-based early warning scores to detect impending critical illness predict in-hospital and overall survival in patients undergoing allogeneic stem cell transplantation. Biology of Blood and Marrow Transplantation. 2007;**13**(5):568-576

[16] Smith GB et al. The ability of the National Early Warning Score (NEWS) to discriminate patients at risk of early cardiac arrest, unanticipated intensive care unit admission, and death. Resuscitation. 2013;**84**(4):465-470

[17] Parshuram CS, Hutchison J, Middaugh K. Development and initial validation of the Bedside Paediatric Early Warning System score. Critical Care. 2009;**13**(4):R135

[18] Parshuram CS et al. Implementing the Bedside Paediatric Early Warning System in a community hospital: A prospective observational study. Paediatrics & Child Health. 2011;**16**(3):e18-e22

[19] Estabrooks PA et al. Harmonized patient-reported data elements in the electronic health record: Supporting meaningful use by primary care action on health behaviors and key psychosocial factors. Journal of the American Medical Informatics Association. 2012;**19**(4):575-582

[20] Mohan R et al. Deriving a de-identified dataset from EPIC-derived data for use in clinical research: Pearls and pitfalls in database creation and analysis. Pediatrics. 2021;**147**(3_MeetingAbstract):7-8. DOI: 10.1542/peds.147.3MA1.7

[21] Introduction to Bayesian Linear Regression. Available from: https://www.simplilearn.com/tutorials/data-science-tutorial/bayesian-linear-regression

[22] Decision Forest Regression component. Available from: https://learn.microsoft.com/en-us/azure/machine-learning/component-reference/decision-forest-regression

[23] RS. A Walk-through of Regression Analysis Using Artificial Neural Networks in Tensorflow. Available from: https://www.analyticsvidhya.com/blog/2021/08/a-walk-through-of-regression-analysis-using-artificial-neural-networks-in-tensorflow/

[24] Epicshare, <h1 data-v-6822abc2="" id="PostTitle" style="box-sizing: border-box; margin-bottom: 0.5rem; margin-top: 0px; line-height: 1.2; font-size: 2rem; scroll-margin-top: 9.75rem; color: rgb(58, 41, 46); font-family: Program, sans-serif;">Saving Lives with AI: Using the Deterioration Index Predictive Model to Help Patients Sooner. Available from: https://www.epicshare.org/share-and-learn/saving-lives-with-ai

[25] Goh KH et al. Artificial intelligence in sepsis early prediction and diagnosis using unstructured data in healthcare. Nature Communications. 2021;**12**(1):711

[26] Nadkarni PM, Ohno-Machado L, Chapman WW. Natural language processing: An introduction. Journal of the American Medical Informatics Association. 2011;**18**(5):544-551

[27] Ruminski CM et al. Impact of predictive analytics based on continuous cardiorespiratory monitoring in a surgical and trauma intensive care unit. Journal of Clinical Monitoring and Computing. 2019;**33**(4):703-711

[28] Stats of the States- Septicemia Mortality. Available from: https://www.cdc.gov/nchs/pressroom/sosmap/septicemia_mortality/septicemia.htm

Chapter 15

A New Liver Segmentation Based on Digital Liver Portal Vein Ramification Using Computer-Assisted Surgery System: Exploring Artificial Intelligence

Xianjun Zhou, Chengzhan Zhu, Bin Wei, Nan Xia, Yongjian Chen and Qian Dong

Abstract

A good understanding of liver anatomy is required for performing precise liver resection. However, the currently described methods of liver segmentation based on portal and hepatic veins are inconclusive. We proposed a system of liver segmentation based on previous reports and our data. Three-dimensional computed tomography software based on artificial intelligence was used to analyze the portal vein branching pattern in 759 patients. We analyzed four different types of liver segmentation and measured their respective segmental liver volumes. We classified four types of liver segmentation based on the right portal vein. Median segmental liver volumes were variable for the different types of segmentation. Our system of liver segmentation enables a better classification of individual patients into one of the different types, thus assisting in preoperative surgical planning. Segmental liver volume is useful for the preoperative evaluation of remnant liver volume.

Keywords: liver anatomy, portal vein, segmentation, liver volume, computer-assisted surgery

1. Introduction

An accurate understanding of liver anatomy is important for surgical safety [1]. This is particularly relevant to the progression of modern surgery toward individualized treatment and the advent of partial hepatectomy and living liver transplantation technology [2, 3]. Initial liver segmentation studies were based on the cadaver liver specimen perfusion model and were limited by the number of specimens and the research techniques available at the time [4–6]. With the development of artificial

IntechOpen

intelligence, the development of modern imaging and digital medical research enabled the analysis of dimensional anatomical relationships and spatial vascular variations by three-dimensional (3D) visualization technology from all directions in a transparent and interactive manner [1, 3, 7, 8]. This has particularly helped with the performance of *in vivo* liver segmentation and liver volume measurement [9, 10]. In recent years, several studies have used digital imaging technology for liver segmentation, although these were often confined to liver lobe variations [11–13] and did not involve systematic research. None of the existing liver segmentation methods includes all possible variations in the liver anatomy. The portal vein branches are relatively consistent in the left hepatic lobe, which is divided into segments II, III, and IV. However, none of the existing single segmentation methods describes the different variations in the right liver. We describe a new liver segmentation system based on 3D reconstruction studies of digital liver models.

We used the 3D U-Net framework. In the field of machine learning, the U-Net is a successful encoder-decoder network that has received a lot of attention in recent years. Its encoder part works similarly to a traditional classification CNN in that it successively aggregates semantic information at the expense of reduced spatial information.

2. Materials and methods

A total of 759 patients without liver disease were enrolled in this study from July 2013 to November 2017. Upper abdominal contrast-enhanced computed tomography (CT) image data were collected for all patients. Patient selection criteria were as follows: (1) no liver lesions or other diseases affecting the portal vein arrangement; (2) availability of high-quality CT imaging that clearly displayed the portal vein up to its fourth-level branch; (3) no history of liver surgery; and (4) CT layer thickness less than 1 mm. This study was approved by the research ethics committee of the affiliated hospital of Qingdao University, and written informed consent was obtained from all parents.

All included patients underwent upper abdomen contrast-enhanced CT (Discovery HD 750; GE Healthcare, Milwaukee, WI, USA and Definition Flash; Siemens Healthcare, Forchheim, Germany). The scan parameters were set as follows: nonionic contrast agent (Iopromide 350 mg I/mL; Schering Ultravist, Berlin, Germany) was injected via the forearm elbow vein or the hand vein with a double-tube high-pressure syringe (Stellant; Medrad, Indianola, PA, USA). Approximately 1.5–2.0 mL/kg body weight of contrast was injected at a rate of 1.0–3.0 mL/s. For Definition Flash CT, the tube rotation time was 0.28 s, detector collimation was 2*64*0.6 mm, and pitch was 1.0. For Discovery HD 750 CT, the tube rotation time was 0.5 s, detector collimation was 64*0.625 mm, pitch was 0.984, and noise index was 10.

2.1. Image processing and 3D reconstruction based on artificial intelligence

DICOM data of the upper abdomen CT were uploaded into the Hisense Computer Aided Surgery System (Hisense CAS, version 2.1.3; Qingdao, China) for 3D reconstruction [3–5]. The following steps were performed: liver image extraction (liver segmentation was performed automatically through the artificial intelligence automatic adjustment of the window width and window level); extraction of intrahepatic vascular system (the scope of blood vessel formation was determined through the selection of intrahepatic vascular markers, followed by automatic extraction of intrahepatic vascular information); and integration (with integration of the liver and intrahepatic vascular system, 3D reconstruction was used to display the portal vein trunk, branch arrangement, and dominated region clearly from all directions in 3D).

2.2. Segmental volume measurement

By using the surgical simulation module of Hisense CAS, watershed analysis was performed based on the portal vein arrangement, radius, and supply area. The volumes of liver segments for types A, B, and C were calculated based on the fourth-level branch of the portal vein. Type D varied greatly and the number of each variant was small.

2.3. Basic principle for Dong's liver segmentation

Based on statistical analysis, approximately 10% of cases were selected for pre-verification. Preliminary segmentation was performed and segmentation principles were proposed; these were verified by using the larger sample. The following basic principles for liver segmentation were developed based on the statistical analysis of preexperimental results obtained by the 3D reconstruction of the normal liver and vascular system of 120 humans.

a. The 3D model of the digitalized liver and vascular system was utilized to describe Dong's liver segmentation based on the portal vein branch. The area supplied by the fourth-level portal vein is often considered the basic unit for precision liver resection. Therefore, the dominant area of the fourth level portal vein was identified as the criterion for liver segmentation in Dong's liver segmentation system.

b. The caudate lobe region of the liver (segment I) has a relatively special portal vein blood supply with large variations. Following the primary portal vein branch, three to six small blood vessel branches are derived directly from the left and right main branches of the secondary portal vein to supply the caudate lobe area. Generally, five to eight short hepatic veins allow for backflow of blood. During precision liver surgery, portal vein bleeding cannot be solved by blocking a third-level or fourth-level portal vein, as performed for other liver segments.

c. We defined the caudate lobe as segment I to respect tradition and to enable easy recall. The subsequent lobes, starting from the left lobe of the liver, were numbered segments II–IX in a clockwise direction.

2.3.1 I 3D reconstruction and intrahepatic vascular system Based on Artificial Intelligence

The 3D reconstruction of the liver and intrahepatic vascular system was performed for 759 patients of different ages. The reconstructed digital liver by use of machine learning appeared to have a clear structure (**Figure 1**). The spatial distribution and variation of the portal vein were observed in rotated directions, leading to the observation of the spatial anatomical relationships of the portal vein within the liver from different angles.

2.3.2 II Dong's liver segmentation

Type A is similar to Couinaud or Cho's segmentation, with the liver containing eight segments (365 cases, 48.09%). Type B contains nine segments because of the three branches of the right-anterior portal vein (203 cases, 26.75%). Type C (76 cases, 10.01%) has two variations, type C-a, wherein the right-posterior portal vein is sector-shaped and the right-anterior portal vein is similar to that in type A, and type C-b, wherein the right-posterior portal vein is sector-shaped and the right-anterior portal vein is similar to that in type B. Type D contains special portal vein variations that need three-dimensional simulation to design individualized liver resection plans (115 cases, 15.15%).

2.3.2.1 Type A

Segment I is the caudate lobe, which is supplied by three to six small portal vein branches derived directly from the left and right main portal veins. Segments II and III are supplied by fourth-level portal vein branches derived from the superior and inferior outer aspects of the umbilical part of the left main portal branch. Segment IV is supplied by the fourth-level branch of the left portal vein.

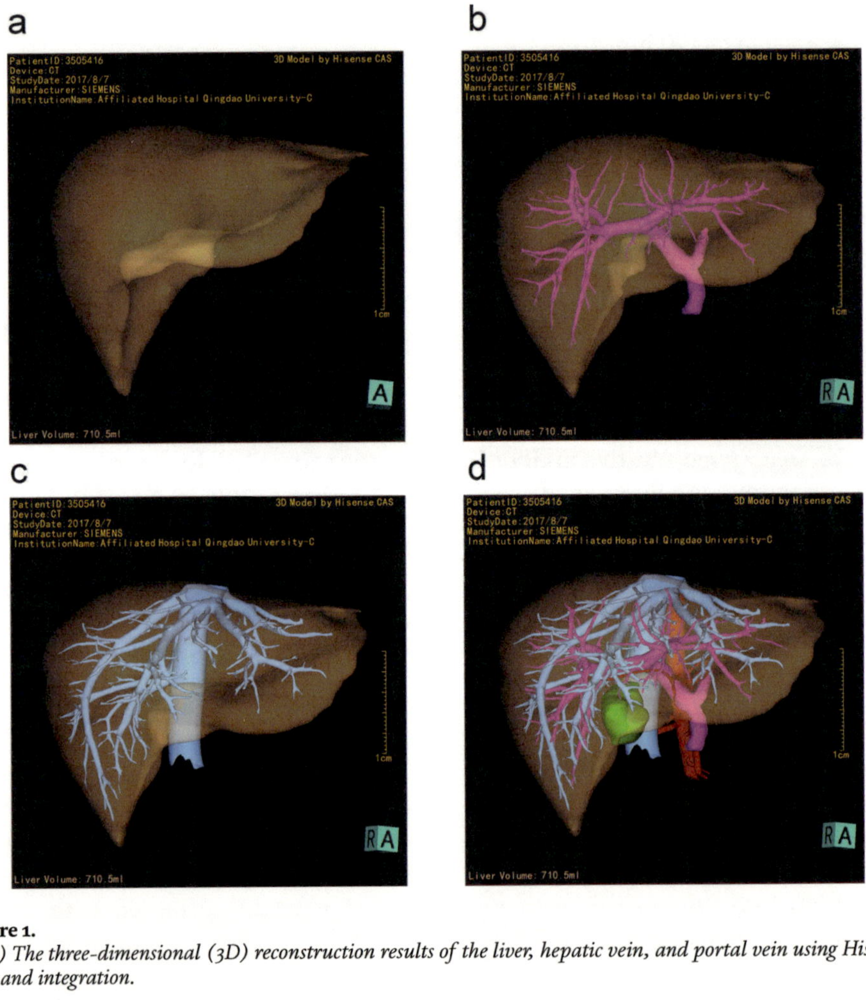

Figure 1.
(a–d) The three-dimensional (3D) reconstruction results of the liver, hepatic vein, and portal vein using Hisense CAS and integration.

The left lobe nomenclature, including segments I to IV, is similar for all four types (**Figure 2**). The right portal vein divides into the right anterior and the right posterior branches. The right anterior branch further divides into two main branches, the cephalic and caudal branches, or the ventral and dorsal branches, depending on the angle of their branching. The caudal or ventral branch supplies segment V, whereas the cephalic or dorsal branch supplies segment VIII (**Figure 3a**).

Segment VI is the area supplied by the fourth-level portal vein derived from the outer inferior aspect of the right liver following the third-level branch of the right portal vein branch. Segment VII is the area supplied by fourth-level portal vein derived from the superior outer aspect of the right liver following the third-level branch of the right portal vein branch (**Figure 3b**).

2.3.2.2 Type B

According to the portal vein branches and the dominant areas, the liver was divided into nine segments for type B. A total of 203 (26.75%) cases were type B. Segments I to IV are similar to that of type A.

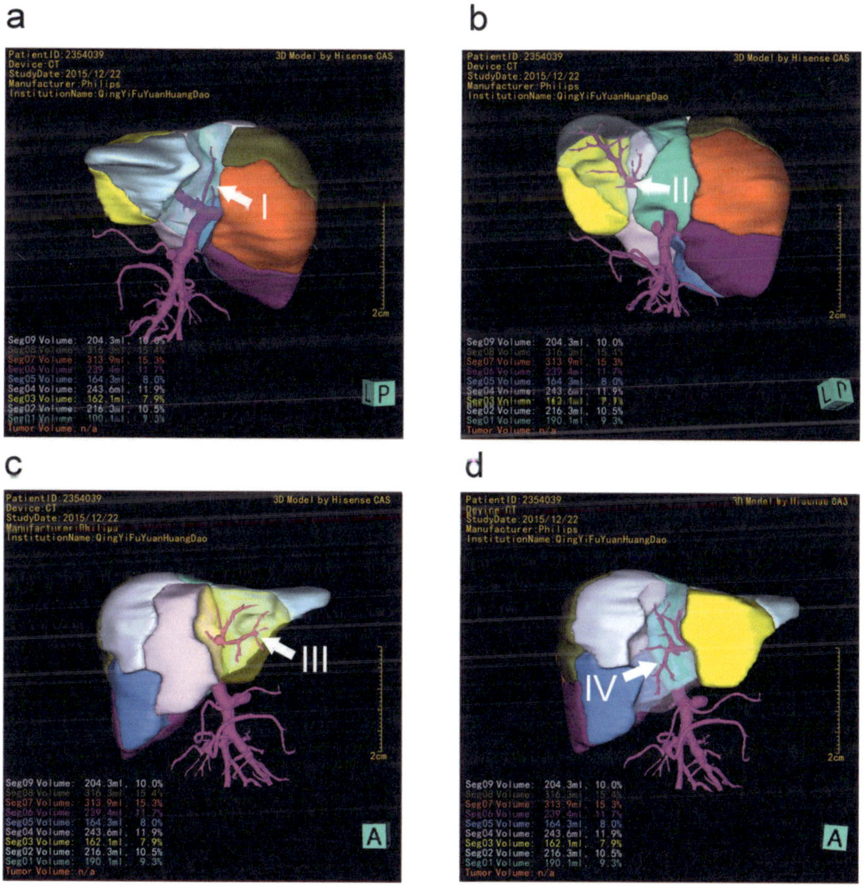

Figure 2.
(a–d) Liver segments I, II, III, and IV and their respective portal venous blood supply.

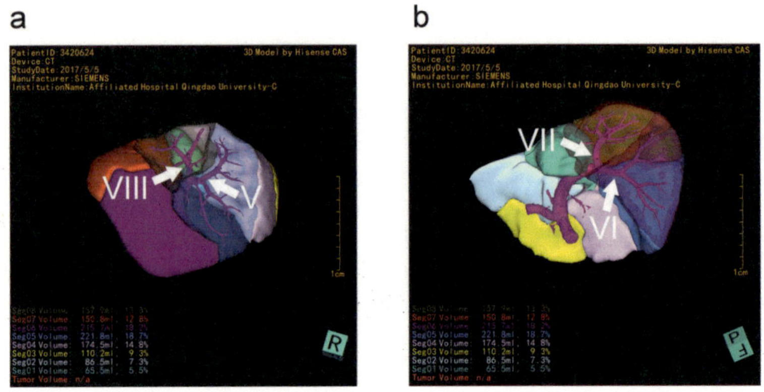

Figure 3.
(a) Branches of the right anterior portal vein and the liver segments supplied by them for type A. (b) Branches of the right posterior portal vein and the liver segments supplied by them for type A.

The right portal vein divides into the right anterior and the right posterior branches. Segments V, VIII, and IX are the areas supplied by the three main branches of the right anterior branch: the caudal (portal branches of segment V, P5), dorsal (portal branches of segment VIII, P8), and ventral branches (portal branches of segment IX, P9), respectively (**Figure 4a**). Segments VI and VII are the areas supplied by the fourth-level portal vein derived from the outer inferior and superior aspects of the right liver, respectively, of the right posterior branch (**Figure 4b**).

2.3.2.3 Type C

The right posterior area of the liver is supplied by 5–11 sector-shaped branches of the portal vein branches that are derived from an arched main vessel (**Figure 5**). It is not possible for segments VI and VII to be resected individually with precision (but is possible for types A and B). The proportion of livers with type C is small but significant from the point of view of precision liver resections. Type C has two variations, type C-a (6.59%), wherein the right-posterior portal vein is sector-shaped and the right-anterior portal vein is similar to that of type A (P8), and type C-b (3.42%),

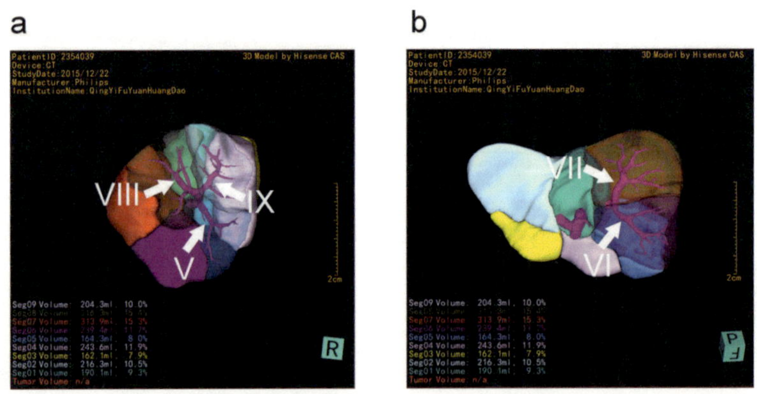

Figure 4.
(a) Branches of the right anterior portal vein and the liver segments supplied by them for type B. (b) Branches of the right posterior portal vein and the liver segments supplied by them for type B.

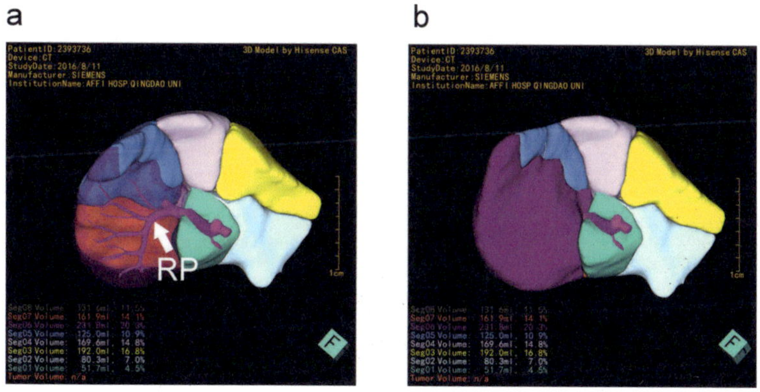

Figure 5.
The right posterior portal vein and its branches supply the segments for type C.

wherein the right-posterior portal vein is sector-shaped and the right-anterior portal vein is similar to that of type B (P8 and P9).

2.3.2.4 Type D

Type D is a special group of variants that included 115 cases (15 15%). The various portal vein configurations identified were as follows. Among the common type, the portal vein divides into right and left branches and the right anterior portal vein branch is derived from the left portal vein (74 cases, 64 35%) (**Figure 6a**). The P6 portal vein is derived from the right anterior portal vein distal to the branching of the P7 portal vein from the right portal vein (19 cases, 16 52%) (**Figure 6b**). The portal vein trunk is trifurcation at the porta hepatis; it divides into the left, right anterior, and right posterior branches (8 cases, 6 96%) (**Figure 6c**). The right anterior portal vein is derived from the saccule of the left portal vein (4 cases, 3 48%) (**Figure 6d**). Approximately four to eight branches with similar thickness are derived from the right anterior portal vein supplying the right anterior liver (**Figure 6e**). The P2 and P3 branches share a common trunk (**Figure 6f**) that leads to several branches that supply liver segments II and III. The right anterior portal vein has a trunk that divides into several sector-shaped small branches.

The different types of liver segmentations in the different sexes are shown in **Table 1**. There was no difference between the sexes in terms of the different types of liver segmentation ($\chi^2 = 2.823$, $p = 0.420$) (**Table 1**). Similarly, there was no difference between the pediatric (3 months to 15 years) and adult groups (>15 years) ($\chi^2 = 1.095$ and $p = 0.778$) (**Table 2**).

2.3.3 III Segmental volumes for types A, B, and C of Dong's liver segmentation system

The volumes of each of the liver segments of the different types are presented in **Tables 3–6**. For type A, segments V and VIII account for 15.78% (±5.12) and 16.43% (±5.18) of the total liver volume, respectively. For type B, the volumes of segments V, VIII, and IX account for 10.36% (±3.72), 11.84% (±3.28), and 12.69% (±3.70), respectively. The volume of the right-posterior (RP) segment of type C was smaller than that of segments VI and VII of type A and type B (26.379% [±5.613] and 24.447 [±5.025], $p < 0.01$).

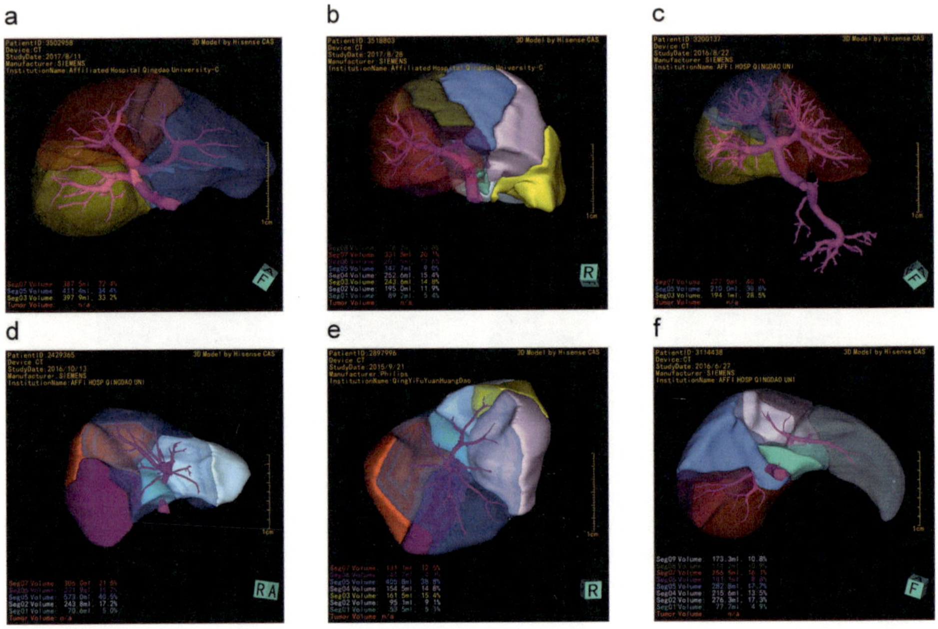

Figure 6.
(a) The right anterior portal vein is derived from the left portal vein main trunk. (b) The P6 portal vein is derived from the right anterior portal vein. (c) The portal vein trunk has trifurcation at the porta hepatis and divides into the left, right anterior, and right posterior branches. (d) The right anterior portal vein is derived from the saccule of the left branch. (e) The right anterior lobe has a dominant supply from seven branches that are simultaneously derived from the right anterior portal vein. (f) The P2 and P3 branches of the left portal vein share a common trunk.

Segmentation	Sex		Total
	Male	Female	
Type A	118 (46.27%)	247 (49.01%)	365 (48.09%)
Type B	77 (30.20%)	126 (25.00%)	203 (26.75%)
Type C	26 (10.20%)	50 (9.92%)	76 (10.01%)
Type D	34 (13.33%)	81 (16.07%)	115 (15.15%)
Total	255 (100%)	504 (100%)	759 (100%)

Male vs. female: $\chi^2 = 2.823$, $p = 0.420$.

Table 1.
Distribution of liver segmentation in different sexes.

Accurate preoperative knowledge of the liver anatomy and volume is essential for performing safe liver resections [1, 10, 14, 15]. We proposed a liver segmentation system to enable better classification of the different types for individual patients to assist with their preoperative surgical planning. Segmental liver volume, which is useful for the preoperative evaluation of remnant liver volume, was also predicted.

Recently, many studies have proposed different methods of liver segmentation based on variations in the vascular anatomy of the liver [11–13]. Functional liver segmentation that included eight segments based on portal vein blood supply and hepatic venous drainage was most well-known and applied in clinical work [4]. However, the actual anatomical segmentation of the liver varied substantially in some cases.

DOI: http://dx.doi.org/10.5772/intechopen.111542

Segmentation	Age		Total
	3 months–15 years	>15 years	
Type A	22 (50.00%)	343 (47.97%)	365 (48.09%)
Type B	9 (20.45%)	194 (27.13%)	203 (26.75%)
Type C	5 (11.36%)	71 (9.93%)	76 (10.01%)
Type D	8 (18.18%)	107 (14.97%)	115 (15.15%)
Total	44 (100%)	715 (100%)	759 (100%)

Pediatric vs. adult age groups: χ^2 = 1.095, p = 0.778.

Table 2.
Distribution of liver segmentation in pediatric and adult groups.

Liver segment classification	% of total liver volume (range)							
	I	II	III	IV	V	VI	VII	VII
Type A (n = 365)	4.86 ± 1.89	10.16 ± 3.07	11.60 ± 3.52	14.27 ± 3.40	15.78 ± 5.12	11.65 ± 4.23	15.28 ± 4.83	16.43 ± 5.18

Table 3.
Volume ratio for each type A segment of Dong's liver segmentation (%).

Liver segment classification	% of total liver volume (range)								
	I	II	III	IV	V	VI	VII	VII	IX
Type B (n = 203)	4.79 ± 2.05	9.55 ± 3.02	11.70 ± 3.43	13.71 ± 3.49	10.36 ± 3.72	10.61 ± 4.17	14.77 ± 4.48	11.84 ± 3.28	12.69 + 3.70

Table 4.
Volume ratio for each type B segment of Dong's liver segmentation (%).

Liver segment classification	% of total liver volume (range)						
	I	II	III	IV	V	RP	VII
Type C-a (n = 50)	4.99 ± 2.42	10.33 ± 3.31	12.32 ± 4.05	14.08 ± 3.06	16.88 + 4.59	24.61 ± 4.70	16.69 ± 4.59

Table 5.
Volume ratio for each type C-a segment of Dong's liver segmentation (%).

Liver segment classification	% of total liver volume (range)							
	I	II	III	IV	V	RP	VII	IX
Type C-b (n = 26)	5.19 ± 1.98	9.70 ± 3.44	11.39 ± 3.66	14.03 ± 3.58	11.47 ± 3.82	24.14 ± 5.69	11.50 ± 3.52	12.50 ± 3.47

Table 6.
Volume ratio for each type C-b segment of Dong's liver segmentation (%).

Based on artificial intelligence, the development of imaging technology has enabled 3D reconstruction of the digital liver model in a CT DICOM file by using simulation software [16, 17]. The possibility of observing the anatomical relationship of the portal vein and hepatic vein in the liver from different angles allows for individualized evaluation of liver segmentation and subsequent surgical planning [18–23]. Based on pediatric patients' CT DICOM data, we developed software called Hisense CAS [17, 24, 25], which could accurately reconstruct the intrahepatic portal vein branches up to their fourth level. In the present study, we analyzed 759 digital livers; based on the variation of the fourth-level portal vein branch, we proposed Dong's liver segmentation system. This system attempts to include all types of anatomical variations in the liver.

We found that the portal vein branches in the left hepatic lobe, which was divided into segments II, III, and IV, were relatively consistent. However, there were several variations in the right liver that cannot be described by a single segmentation method. Consequently, we classified them into four types: A, B, C, and D. For types A and B, segments VI and VII are supplied by a fourth-level portal vein derived from the outer, inferior, and superior aspects of the right posterior portal vein branches.

Couinaud divided cephalic segment VIII and caudal segment V based on the right anterior portal vein. This was disputed by a recent study that proposed that the right anterior divides into ventral and dorsal branches [11, 13]. Our study findings demonstrated that in some livers, the right anterior usually divides into two main branches, either cephalic and caudal or ventral and dorsal. We classified this as type A. Our observations suggest that a preoperative understanding of the angle of the portal vein branch is necessary for the right-anterior branch to avoid intraoperative injuries. Furthermore, the right anterior portal vein branch may also divide into three main branches, including the caudal (P5), cephalic-dorsal (P8), and cephalic-ventral (P9) branches. We classified this as type B.

The right posterior portal vein branch of type C is a single main branch with several small sector-shaped branches that supply the right-posterior lobe. These anatomical variations are important for segmental, subsegmental, and combined-segmental precision resections of the right liver.

A variety of special variations that could not be categorized into the first three types were included as type D. This strategy of grouping the special variants into one type may facilitate a full understanding of the complexity of liver anatomy. A higher proportion of such variance also supported the need for individualized precision surgery. To perform precision hepatectomy, liver segmentation should be performed based on individual liver models established using each patient's imaging data preoperatively so that virtual surgery and remnant liver volume may be evaluated by using the 3D simulation software.

According to Kumon's criteria, the caudate lobe (segment I) comprises three parts: the Spiegel lobe, the paracaval portion, and the caudate carina. Because of the uniqueness of the caudate lobe blood supply, the Spiegel lobe is supplied by one or two caudate lobe portal branches. Variations in the portal blood supply to the caudate lobe are very common. In our study, a considerable proportion of subjects were found to have two to five branches that were derived from the left and right portal veins supplying the caudate lobe. However, the actual number of such branches could not be accurately determined because of their tiny size and inadequate CT resolution. Because of these tiny vessels, we suggest that surgeons should demonstrate extra care during caudate lobe surgery.

We did not find any significant differences in sex and age using Dong's liver segmentation. Because our data were from the Chinese population, the differences in the liver anatomy of people from various races and regions need further exploration.

The average volume of each segment of the different segmentation types can be used for predicting remnant liver volume to ensure safe anatomic hepatectomy.

However, because of the large diversity in portal vein anatomy, it is our opinion that individualized volume measurements are critical for the safety of anatomic hepatectomy, especially in patients with large tumors, impaired liver function, or atypical portal vein branching.

Artificial intelligence technology has made significant breakthroughs and clinical applications in the field of precision surgery. The development of digital medicine has provided new perspectives regarding liver segmentation. We believe that Dong's liver segmentation system and segmental liver volume will enable a better understanding of liver anatomy and will be useful for liver surgeons.

Author details

Xianjun Zhou[1,2], Chengzhan Zhu[2,3], Bin Wei[2], Nan Xia[2], Yongjian Chen[2] and Qian Dong[1,2]*

1 Department of Pediatric Surgery, The Affiliated Hospital of Qingdao University, Qingdao, China

2 Shandong Provincial Key Laboratory of Digital Medicine and Computer-Assisted Surgery, Shandong College Collaborative Innovation Center of Digital Medicine Clinical Treatment and Nutrition Health, Qingdao University, Qingdao, China

3 Department of Hepatobiliary and Pancreatic Surgery, The Affiliated Hospital of Qingdao University, Qingdao, China

*Address all correspondence to: 13608968352@163.com

References

[1] Sakamoto Y, Kokudo N, Kawaguchi Y, Akita K. Clinical anatomy of the liver: Review of the 19th Meeting of the Japanese Research Society of Clinical Anatomy. Liver Cancer. 2017;**6**:146-160

[2] Nelson RC, Chezmar JL, Sugarbaker PH, Murray DR, Bernardino ME. Preoperative localization of focal liver lesions to specific liver segments: Utility of CT during arterial portography. Radiology. 1990;**176**:89-94

[3] Uchida M. Recent advances in 3D computed tomography techniques for simulation and navigation in hepatobiliary pancreatic surgery. Journal of Hepato-Biliary-Pancreatic Sciences. 2014;**21**:239-245

[4] Couinaud C. Anatomic principles of left and right regulated hepatectomy: Technics. Journal of Chir (Paris). 1954;**70**:933-966

[5] Couinaud C. The anatomy of the liver. Annals of Italian Chir. 1992;**63**:693-697

[6] Bismuth H. Surgical anatomy and anatomical surgery of the liver. World Journal of Surgery. 1982;**6**:3-9

[7] Mise Y, Tani K, Aoki T, et al. Virtual liver resection: Computer-assisted operation planning using a three-dimensional liver representation. Journal of Hepato-Biliary-Pancreatic Sciences. 2013;**20**:157-164

[8] Seyama Y, Kokudo N. Assessment of liver function for safe hepatic resection. Hepatology Research. 2009;**39**:107-116

[9] Kubota K, Makuuchi M, Kusaka K, et al. Measurement of liver volume and hepatic functional reserve as a guide to decision-making in resectional surgery for hepatic tumors. Hepatology. 1997;**26**:1176-1181

[10] Simpson AL, Geller DA, Hemming AW, et al. Liver planning software accurately predicts postoperative liver volume and measures early regeneration. Journal of the American College of Surgeons. 2014;**219**:199-207

[11] Kobayashi T, Ebata T, Yokoyama Y, et al. Study on the segmentation of the right anterior sector of the liver. Surgery. 2017;**161**:1536-1542

[12] Kogure K, Kuwano H, Fujimaki N, Ishikawa H, Takada K. Reproposal for Hjortsjo's segmental anatomy on the anterior segment in human liver. Archives of Surgery. 2002;**137**:1118-1124

[13] Cho A, Okazumi S, Miyazawa Y, et al. Proposal for a reclassification of liver based anatomy on portal ramifications. American Journal of Surgery. 2005;**189**:195-199

[14] Dong Q, Jiang B, Lu Y, Zhang H, Jiang Z, Lu H, et al. Surgical management of giant liver tumor involving the hepatic hilum of children. World Journal of Surgery. 2009;**33**:1520-1525

[15] Dong Q, Xu W, Jiang B, et al. Clinical applications of computerized tomography 3-D reconstruction imaging for diagnosis and surgery in children with large liver tumors or tumors at the hepatic hilum. Pediatric Surgery International. 2007;**23**:1045-1050

[16] van der Vorst JR, van Dam RM, van Stiphout RS, et al. Virtual liver resection and volumetric analysis of the future liver remnant using open source image processing software. World Journal of Surgery. 2010;**34**:2426-2433

[17] Zhang G, Zhou XJ, Zhu CZ, Dong Q, Su L. Usefulness of three-dimensional(3D) simulation software in hepatectomy for pediatric hepatoblastoma. Surgical Oncology. 2016;**25**:236-243

[18] Hallet J, Gayet B, Tsung A, Wakabayashi G, Pessaux P. Systematic review of the use of pre-operative simulation and navigation for hepatectomy: Current status and future perspectives. Journal of Hepato-Biliary-Pancreatic Sciences. 2015;**22**:353-362

[19] Beller S, Hunerbein M, Eulenstein S, Lange T, Schlag PM. Feasibility of navigated resection of liver tumors using multiplanar visualization of intraoperative 3-dimensional ultrasound data. Annals of Surgery. 2007;**246**:288-294

[20] Wigmore SJ, Redhead DN, Yan XJ, et al. Virtual hepatic resection using three-dimensional reconstruction of helical computed tomography angioportograms. Annals of Surgery. 2001;**233**:221-226

[21] Guiney MJ, Kruskal JB, Sosna J, Hanto DW, Goldberg SN, Raptopoulos V. Multi-detector row CT of relevant vascular anatomy of the surgical plane in split-liver transplantation. Radiology. 2003;**229**:401-407

[22] Kurimoto A, Yamanaka J, Hai S, et al. Parenchyma-preserving hepatectomy based on portal ramification and perfusion of the right anterior section: Preserving the ventral or dorsal area. Journal of Hepato-Biliary-Pancreatic Sciences. 2016;**23**:158-166

[23] Okamoto E, Kyo A, Yamanaka N, Tanaka N, Kuwata K. Prediction of the safe limits of hepatectomy by combined volumetric and functional measurements in patients with impaired hepatic function. Surgery. 1984;**95**:586-592

[24] Su L, Zhou XJ, Dong Q, et al. Application value of computer assisted surgery system in precision surgeries for pediatric complex liver tumors. International Journal of Clinical and Experimental Medicine. 2015;**8**:18406-18412

[25] Zhao J, Zhou XJ, Zhu CZ, et al. 3D simulation assisted resection of giant hepatic mesenchymal hamartoma in children. Computational Assistant Surgery (Abingdon). 2017;**22**:54-59

Chapter 16

Fuzzy Expert System for Rectal Cancer Based on Possibility Measure

Latafat A. Gardashova, Yusif R. Aliyarov and Shamil A. Ahmadov

Abstract

Intestinal infections in common and colorectal cancer in particular are quite widely spread and affect modern population in a significant manner. Therefore, they have been objects of intensive scientific research for quite a long time. It is known that the colorectal cancer's diagnostics can face some difficulties caused by the uncertainties in patients' health status and disease data. The uncertainty, in common, can be classified as probabilistic or possibilistic (fuzzy). The goal of this chapter is to analyze a fuzzy-rule-based medical expert system for the colorectal cancer's diagnostics. In the modeling, fuzzy inference based on possibility measure and knowledge extraction based on fuzzy clustering are applied. During the initial stage of the system's modeling, the applied parameters of colorectal cancer were defined by using clinical data. During the next stage, the soft-computing-based evaluation of the cancer's factors is performed. During the third stage, the applied fuzzy inference, based on possibility measure, is introduced and supported by the examples. The knowledge base of the modeled system consists of the case data obtained from 100 patients in the course of 3 years by the National Center of Oncology. The effectiveness of the modeled system was checked on the testing subset of 30 diagnoses, and 22 predictions by the expert system were defined as correct.

Keywords: colorectal cancer, IF-THEN rules, possibility measure-based inference system, tumor response, fuzzy logic, fuzzy inference, fuzzy clustering

1. Introduction

Cancer has a long and complicated history: it appeared and was recognized even in the ancient times. Modern science has carried out some significant amounts of research on tumors and their treatment. The classic triplet of the disease's treatments is surgery, radiation, and chemotherapy, which are constantly supplemented by more and more advanced methods. Modern oncology has, at its disposal, a wide arsenal of tools and methods for treating cancer: for saving human life, they help to prevent its occurrence and development; in hopeless cases, they prevent the maximum extension and ease the painful symptoms.

Due to the wide spread of oncological diseases, it is especially important to be able to detect cancer at the early stage, when it is more possible to completely heal the patient. Nowadays, cancer is the second leading cause of death in the world, after cardiovascular diseases. Cancer causes almost one in six deaths worldwide. According to the World Health Organization, the incidence of cancer in the next 20 years will increase by 70%. The State Statistical Committee also reports that in Azerbaijan, for every 100,000 people, there are over 400 patients with a malignant tumor; most of them are women. The conducted statistical data demonstrate that in our country, there is an increase in the number of patients diagnosed with cancer. Many experts believe that in a few years, malignant neoplasms will become the main cause of death worldwide, leaving cardiovascular diseases far behind. The worst thing is that the incidence of cancer is growing, but the survival rate is not increasing. In most cases, this occurs because of the late detection of the disease, as success in recovery strongly depends on the early diagnosis of asymptomatic cancer. The problem with the growing number of cancer patients should be solved not only by medicine but also by all sciences that can help in the fight against this cruel disease. This work is specifically aimed at helping oncologists in making an accurate diagnosis at early stages and possibly saving someone's life.

Nowadays, one of the most spread cancer-related infections is colorectal cancer (CRC). The statistics of this illness is studied in [1], and it has been found that CRC should be more investigated among the young generation.

In the other research [2], risk factors that affect development of CRC are analyzed. In the research, the risk for growth of cancer is defined, but patients' gender wasn't taken into consideration. Thus, a more accurate analysis of colorectal cancer is required.

Information about the illness is discussed in [3–9]. The authors used two data-driven approaches: logistic regression and neural network. The effectiveness of logistic regression in the study appeared to be near 66%; the effectiveness of neural approach was 78%. The study was performed on the data obtained from 403 patients. The results demonstrate superior effectiveness of neural networks in comparison with logistic regression when applied to cancer diagnostics. In general, neural networks have several advantages: ability to process vast amounts of information, fault tolerance, generalization ability, adaptability, and learning. In the discussed studies and applied methods, crisp statistic information was used; but data on patients are always rather inaccurate, which enables the applicability of fuzzy data.

There are several research studies on medical expert systems reported in scientific literature [10–14]. These research studies are based on linguistic information, fuzzy inference reasoning, and probability-based reasoning. However, these systems' performance is accompanied by the collateral information loss; thus, these studies possess some effectiveness limits. From this viewpoint, a possibility-measure-based fuzzy inference method seems to be more effective [15–19]. This measure-based algorithm is a kernel of information processing of the software system ESPLAN [20]. Possibility measure is a fuzzy measure and can partially operate Z number-based information. Zadeh's last theory [21] is an extension of fuzzy logic and able to represent different types of information uncertainties. Processing of information based on possibility measure might be quite effective in medicine.

The purpose of this study is to design a fuzzy rule-based expert system for diagnosis of colorectal cancer based on possibility measure and data extracted from Big Data. The rest of the paper is organized as follows. Section 2 briefly describes fuzzy c-means algorithm and the possibility-measure-based inference algorithm. Statement of the problem and its solution are given in Section 3. Finally, Section 4 concludes the paper.

2. Preliminaries

2.1 Representation of fuzzy if: then rules and possibility-measure-based inference algorithm

The framework of the knowledge base relies on the fuzzy interpretation of production rules [20]:

$$\begin{aligned} &R^k : IF \ \mathrm{x}_1 \text{ is } \tilde{\mathrm{A}}_{\mathrm{k1}} \text{ and } \mathrm{x}_2 \text{ is } \tilde{\mathrm{A}}_{\mathrm{k2}} \text{ and ... and } \mathrm{x}_\mathrm{m} \text{ is } \tilde{\mathrm{A}}_{\mathrm{km}} \text{ THEN} \\ &\mathrm{y}_1 \text{ is } \tilde{\mathrm{B}}_{\mathrm{k1}} \text{ and } \mathrm{y}_2 \text{ is } \tilde{\mathrm{B}}_{\mathrm{k2}} \text{ and ... and } \mathrm{y}_{\mathrm{kl}} \text{ is } \tilde{\mathrm{B}}_{\mathrm{kl}}, k = \overline{1, K} \end{aligned} \tag{1}$$

where $x_i, i = \overline{1, m}$ and $y_j, j = \overline{1, l}$ are input and output variables, rule antecedents $\tilde{A}_{kj}$ and consequents $\tilde{B}_{kj}$ are defined by using fuzzy sets, and k is the number of rules.
Inputs and outputs of the rule are linguistic data.
Main steps of the applied fuzzy-measure-based reasoning algorithm are as follows:

1. Fuzzification: inputs and outputs are defined in a linguistic manner by using trapezoidal fuzzy numbers.

2. The firing levels of the rules are calculated by using possibility measure (*Poss*):

$$\text{If the sign is “ = ” and } \lambda_k = \left(1 - Poss\left(\tilde{v}_k | \tilde{a}_{jk}\right)\right) \cdot cf_k, \text{ then} \tag{2}$$

$$\lambda_{jk} = \left(1 - Poss\left(\tilde{v}_k | \tilde{a}_{jk}\right)\right) \ cf_k. \tag{3}$$

If the sign is “≠”, then *Poss* is determined as

$$Poss(\tilde{v}|\tilde{a})) = \max_y \min(\mu_{\tilde{v}}(y), (\mu_{\tilde{a}}(y)) \in [0, 1], \tau_j = \min(\lambda_{jk}). \tag{4}$$

Here, one of the main elements of logistic inference is demonstration of the object. Value of each w_i object consists of its linguistic value and the confidence degree of the linguistic value. Together, they constitute a pair, (v_i, cf_i).

3. For each rule, the following computation is performed

$$R_j = \left(\min_j \lambda_{jk}\right) * CF_j/100 \tag{5}$$

where CF is the confidence degree of a rule, j is the index of a rule, k is the index of the relation, and λ_{jk} is the truth degree of the kth elementary antecedent.

4. This step is to define the firing level (π) and to check $R_j \geq \pi$. If the condition holds true, then the consequent part of the rule is calculated.

5. The evaluated w_i objects have S_i value: w_i, (v_i^1, cf_i^1), ..., ..., $\left(v_i^{S_i}, cf_i^{S_i}\right)$. S_i is the number of the rules in the fuzzy inference process

6. Calculation of the resulting value by using the fuzzy average value is performed as follows

$$\overline{v}_i = \frac{\sum_{n=1}^{S_i} v_i^n \cdot cf_i^n}{\sum_{n=1}^{S_i} cf_i^n} \tag{6}$$

IF $x_1 = \tilde{a}_1^j$ AND $x_2 = \tilde{a}_2^j$ AND ... THEN $y_1 = \tilde{b}_1^j$ AND $y_2 = \tilde{b}_2^j$ AND ...
IF ... THEN $Y_1 = AVR\,(y_1)$ AND $Y_2 = AVR\,(y_2)$ AND ...
This model has a built-in function, AVRG, which calculates the average value.

2.2 Fuzzy C-means algorithm

Fuzzy C-Means algorithm attempts to minimize the sum of squared errors. The algorithm is based on the iterative minimization of the following objective function [22, 23]:

$$J(W, C) = \sum_{j=1}^{k} \sum_{i=1}^{n} w_{i,j}^{p} dist\left(x_i, c_j\right)^2 \tag{7}$$

The following condition is satisfied for the sum of degrees of membership of a given element xi to all clusters:

$$\sum_{j=1}^{k} w_{i,j} = 1 \tag{8}$$

The following condition is satisfied for the sum of membership degrees of all elements in each cluster:

$$0 < \sum_{i=1}^{n} w_{i,j} < n \tag{9}$$

The corresponding c_j centroid for a C_j cluster is defined as:

$$c_j = \frac{\sum_{i=1}^{n} w_{i,j}^{p} x_i}{\sum_{i=1}^{n} w_{i,j}^{p}} \tag{10}$$

The fuzzy partition update formula can be obtained by minimizing the objective function with the constraint that the sum of the weights equals 1:

$$w_{i,j} = \frac{\left(1/dist\left(x_i, c_j\right)^2\right)^{\frac{1}{p-1}}}{\sum_{q=1}^{k}\left(1/dist\left(x_i, c_q\right)^2\right)^{\frac{1}{p-1}}} \tag{11}$$

3. Problem description and possible solution

Nowadays, as was previously mentioned, CRC is the second most frequent malignancy in the case of both men and women. The tumor is localized in the rectum, the farthest portion of the digestive tract, in around one-third of cases. Patients' quality of life is severely impacted by surgical therapy for rectal cancer, which results in dysfunctions that include fecal incontinence, urinary problems, and sexual issues. Increasing the number of sphincter-preserving surgeries was the primary goal of rectal cancer treatment for the past 20 years; today, the focus is on organ preservation strategies.

Neoadjuvant radiotherapy and chemotherapy are used to increase local control and overall survival in around 75–80% of instances for individuals with rectal cancer, making their care complicated. However, only 20–30% of patients who receive neoadjuvant therapy gets a full pathological response; the other 70–80% experiences a poor or ineffective response. How we can anticipate tumor response in people with rectal cancer is the key issue right now.

This variance is assumed to be influenced by the tumor's size, height from the anal margin, depth of invasion, differentiation and, of course, genetic variables such as the KRAS and BRAF mutation. The purpose of this work is to create an expert system to forecast tumor response value following neoadjuvant chemoradiation. A crucial issue is how to define the predict value of the tumor response following neoadjuvant chemoradiation. To assess tumor response using pertinent parameters is the fundamental problem. Using fuzzy rules, we can calculate the tumor response value. A compound index made up of five characteristics, each of which is judged by an expert, makes up the tumor response value following neoadjuvant chemoradiation, abbreviated as R.

The five components are: V—age, LO—localization of tumors, T—infestation rate, N—state of lymph nodes, G—mutation in the genes, and R—predict value of tumor response.

Using the abovementioned parameters, the tumor response value model can be expressed as a set of 21 rules obtained by using fuzzy C-means algorithm:

1. *If* $Age(V) = about\ 80$ *and* $Localization\ tumor(LO) = about\ 2$ *and* $Infestation\ rate(T) = about\ 2$ *and* $State\ of\ lymph\ nodes(N) = about\ 1$ *and* $Mutation\ in\ the\ genes(G) = about\ 0$, *THEN predict value of tumor response* $(R) = about\ 0$;

2. *If* $Age(V) = about\ 40$ *and* $Localization\ tumor(LO) = about\ 2$ *and* $Infestation\ rate\ (T) = about\ 2$ *and* $State\ of\ lymph\ nodes(N) = about\ 3$ *and* $Mutation\ in\ the\ genes\ (G) = about\ 0$, *THEN predict value of tumor response* $(R) = about\ 0$;

… … …

3. *If* $Age(V) = about\ 20$ *and* $Localization\ tumor(LO) = about\ 92$ *and* $Infestation\ rate(T) = about\ 2$ *and* $State\ of\ lymph\ nodes(N) = about\ 3$ *and* $Mutation\ in\ the\ genes(G) = about\ 1$, *THEN predict value of tumor response* $(R) = about\ 100$

Our goal is to use five parameters represented by fuzzy linguistic terms to describe the level of the tumor response value. Values of linguistic terms are given below as intervals. In addition, they are expressed as fuzzy data in diagrams.

Age (V):
Positive [0–40]
Medium positive [30–50]
Medium negative [40–60]

Negative [60–100]
Localization of tumors (LO):
Negative [0–5]
Weak negative [3–8]
Medium positive [6–11]
Positive [10–15]
Infestation rate (T):
Early form [0–1]
Localized [1 – 2]
Early locally developed [2 – 3]
Late locally developed [3 – 4]
Metastasized [4–4<]
Status of lymph nodes (N):
Negative [0–2]
Medium Positive [1–4]
Positive [4–20]
Mutation in genes (G):
Negative [0–0.5]
Positive [0.5–1]
TRG (tumor regression grade) (R):
Very bad [0–10]
Bad [10–20]
Sufficient [50–60]
Good [70–80]
Excellent [90–100]
Graphical representation of these linguistic terms is as shown (**Figures 1–6**):

From the defined linguistic terms, a knowledge base of interpretable rules is created. For instance:

Rule. *If age is about 35 and localization of tumors is middle positive and infestation rate is middle positive and state of lymph nodes is middle positive and mutation in the genes is positive, THEN predict value of tumor response is bad.*

ESPLAN shell is used for creating an expert system for rectal cancer. Below, the computer simulation is discussed.

Computer simulation. ESPLAN shell has the following modules: the module that manages all the procedure of the system; read-in and interpretation of knowledge; inference; explanation generator; knowledge base and work are service; environment interface; user interface. ESPLAN shell is realized using Prolog Artificial Intelligence language. There are functional constructions that Prolog predicates in this system. This possibility of system gives it a chance for including new functions to the program.

Representation objects and linguistic terms by using ESPLAN are given in **Figure 7**.

For example: Parameters about 50 are represented as: *about K: (D, K,1.1*K, D) = about 50:(D = 7.5, K = 47.5, 1.1 K = 52.5, D = 7.5).*

Given linguistic terms are used in ESPLAN system:
much: (D, F – D, F, 0);
more than a: (D, K + D, F, 0);
about K: (D, K,1.1*K, D);
neutral: (D, M + 2 * D, M + 3*D, D);
less than K: (0, M, K – D, D).

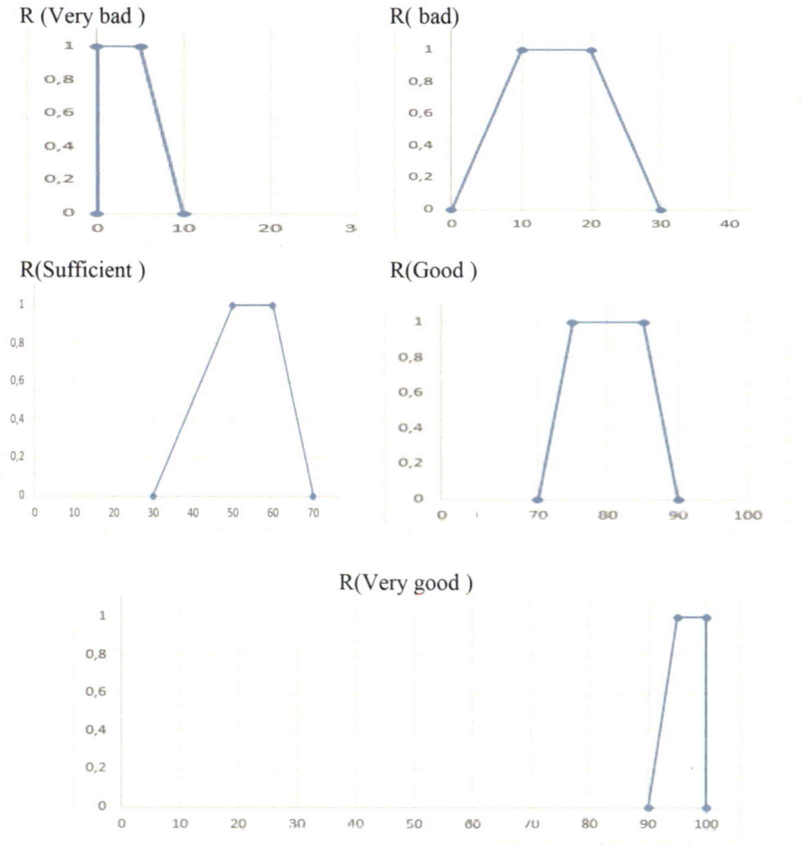

Figure 1.
Linguistic terms for Predict value of tumor response(R).

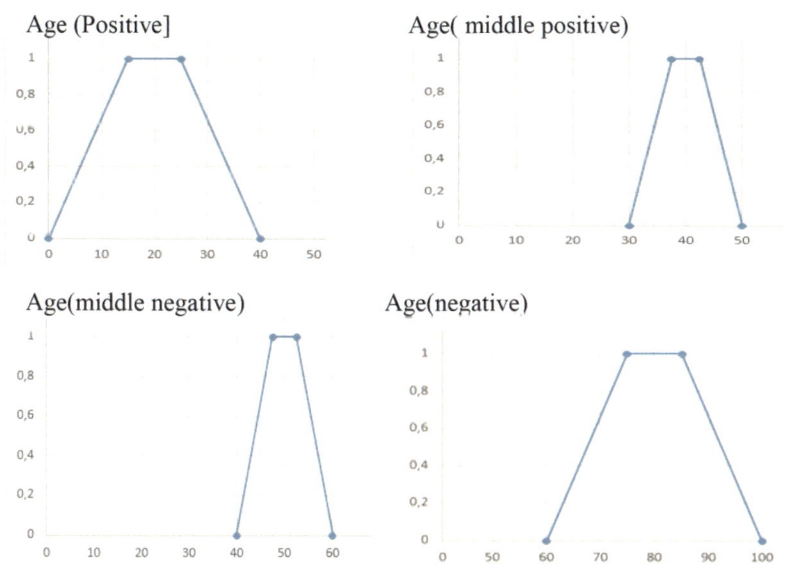

Figure 2.
Linguistic terms for Age(V).

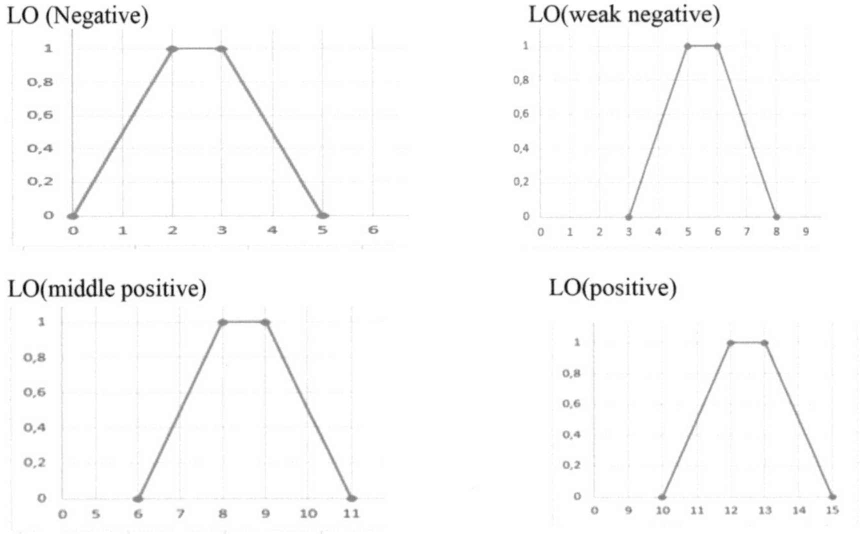

Figure 3.
Linguistic terms for Localization of tumors(LO).

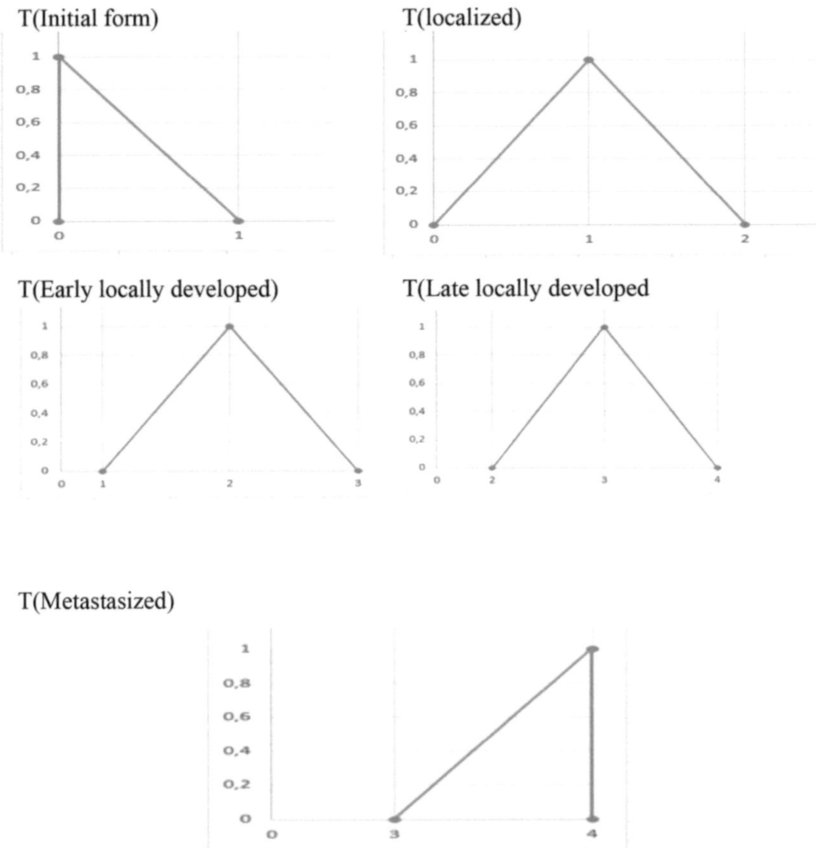

Figure 4.
Linguistic terms for Infestation rate(T).

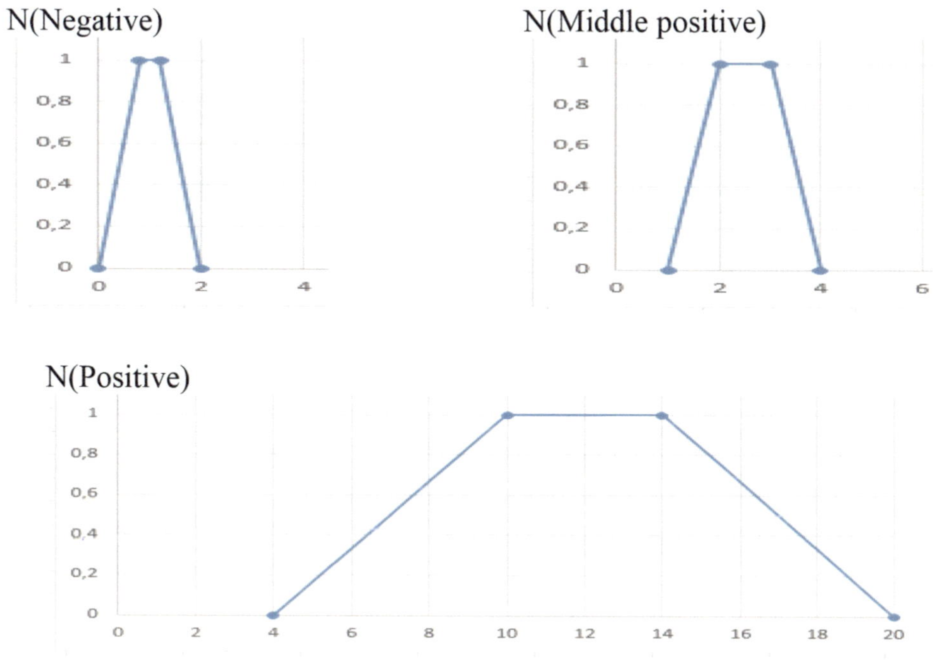

Figure 5.
Linguistic terms for State of Lymph nodes(N).

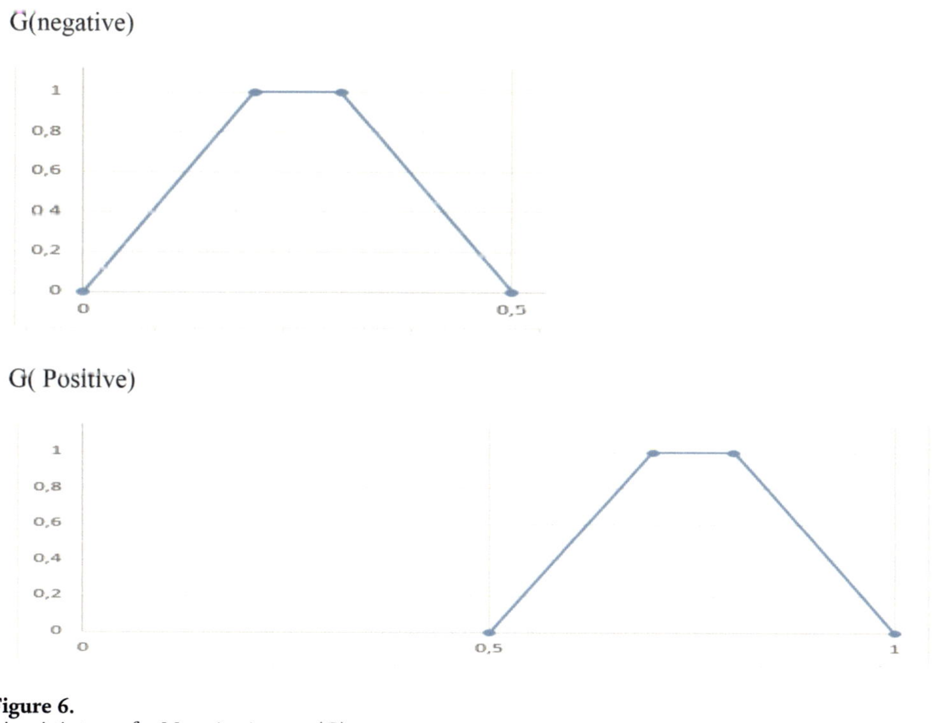

Figure 6.
Linguistic terms for Mutation in genes(G).

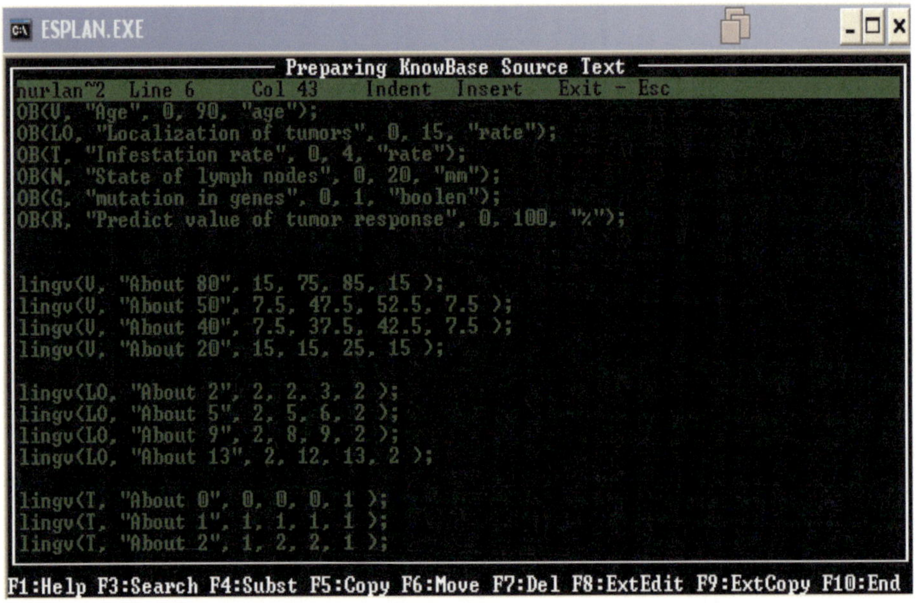

Figure 7.
Values of parameters for tumor response.

Here, minimum value is M, and the maximum value of the universe is F; D = (F-M)/5.

Demonstration of the rule is given below (**Figure 8**):

Fragment of the knowledge translation process is represented in **Figure 9**, and Fuzzy inference process is in **Figures 10–13**.

For instance,

object= "localization of tumors",

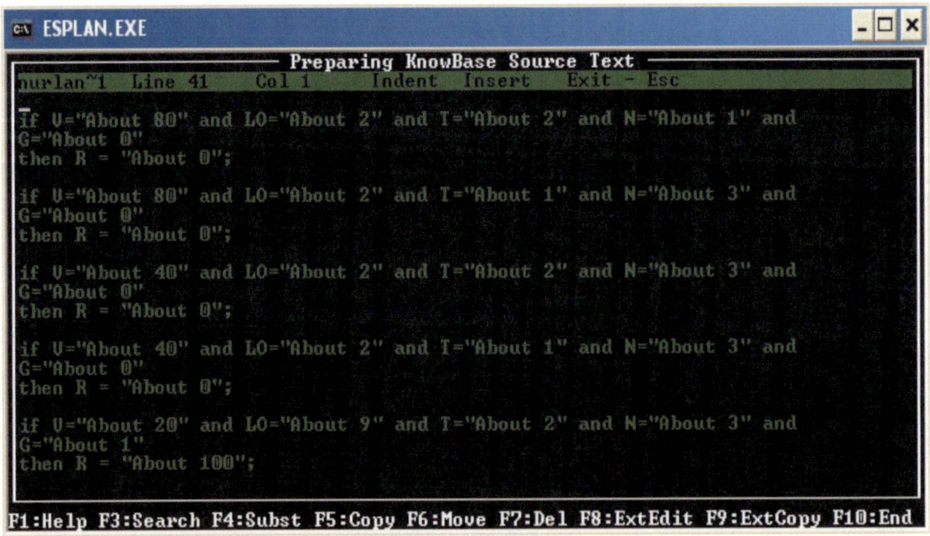

Figure 8.
Representation of the rule.

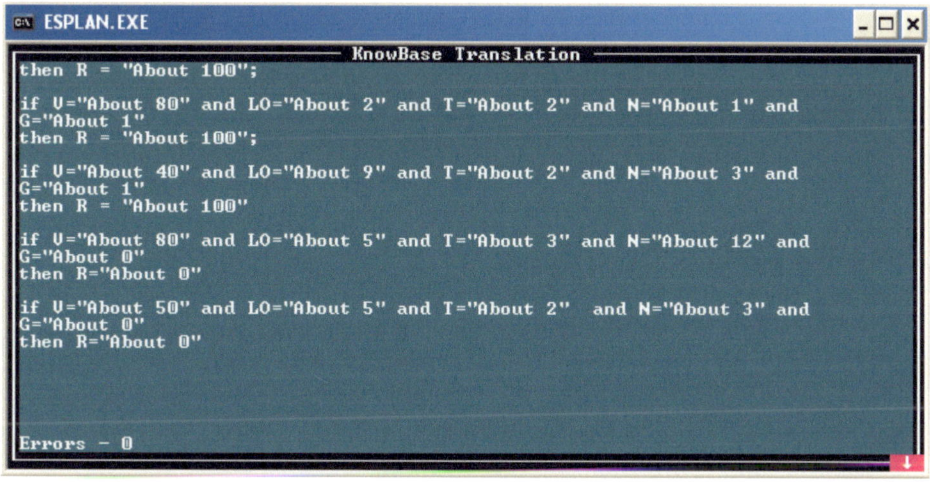

Figure 9.
Knowledge translation process.

M = minimum = 0, F = maximum = 15,

linguistic term = "about 5": About 5 = (D, M + 2*D, M + 3*D, D)

The abovementioned model is created using knowledge representation language and implemented in ESPLAN shell. Results of the performed test are:

Test 1: If age = about 38 and localization of tumors = about 4 and infestation rate = about 2 and state of lymph nodes = abou11 and mutation in the genes = about 0, THEN predict value of tumor response =?

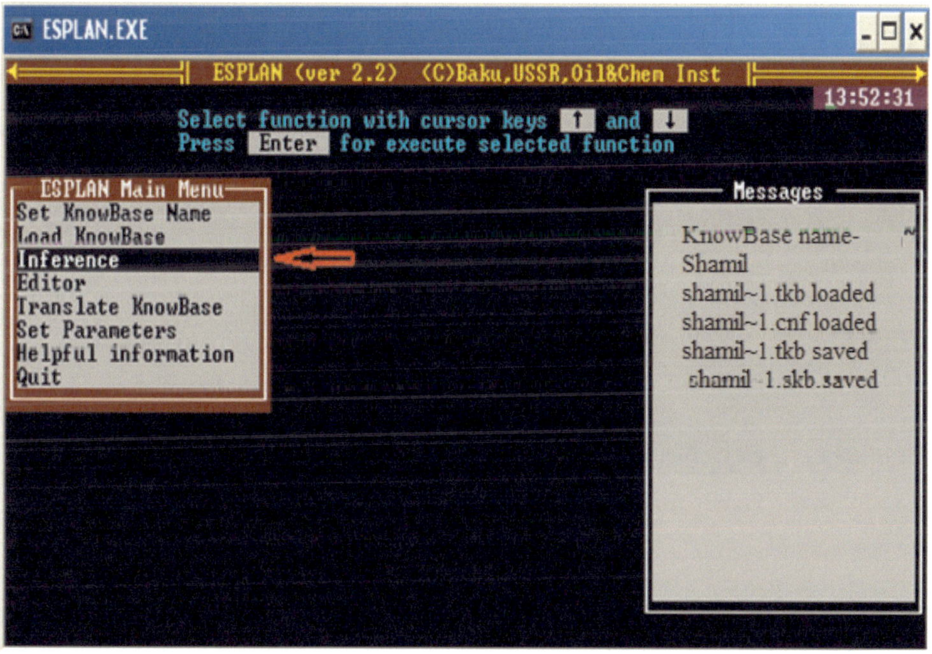

Figure 10.
Fuzzy inference process (1).

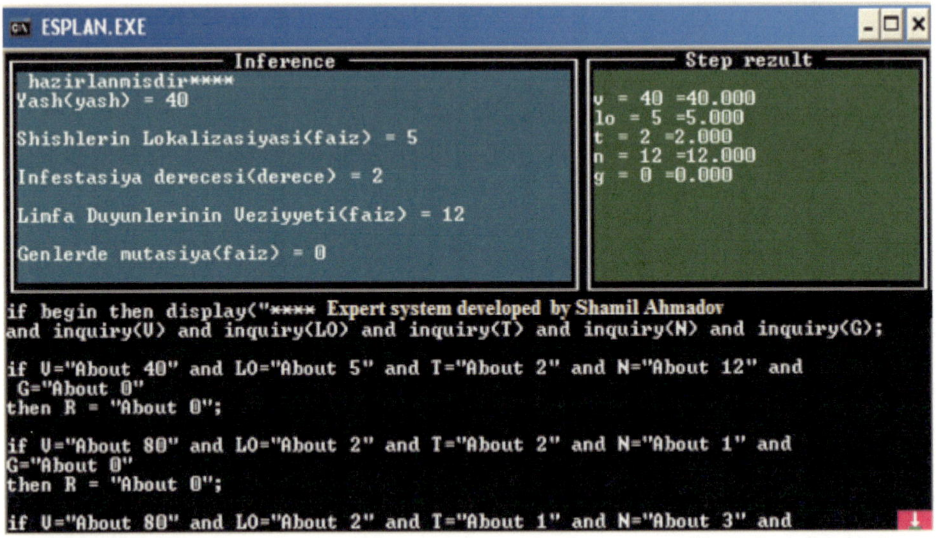

Figure 11.
Fuzzy inference process (2).

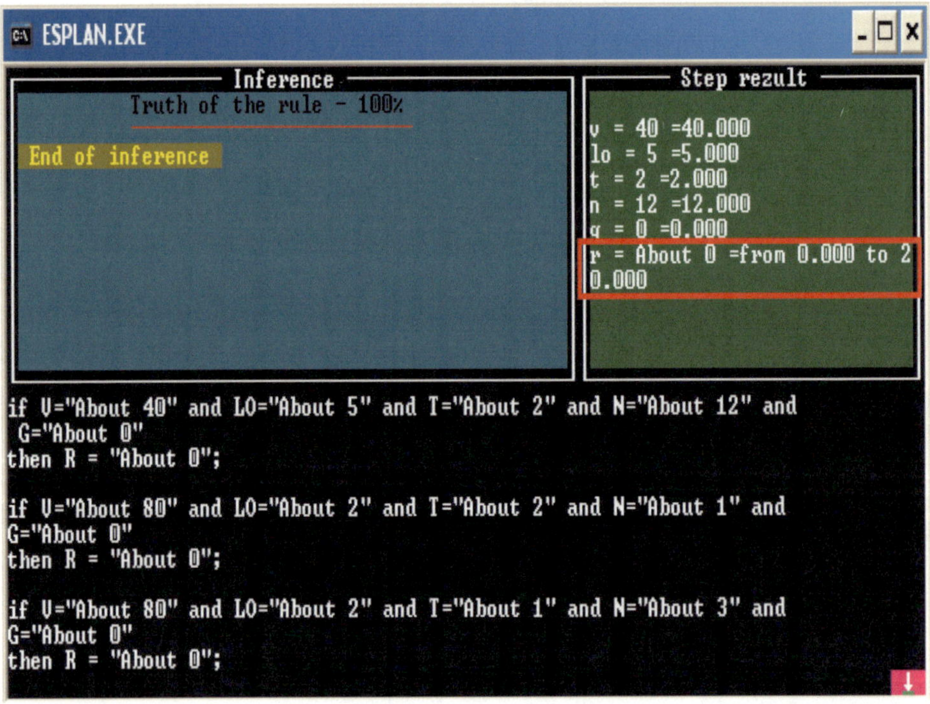

Figure 12.
Fuzzy inference result.

Result: predict value of tumor response is from 0 to 2.

The results of tests are shown in **Figures 12** and **13**.

Test 2: *Test 1: If age = middle positive and localization of tumors = weak negative and infestation rate = middle positive and state of lymph nodes = positive and mutation in the genes = negative, THEN predict value of tumor response =?*

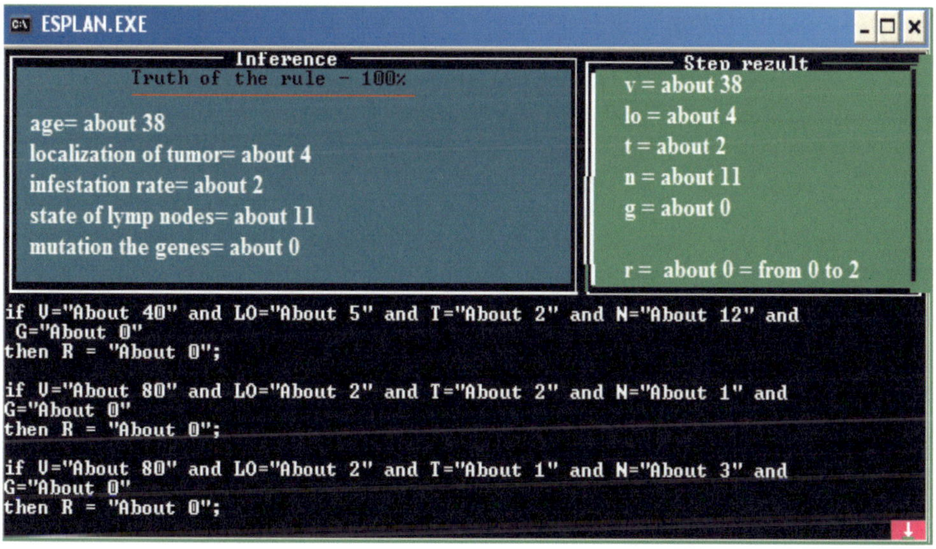

Figure 13.
Fragment of results.

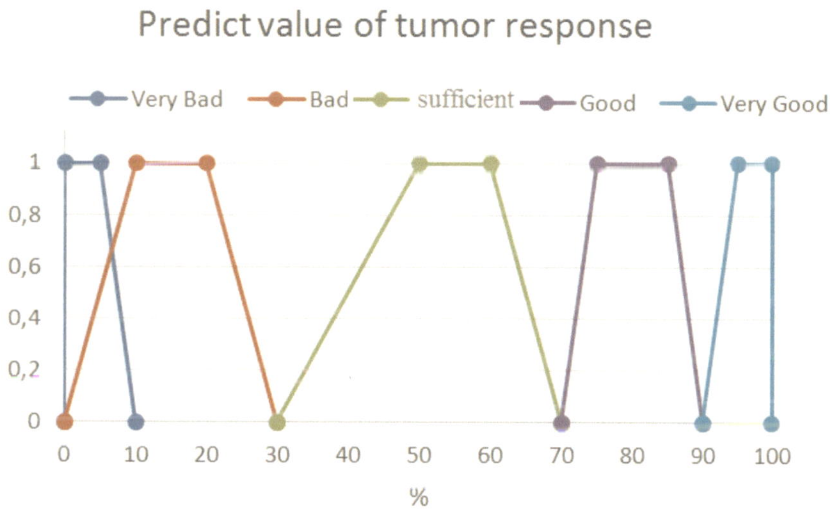

Figure 14.
Linguistic terms of tumor response.

FOR TEST 2. ANSWER:

predict value of tumor response =? ***very good.***

Representation of linguistic terms of tumor response is given in **Figure 14**.

Knowledge base is realized using possibility measure-based algorithm in ESPLAN. In this system, fuzzy logic theory is used in demonstration and operation of the linguistic terms. After fulfilling of the knowledge base of the system by adding values of several objects (for example, age is about 50), searching the solution in knowledge base is done by logical inference procedure.

There is the following opportunity of the ESPLAN shell: creating an expert system for several applications, relation with applied software package, explanation of the advices, demonstration of the results, interface with user, and so on.

The advantages of the created expert system are: working with linguistic values; possibility measure-based reasoning; realization of composition rule of inference, including knowledge base as dialog; storing knowledge about different areas in the knowledge base of the system; setting of a confidence degree for any rule (in percentage); application of external programs; and data interchange by using a file system.

4. Conclusion

The data used in this study are from the Database of National Center of Oncology. Three years of case data of 100 patients are implemented for extracting the knowledge-based rule using clustering method. Veracity of 30 diagnoses of patients was checked, and 22 from them were defined as correct. In this chapter, for the evaluation of value of tumor response, a possibility-measure-based method is used. The created expert system for rectal cancer was implemented in the ESPLAN. Several tests were performed, and the outcomes were compared to the actual patient data.

The presentation of the developed system and samples of its use in medicine demonstrate that it has a wide range of potential capabilities for making decisions based on fuzzy information under uncertain circumstances. Experimental findings demonstrate the effectiveness of the proposed intelligent system.

In the future, we are planning to study and compare different types of cancer illnesses by using soft computing tools-neural network, genetic algorithm, evolutionary computing, chaos theory, Zadeh last theory-Z-number theory, and real-life results for giving help and advice to doctors for decision-making during the treatment process. For the future works, the data that have been used in computations will be gathered from different hospitals and centers of oncology from all over the world by using internet resources.

Conflict of interest

The authors declare no conflict of interest.

Author details

Latafat A. Gardashova[1*], Yusif R. Aliyarov[2] and Shamil A. Ahmadov[1,3]

1 Azerbaijan State Oil and Industry University, Baku, Azerbaijan

2 National Center of Oncology, Azerbaijan

3 French-Azerbaijani University, Baku, Azerbaijan

*Address all correspondence to: latsham@yandex.ru

References

[1] Siegel RL, Miller KD, Goding Sauer A, Fedewa SA, Butterly LF, Anderson JC, et al. Colorectal cancer statistics, 2020. CA: a Cancer Journal for Clinicians. 2020;**70**:145-164

[2] Amersi F, Agustin M, Ko CY. Colorectal cancer: Epidemiology, risk factors, and health services. Clinics in Colon and Rectal Surgery. 2005;**18**(3): 133-140

[3] Grumett S, Snow P, Kerr D. Neural networks in the prediction of survival in patients with colorectal cancer. Clinical Colorectal Cancer. 2003;**2**(4): 239-244

[4] Phan K, Kahlaee HR, Kim SH, Toh JWT. Laparoscopic vs. robotic rectal cancer surgery and the effect on conversion rates: a meta-analysis of randomized controlled trials and propensity-score-matched studies. Techniques in Coloproctology. 2019; **23**(3):221-230

[5] Araghi M, Soerjomataram I, Jenkins M, Brierley J, Morris E, Bray F, et al. Global trends in colorectal cancer mortality: Projections to the year 2035. International Journal of Cancer. 2019; **144**(12):2992-3000

[6] Bartos A, Bartos D, Stoian R, Szabo B, Cioltean C, Iancu I, et al. Short-term outcome and survival after multiorgan resection for locally advanced colo-rectal cancer. Identification of risk factors. Annali Italiani di Chirurgia. 2018;**89**: 229-236

[7] Tharin Z, Blanc J, Alaoui IC, Bertaut A, Ghiringhelli F. Influence of primary tumor location and resection on survival in metastatic colorectal cancer. World Journal of Gastrointestinal Oncology. 2020;**12**(11):1296-1310

[8] Ngan TT, Lan LTH, Tuan TM, Son LH, Tuan LM, Minh NH. Colorectal cancer diagnosis with complex fuzzy inference system. In: Satapathy S, Bhateja V, Nguyen B, Nguyen N, Le DN, editors. Frontiers in Intelligent Computing: Theory and Applications. Advances in Intelligent Systems and Computing. Vol. 1013. Singapore: Springer; 2020. DOI: 10.1007/978-981-32-9186-7_2

[9] Silva A, Oliveira T, Julian V, Neves J, Novais P. A mobile and evolving tool to predict colorectal cancer survivability. In: IFIP International Conference on Artificial Intelligence Applications and Innovations, Sep 2016. Springer, Cham. 2016. pp. 14-26

[10] Amato F, López A, María E, Peña-Méndez PV, Hampl A, Havel J. Artificial neural networks in medical diagnosis. Journal of Applied Biomedicine. 2013;**11**: 47-58

[11] Echeverría FR, Echeverría CR. Application of expert systems in medicine. In: Proceedings of the 2006 Conference on Artificial Intelligence Research and Development. Amsterdam, The Netherlands: IOS Press; 2006. pp. 3-4

[12] De Medeiros IB, Machado MAS, Damasceno WJ, Caldeira AM, dos Santos RC, da Silva Filho JB. A fuzzy inference system to support medical diagnosis in real time. Procedia Computer Science. 2017;**122**:167-173

[13] Fathy SK. A predication survival model for colorectal cancer. In: Proceedings of the 2011 American Conference on Applied Mathematics and the 5th WSEAS International Conference on Computer Engineering and

Applications, Jan 2011. World Scientific and Engineering Academy and Society (WSEAS). 2011. pp. 36-42

[14] Prasath V, Lakshmi N, Nathiya M, Bharathan N, Neetha P. A survey on the applications of fuzzy logic in medical diagnosis. International Journal of Scientific and Engineering Research. 2013;**4**(4):1199-1203

[15] Aliev RA, Aliev BF, Gardashova LA, Huseynov OH. Selection of an optimal treatment method for acute periodontitis disease. Journal of Medical Systems. 2012;**36**(2):639-646. DOI: 10.1007/s10916-010-9528-6

[16] Gardashova LA, Allahverdiyev RA, Saner T, Eyupoglu SZ. Analysis of the job satisfaction index problem by using fuzzy inference. Procedia Computer Science. 2016;**102**:45-50. DOI: 10.1016/j.procs.2016.09.368

[17] Mirzakhanov VE, Gardashova LA. Modification of the Wu-Mendel approach for linguistic summarization using IF-THEN rules. Journal of Experimental & Theoretical Artificial Intelligence. 2019;**31**(1):77-97. DOI: 10.1080/0952813X.2018.1518998

[18] Gardashova LA, Aliyev BF. Dental disease detection using Fuzzy logic. In: Advances in Intelligent Systems and Computing Series, ICAFS 2020. Vol. 1306. Springer. pp. 126-132. Available from: https://www.springer.com/gp/book/9783030640576

[19] Aliev BF, Gardashova LA. Selection of an optimal treatment method for acute pulpitis disease. Procedia Computer Science. 2017;**120**:539-546

[20] Aliev RA, Aliev RR. Soft Computing and its Application. New Jersey, London, Singapore, Hong Kong: World Scientific; 2001. p. 444

[21] Zadeh LA. A note on Z-numbers. Information Science. 2011;**181**(14): 2923-2932. DOI: 10.1016/j.ins.2011.02.022

[22] Dunn JC. A fuzzy relative of the ISODATA process and its use in detecting compact well-separated clusters. Journal of Cybernetics. 1973;**3**:32-57. DOI: 10.1080/01969727308546046

[23] Bezdek JC, Ehrlich R, Full W. FCM: The fuzzy c-means clustering algorithm. Computers & Geosciences. 1984;**10**(2-3): 191-203. DOI: 10.1016/0098-3004(84)90020-7